Respiratory Care Principles

A Programmed Guide to Entry-Level Practice

Third Edition

Respiratory Care Principles

A Programmed Guide to Entry-Level Practice

Third Edition

THOMAS A. BARNES, EdD, RRT
Director of Clinical Education
Respiratory Therapy Program
Associate Professor of Respiratory Therapy
College of Pharmacy and Allied Health Professions
Northeastern University
Boston, Massachusetts

In consultation with
JAN KAREL SCHREUDER, MD
Department of Anesthesiology
North Central Bronx Hospital
Bronx, New York

and

JACOB S. ISRAEL, MD
Department of Anesthesiology
North Central Bronx Hospital
Bronx, New York

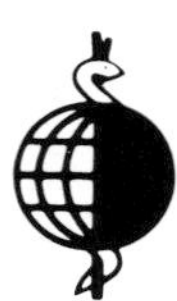

F. A. DAVIS COMPANY • Philadelphia

Printed in the United States of America

Last digit indicates print number: 10 9 8 7 6 5 4 3 2 1

As new scientific information becomes available through basic and clinical research, recommended treatments and drug therapies undergo changes. The author(s) and publisher have done everything possible to make this book accurate, up to date, and in accord with accepted standards at the time of publication. The authors, editors, and publisher are not responsible for errors or omissions or for consequences from application of the book, and make no warranty, expressed or implied, in regard to the contents of the book. Any practice described in this book should be applied by the reader in accordance with professional standards of care used in regard to the unique circumstances that may apply in each situation. The reader is advised always to check product information (package inserts) for changes and new information regarding dose and contraindications before administering any drug. Caution is especially urged when using new or infrequently ordered drugs.

Library of Congress Cataloging in Publication Data

Barnes, Thomas A.
Respiratory care principles : a programmed guide to entry-level practice / Thomas A. Barnes, in consultation with Jan Karel Schreuder, Jacob S. Israel. — 3rd ed.
p. cm.
Rev. ed. of: Brady's programmed introduction to respiratory therapy, c1980.
Includes bibliographical references and index.
ISBN 0-8036-0662-1 (soft)
1. Respiratory therapy—Programmed instruction. I. Schreuder, Jan Karel. II. Israel, Jacob S., 1926– . III. Barnes, Thomas A. Brady's programmed introduction to respiratory therapy. IV. Title.
[DNLM: 1. Respiration—programmed instruction. 2. Respiratory Therapy—programmed instruction. 3. Respiratory Tract Diseases--programmed instruction. WF 18 B261b]
RC735.I5B375 1991
615.8'36'077—dc20
DLC
for Library of Congress 91-9456
CIP

Dedication

This book is dedicated to my father, Ernest H. Barnes, who taught me the value of hard work, and to my mother, Barbara Beckendorf Barnes, who taught me the value of laughter.

Preface

The third edition of this book has been expanded and redesigned to cover the principles needed to practice safely upon entry into the field of respiratory care. The book will be useful to students reviewing for the National Board for Respiratory Care (NBRC) CRTT Self-Assessment Exam given just prior to graduation by most respiratory therapy schools. It will also be helpful to those studying for the NBRC Entry-Level CRTT Exam. A successful score on the Self-Assessment Exam is the criterion many states use to award a license to practice respiratory care. The book is appropriate too for learners for whom individual differences in style, time, place, and pace of learning are important considerations. It should also be useful to programs with respiratory care curricula that emphasize directed independent study units.

This book should be of interest to anyone actively involved in administering respiratory care. Besides respiratory therapy students, it should be used by students in nursing, physical therapy, emergency paramedical, and physician assistant schools if their career plans involve treating patients with respiratory disorders.

The book is organized into 242 instructional frames divided into 16 chapters that include pretests and posttests, learning exercises, and a bibliography. The end-of-chapter exams and the summative exam in Chapter 17 are designed to evaluate the reader's understanding of the respiratory care principles needed for entry-level practice and to direct attention to areas of weakness. The first three chapters cover basic principles in respiratory and acid-base physiology and medical physics, which are the foundation of many concepts covered later in the book. Medical asepsis and initial assessment and diagnosis are covered next, since they also are fundamental to all of the respiratory care modalities. Oxygen therapy, humidity and aerosol therapy, airway care, mechanical ventilation, and cardiopulmonary resuscitation are covered with an emphasis on principles included on the NBRC entry-level exam matrix. To close the therapeutic loop, monitoring and pulmonary rehabilitation are covered in Chapters 11 and 12. The last five chapters cover respiratory care equipment and the summative exam. The four chapters on equipment emphasize performance characteristics, proper adjustment, and troubleshooting malfunctions. The summative exam comprises 200 multiple-choice and multiple true-false questions that are referenced to the frames in the other 16 chapters.

The exam provides the reader a means to assess comprehensively his or her understanding of entry-level principles of practice.

My appreciation is extended to my wife, Diane, for her support over the 15 months during which the third edition of this text was planned and written. The contribution of Dr. Jan Karel Schreuder is gratefully acknowledged for his critical and timely review of the manuscript as a medical consultant to the author. I also wish to thank a good friend, Dr. Jacob S. Israel, for his help with the first two editions of the book and for his review of this most recent edition. Special thanks go to Jean-François Vilain, Senior Editor, F.A. Davis Publishers, for support in the critical early stages and for his great enthusiasm for this book. I am indebted to Philip Geronimo at the University of Toledo Community and Technical College, Allen Marangoni at Wheeling Jesuit College, and Anna Parkman at the University of Charleston for the time and energy they spent reviewing the third edition; their comments added greatly to the final manuscript. It is my sincere hope that this text will help new practitioners to understand the principles that will make them safe and competent respiratory care professionals.

Thomas A. Barnes

Instructions to the Reader

This is a programmed book in which the subject matter is divided into 242 frames of information that can be modified and completed at your own pace to meet your individual needs. Although its pages are numbered in the usual way, you should not try to read them consecutively. When you have completed one frame you must either (1) read the following question and refer to the page and section listed beside your answer or (2) if there is no question, follow the directions at the bottom of the page. To help you retain the information, the book will continually ask you questions, and your progress will depend upon your ability to select the right answers. If you do select a wrong answer, additional information provided on the answer page or a review of the frame of instruction should clarify any misunderstandings you may have. You will find that reading this book is like having an individual tutor.

Each chapter has 40 multiple-choice questions designed to measure what you know about the principles being covered. The 20-question pretest should be taken before starting the chapter to identify areas of strength and weakness. The 20-question posttest should be completed before leaving the chapter to ensure that you have understood the principles. The answers to the questions are referenced by frame numbers so that you can give special attention to, or review, topics where your answers are incorrect.

The exercises following the last frame in each chapter are designed to reinforce your understanding and retention of the material. It is important to take the time to complete the exercises, using the textbooks listed in the bibliography if necessary.

If you approach programmed learning thoughtfully and cooperate by following instructions, you should arrive at the final page of this text with an entry-level understanding of respiratory care principles. Your last learning activity should be to complete the 200-question summative exam in Chapter 17 and to review the frames where your answer is incorrect.

Contents

1

Respiratory Physiology

1. The respiratory system
2. Respiration
3. Upper airways
4. Lower airways
5. The trachea and larynx
6. Respiratory bronchioles
7. Pulmonary capillaries
8. Gas exchange
9. Thoracic cavity
10. The lungs
11. The pleura
12. The diaphragm
13. Intercostal muscles
14. The respiratory musculature
15. Respiratory rate
16. Components of the respiratory system
17. Pulmonary circulation
18. External and internal respiration
19. Anatomy of the pulmonary circulation
20. The heart
21. The cardiovascular system
22. Normal alveolar ventilation
23. Physiologic dead space
24. Abnormal ventilation
25. The language of respiratory physiology
26. Normal lung volumes and capacities
27. Expiratory reserve and residual volumes
28. Functional residual capacity
29. Vital capacity
30. Inspiratory capacity
31. Primary and secondary physiology symbols
32. Dead-space ventilation
33. Regulation of ventilation
34. Nerve impulses
35. Breathing patterns
36. Oxygen uptake
37. Carbon dioxide output
38. Normal blood gas values
39. Oxygen transport
40. Causes of hypoxia
41. Circulatory, anemic, and histotoxic hypoxia
42. Clinical signs of hypoxemia
43. The oxyhemoglobin dissociation curve

PRETEST

This pretest is designed to measure what you already know about the respiratory and cardiovascular systems. Check your answers on page 4 and then continue on page 5, frame 1.

1. The exchange of oxygen and carbon dioxide between the alveoli and pulmonary capillaries is called
   A. ventilation.
   B. inspiration.
   C. breathing.
   D. internal respiration.
   E. external respiration.

2. Rapid exchange of respiratory gases *first* takes place in the
   A. trachea.
   B. main-stem bronchi.
   C. segmental bronchi.
   D. terminal bronchioles.
   E. respiratory bronchioles.

3. Supplying oxygen to the alveoli and removing carbon dioxide is called
   A. inspiration.
   B. expiration.
   C. ventilation.
   D. metabolism.
   E. respiration.

4. Venous blood flows into pulmonary capillaries from the
   A. superior vena cava.
   B. pulmonary veins.
   C. pulmonary venules.
   D. pulmonary arteries.
   E. pulmonary arterioles.

5. The space between the lungs is called the
   A. mediastinum.
   B. pericardial area.
   C. thoracic cavity.
   D. pleural area.
   E. epigastric area.

6. A healthy adult at rest has a respiratory rate of
   A. 6 to 10/min.
   B. 8 to 12/min.
   C. 12 to 20/min.
   D. 20 to 30/min.
   E. 30 to 40/min.

7. Blood leaving the right ventricle flows into the
   A. aorta.
   B. superior vena cava.
   C. pulmonary artery.
   D. pulmonary veins.
   E. inferior vena cava

8. Alveolar minute ventilation for a 150-lb adult with a tidal volume of 450 mL and a rate of 15/min is
   A. 1.2 L/min.
   B. 1.8 L/min.
   C. 2.4 L/min.
   D. 4.5 L/min.
   E. 5.4 L/min.
9. Adequate alveolar ventilation is indicated by a Pa_{CO_2} of
   A. 35 mm Hg.
   B. 40 mm Hg.
   C. 46 mm Hg.
   D. 75 mm Hg.
   E. 100 mm Hg.
10. A young healthy male has a total lung capacity of
   A. 1200 mL.
   B. 2400 mL.
   C. 3100 mL.
   D. 4800 mL.
   E. 6000 mL.
11. The air remaining in your lungs after a maximal exhalation is the
   A. vital capacity.
   B. functional residual capacity.
   C. expiratory reserve volume.
   D. residual volume.
   E. tidal volume.
12. The regular automatic pattern of ventilation is controlled by the
   A. pons.
   B. medulla.
   C. apneustic center.
   D. pneumotaxic center.
   E. spinal cord.
13. A normal mixed venous oxygen tension is
   A. 30 mm Hg.
   B. 40 mm Hg.
   C. 46 mm Hg.
   D. 75 mm Hg.
   E. 100 mm Hg.
14. A normal P_{AO_2} when breathing air at sea level is
   A. 30 mm Hg.
   B. 40 mm Hg.
   C. 75 mm Hg.
   D. 90 mm Hg.
   E. 104 mm Hg.
15. Moderate hypoxemia is defined as a Pa_{O_2}
   A. 20 to 40 mm Hg.
   B. 30 to 40 mm Hg.
   C. 40 to 60 mm Hg.
   D. 60 to 80 mm Hg.
   E. 80 to 100 mm Hg.

16. All of the following are clinical signs of moderate hypoxemia *except*
    A. restlessness.
    B. cyanosis.
    C. bradycardia.
    D. tachypnea.
    E. decreased cognition.

17. An abnormally slow breathing rate is called
    A. hyperventilation.
    B. hypoventilation.
    C. hypopnea.
    D. tachypnea.
    E. bradypnea.

18. Inadequate alveolar ventilation resulting in a Pa_{CO_2} >45 torr is called
    A. hyperventilation.
    B. hypoventilation.
    C. hypopnea.
    D. tachypnea.
    E. bradypnea.

19. The maximum amount of O_2 held by 15 g of hemoglobin is
    A. 0.3 mL.
    B. 4.5 mL.
    C. 10.0 mL.
    D. 15.0 mL.
    E. 20.1 mL.

20. Carbon dioxide normally diffuses into alveoli across a gradient of
    A. 6 mm Hg.
    B. 40 mm Hg.
    C. 60 mm Hg.
    D. 75 mm Hg.
    E. 100 mm Hg.

ANSWERS TO PRETEST

1. E (F18)
2. E (F6)
3. C (F15)
4. E (F7)
5. A (F11)
6. C (F15)
7. C (F17)
8. D (F32)
9. B (F24)
10. E (F29)
11. D (F27)
12. B (F33)
13. C (F38)
14. E (F36)
15. C (F39)
16. C (F40)
17. E (F35)
18. B (F24)
19. E (F39)
20. A (F37)

FRAME 1. THE RESPIRATORY SYSTEM

There are many physiologic mechanisms involved in supplying the tissues with oxygen and disposing of the excess carbon dioxide produced by metabolism. The respiratory and circulatory systems have primary roles for these functions. The respiratory system is responsible for supplying the lungs, and ultimately the blood, with oxygen and excreting carbon dioxide from the body. The circulatory system is responsible for transporting oxygen to the tissues and removing excess carbon dioxide to the lungs (to be excreted).

Although the terms are sometimes used interchangeably, there is a distinction between breathing (which we will call ventilation) and respiration. *Breathing,* or *ventilation,* is the mechanical process of taking air into the lungs (inhalation or inspiration) and expelling it from the lungs into the atmosphere (exhalation or expiration). Respiration is the exchange of gases providing the blood and tissues with oxygen and removing excess carbon dioxide.

(Q) Ventilation is best defined as

a. supplying oxygen to the tissues and removing excess CO_2. 8 A
b. supplying oxygen to the lungs and removing excess CO_2. 9 a
c. both *a* and *c*. 9 A

FRAME 2. RESPIRATION

Ventilation means breathing. Respiration, on the other hand, refers to the diffusion of oxygen from the lungs into the bloodstream and from the bloodstream into the tissues; and conversely, to the diffusion of carbon dioxide from the tissues into the bloodstream and from the bloodstream into the lungs.

The function of the respiratory system is to supply adequate oxygen and remove excess carbon dioxide. Its airways consist of the mouth, nose, pharynx, larynx, trachea, bronchi, and bronchioles. Approximately one third of a normal tidal volume remains in the airways, and the other two thirds travels to the alveoli, where respiratory gas exchange occurs.

(Q) Although some of the inspired air remains in the airways, most can be found in the

a. alveoli. 9 B
b. bronchi. 9 b
c. trachea. 17 A

FRAME 3. UPPER AIRWAYS

The nose functions to remove impurities from the air breathed in, as well as to begin moistening, warming, or cooling the air before it reaches the lungs. This is accomplished by an air conditioning process that involves passing the inhaled air through a series of curved nasal pathways. These pathways are lined by small hairs in the moist nasal mucosa.

The pharynx is a tubelike structure, commonly called the throat, that extends from the base of the skull to the esophagus. It consists of three parts: (1) the nasopharynx, which serves as the passageway for air from the nose; (2) the oropharynx, which opens into the mouth to serve as a passageway for both food and air; and (3) the laryngopharynx, which opens into the larynx and the esophagus. When food and air enter through the mouth, the food passes into the esophagus and the air enters the trachea. To prevent food from entering the trachea, a small leaf-shaped cartilage (the epiglottis) closes over the opening of the trachea during the act of swallowing.

(Q) Which is the correct statement?

a. During the act of swallowing, food enters the esophagus and air enters the trachea. 8 B

b. During the act of swallowing, the trachea is covered by the epiglottis until the food has entered the esophagus. 9 C

FRAME 4. LOWER AIRWAYS

The right main-stem bronchus enters the right lung at a 25° angle and the left main-stem bronchus enters the left lung at a 40° to 60° angle. Here, they immediately divide into smaller bronchi, which continue branching and eventually form the still smaller bronchioles. The bronchioles also branch until they terminate in the microscopic alveolar ducts. The alveolar ducts terminate in alveolar atria, the walls of which consist of alveoli. It is in the alveoli that the major exchange of gases takes place. Alveolar air and blood are separated by thin layers of tissue and fluid. Oxygen from the alveoli diffuses through these layers into the capillaries that surround the alveoli. Carbon dioxide diffuses from the capillaries into the alveolar air. Even though the alveoli seem to be simply an extension of the bronchioles, they are considered the functional units of the lungs.

(Q) The various tubes making up the bronchial tree serve to

a. form a passageway for air to reach the alveoli. 8 D

b. exchange oxygen for carbon dioxide. 9 d

c. do both of the above. 17 B

FRAME 5. THE TRACHEA AND LARYNX

The trachea (commonly called the windpipe) is a cylindrical cartilaginous tube about 4 to 5 in. long, which descends from the larynx (voice box) to the main-stem bronchi. The larynx consists of a group of cartilages, muscles, and ligaments that keep the airway open during breathing, separate the airway from the digestive tract during swallowing, and allow speech to occur. The cricoid cartilage forms a complete ring and is attached at its posterior lateral surface to the thyroid cartilage (Adam's apple). The lining of the trachea contains hairlike cilia, which sweep most particles that have been inhaled back to the larynx to be coughed up or swallowed. Bacteria and debris from the alveoli and other peripheral parts of the lung similarly are swept upward.

The trachea divides into major branches, the right and left main-stem bronchi, at the level of the fifth thoracic vertebra (Fig. 1–1). Sometimes the trachea may become blocked due to swelling in the larynx, aspiration of foreign substances, or an accumulation of secretions. When this happens, the anterior surface of the trachea may be cut open (an operation called a tracheotomy) to allow adequate ventilation (intake of oxygen and removal of carbon dioxide) and removal of secretions.

(Q) The trachea divides into

a. right and left lung. 8 C
b. right and left main-stem bronchi. 9 D
c. right and left bronchioles. 9 c

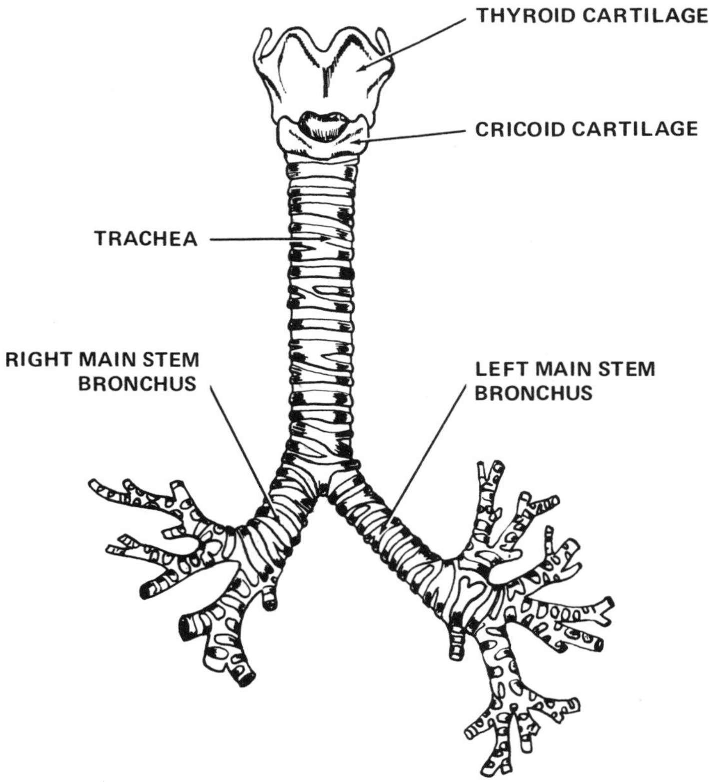

Figure 1–1

ANSWERS TO FRAMES

8A (from page 5, frame 1)
Not quite. This is the end result of ventilation. The actual delivery of oxygen and the removal of excess carbon dioxide from the tissues is accomplished through respiration. Return to page 5, frame 1, and select another answer.

8B (from page 6, frame 3)
Wrong. During the act of swallowing, the opening of the trachea must be blocked so that food and liquids cannot enter the airway. This is accomplished by the epiglottis covering the opening to the trachea, until swallowing is completed. Please continue on page 7, frame 4.

8C (from page 7, frame 5)
Wrong. The trachea divides into the two structures similar to but smaller than the trachea, which are also constructed of cartilaginous rings and covered with epithelial tissue. What are these structures called? Return to page 7, frame 5, and study Figure 1–1; then select another answer.

8D (from page 6, frame 4)
Correct. The main-stem bronchi, smaller bronchi, bronchioles, and alveolar ducts all serve to deliver air to the alveoli, where the gas exchange takes place. Please continue on page 7, frame 5.

8a (from page 54, frame 42)

Moderate hypoxemia: restlessness, tachycardia, cyanosis, diaphoresis
Severe hypoxemia: unconsciousness, apnea, bradycardia, asystole

Some of the other symptoms of acute hypoxia are rapid pulse, impairment of the special senses, headache, loss of appetite, mental disturbances (such as euphoria or delirium), labored breathing, cyanosis, and, in severe cases, muscular twitching, convulsions, and unconsciousness. The effects of acute hypoxemia may last for 48 hours or longer and include headache, lethargy, nausea, vomiting, and in some cases permanent brain damage. Please continue on page 55, frame 43.

9A (from page 5, frame 1)
Wrong. Respiration is the supplying of oxygen to the blood and tissues, and the removal of excess carbon dioxide from the tissues and blood. Return to page 5, frame 1, and select another answer.

9B (from page 5, frame 2)
Correct. Although some of the inspired air (about one third) remains in the airway, most of it reaches the alveoli, where the exchange of gases takes place. Since no rapid exchange of gases takes place in the airways, these structures are considered to be *dead space*. Please continue on page 6, frame 3.

9C (from page 6, frame 3)
Correct. During the act of swallowing, the opening of the trachea must be blocked so food and liquids cannot enter the airway. This is accomplished by the covering of the opening to the trachea (glottis) by the epiglottis until swallowing is completed. Please continue on page 6, frame 4.

9D (from page 7, frame 5)
Correct. At the level of the fifth thoracic vertebra, the trachea divides into two main-stem bronchi, which, in turn, divide several times into smaller bronchi, and then into bronchioles. Please continue on page 10, frame 6.

9a (from page 5, frame 1)
Correct. Ventilation means breathing in fresh air by inhalation, or inspiration, and expelling stale air by exhalation, or expiration. Please continue on page 5, frame 2.

9b (from page 5, frame 2)
Wrong. The bronchi serve simply as airways. Although some of the inspired air remains in the bronchi, the amount is small. Return to page 5, frame 2, and select another answer.

9c (from page 7, frame 5)
Wrong. The bronchioles, which lack cartilage, are one of the subdivisions of the bronchi. Return to page 7, frame 5, and study Figure 1–1; then select another answer.

9d (from page 6, frame 4)
Wrong. The pulmonary exchange of gases takes place in the alveoli and respiratory bronchioles, the functional units of the lungs. Return to page 6, frame 4, and review the material; then select another answer.

FRAME 6. RESPIRATORY BRONCHIOLES

Large bronchi are named after lobes of the lung, and smaller bronchi are identified by the lung segments to which they deliver inhaled gas, for example, *right upper lobe bronchus, right upper lobe posterior segment bronchus* (Fig. 1–2). After dividing several times into progressively smaller branches the airways terminate as respiratory bronchioles and alveolar ducts, which lead into the alveolar atrium. Both the respiratory bronchioles and the alveolar ducts have alveoli on their walls, and gas exchange will occur from these airways.

(Q) The respiratory bronchioles are actually an extension of

a. lobar bronchi. 17 C
b. segmental bronchi. 16 A
c. terminal bronchioles. 16 a

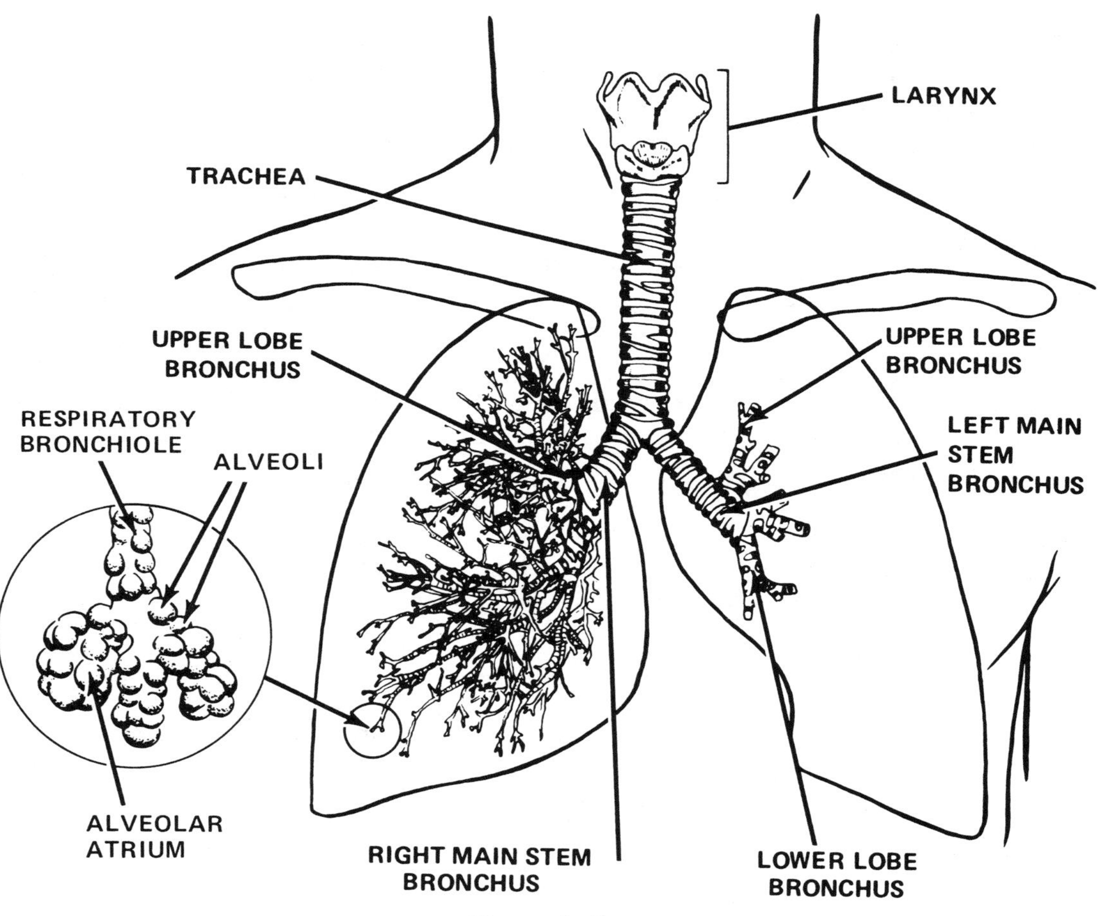

Figure 1–2

FRAME 7. PULMONARY CAPILLARIES

(Q) The exchange of gases in the lungs takes place as follows:

a. Oxygen diffuses from the capillaries into the alveoli. Carbon dioxide diffuses through the alveoli into the capillaries. 17 D

b. Oxygen diffuses from the alveoli into the capillaries. Carbon dioxide diffuses from the capillaries into the alveoli. 17 a

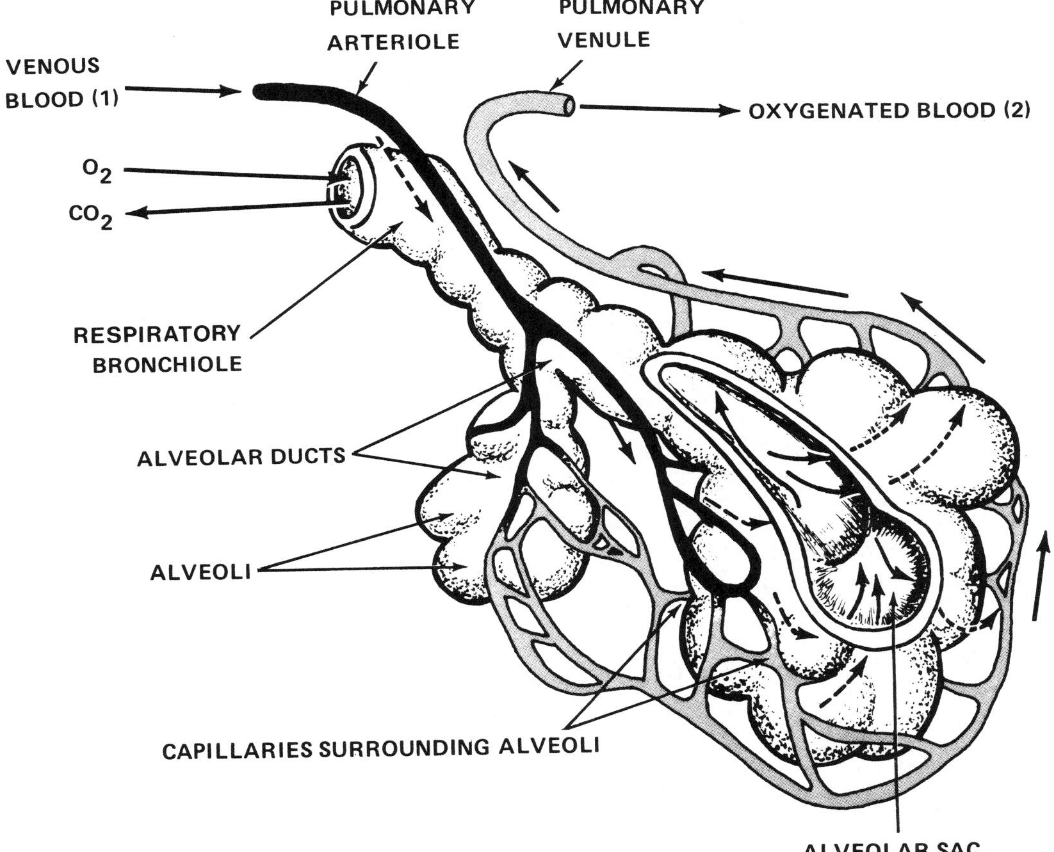

Figure 1–3 (1) Low oxygen content and increased amount of carbon dioxide; (2) increased oxygen content and decreased amount of carbon dioxide.

FRAME 8. GAS EXCHANGE

The function of the lungs is to provide gas exchange between the blood and air. The internal structure of the lung contains millions of thin-walled alveoli enveloped by capillaries, permitting a rapid gas exchange of oxygen and carbon dioxide. Figure 1–3 in frame 7 shows how carbon dioxide diffuses across a small pressure gradient from the pulmonary capillary blood into the alveoli.

The alveoli provide oxygen to the bloodstream to be distributed via the systemic circulation to the cells. This exchange of gases takes place continuously. Additional oxygen is drawn in with each inhalation and carbon dioxide removed with each exhalation. The exchange of gases takes place because of a physical phenomenon called diffusion. When the concentration of certain molecules on one side of a semipermeable membrane differs from the concentration of the same molecules on the other side, the molecules in the greater concentration will diffuse through the membrane. This will continue until there are equal concentrations on both sides of the membrane.

(Q) The exchange of gases through the alveoli occurs because of

a. a greater concentration of carbon dioxide in the pulmonary capillary blood than in the alveoli. 17 b

b. a greater concentration of oxygen in the alveoli than in the pulmonary capillary blood. 16 B

c. both of these reasons. 16 b

FRAME 9. THORACIC CAVITY

The thoracic, or chest, cavity contains the pleural, pericardial, and mediastinal structures. The lungs are housed in the pleural cavity. The mediastinal portion (the space between the two lungs) is occupied by the trachea, esophagus, heart, large blood vessels, various nerves, the thymus, and lymph nodes. The pericardial area is occupied by the heart and its enveloping sac.

(Q) In which area of the thoracic cavity are the lungs situated?

a. the mediastinal area 17 d

b. the pericardial area 16 D

c. the pleural area 16 c

FRAME 10. THE LUNGS

The lungs occupy the lateral cavities of the chest, separated from each other by the heart and the other mediastinal structures. The right lung is composed of three lobes (upper, middle, and lower), and the left lung has two lobes (upper and lower). Each lobe is subdivided into two to five segments, separated by connective tissue septa (partitions). The lungs have a total of 19 lung segments (Fig. 1–4), with 10 segments in the right lung and nine in the left lung. Pulmonary disorders may be confined to or localized in one or more of these segments.

(Q) Which lung contains the most lung segments?

a. the left lung 17 c

b. the right lung 16 C

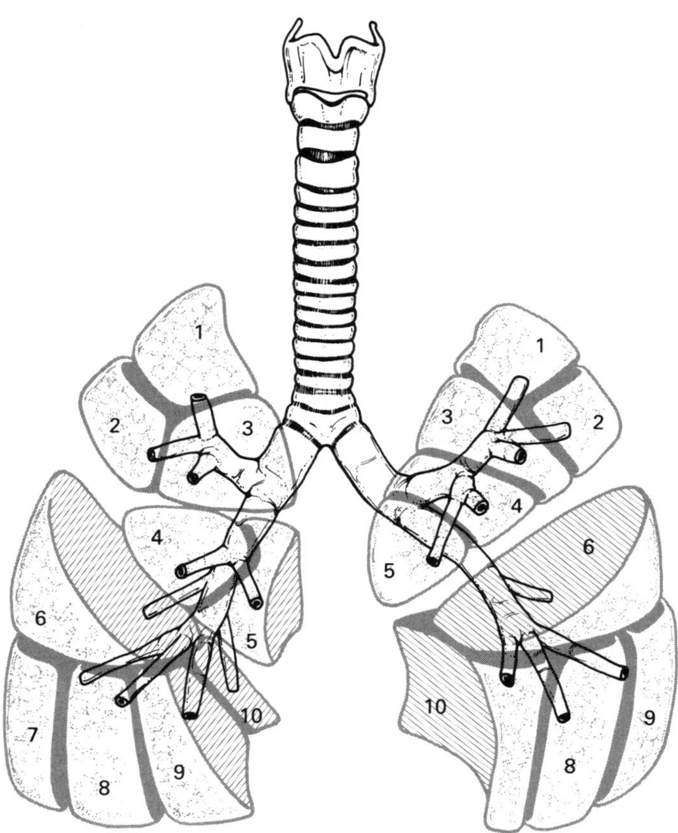

Figure 1–4 Bronchopulmonary segments of the human lung. *Left and right upper lobes:* (1) apical, (2) posterior, (3) anterior, (4) superior lingular, and (5) inferior lingular segments. *Right middle lobe:* (4) lateral and (5) medial segments. *Lower lobes:* (6) superior (apical), (7) medial-basal, (8) anterior-basal, (9) lateral-basal, and (10) posterior-basal segments. There is no medial-basal lobe in the left lung. (Source: Weibel, ER: Design and structure of the human lung. In Fishman, AP [ed]: Pulmonary Diseases and Disorders, Vol 1. McGraw-Hill, New York, 1980. Used with permission.)

FRAME 11. THE PLEURA

The pleura (a serous surface) consists of two membranes. As shown in Figure 1–5, the outer one lines the thoracic cavity (parietal pleura), and the other forms the outer covering of the lungs (visceral pleura). These layers are separated by a small amount of fluid. As the lungs expand with incoming air, the layers glide over each other. Friction is prevented by the lubricant between the layers. Sometimes the layers become inflamed (as in pleurisy), and inhalation is very painful.

The mediastinum separates the two lungs, between the sternum in the front and the vertebral column behind and from the thoracic inlet above to the diaphragm below. It contains the heart and its large vessels, the trachea, esophagus, thymus, and lymph nodes.

Please continue on page 15, frame 12.

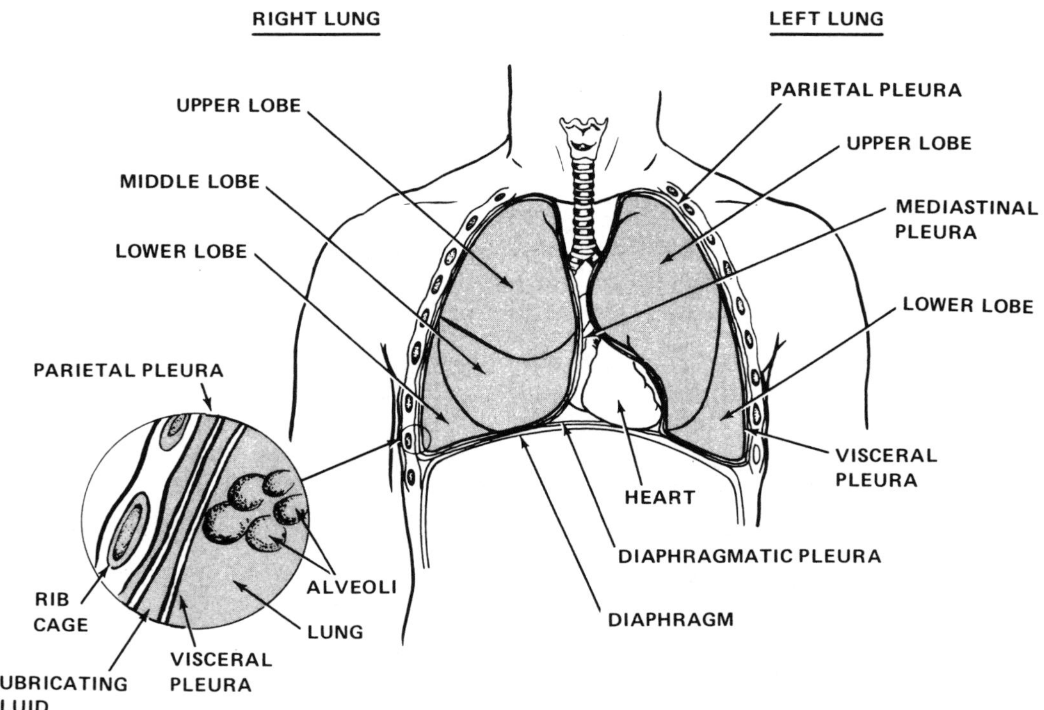

Figure 1–5

FRAME 12. THE DIAPHRAGM

Although there are many muscles that assist inspiration, the two major groups involved are the muscles of the diaphragm and the external intercostal muscles. The musculomembranous sheet separating the abdominal and thoracic cavities is the diaphragm. The pericardium (the sac surrounding the heart) adheres to part of the diaphragm's domed surface. On either side of the heart, the base of each lung also rests upon its upper surface (Fig. 1–6). The parietal and visceral membranes of the pleura separate the lungs and the diaphragm. Three major openings in the diaphragm allow the esophagus, blood vessels, and nerves to pass from the thoracic cavity to the abdominal cavity.

(Q) The diaphragm at rest has a shape that is

a. flat. 16 d

b. domed. 21 A

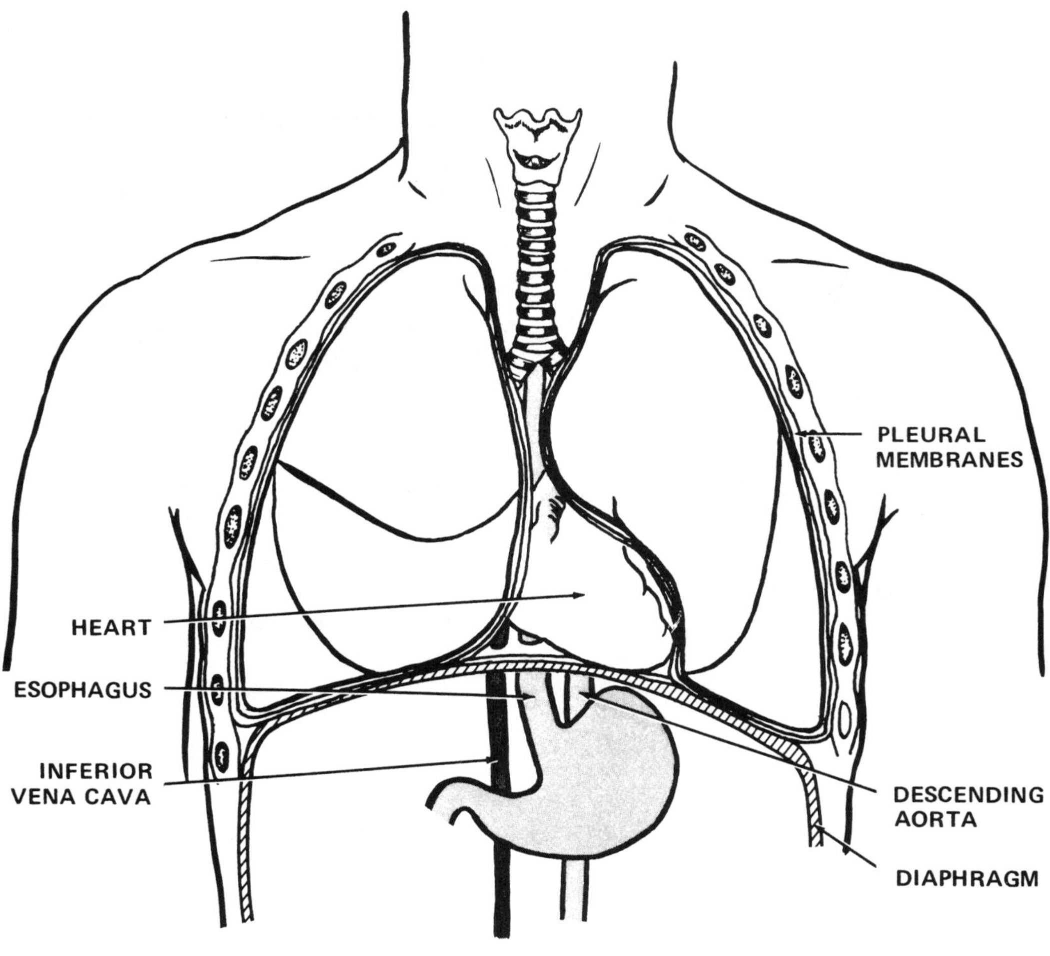

Figure 1–6

16A (from page 10, frame 6)
Wrong. The segmental bronchi divide several times and the smaller branches are called bronchioles. Return to page 10, frame 6, review the material; then try the question again.

16B (from page 12, frame 8)
Wrong. This would account for the oxygen diffusing into the bloodstream, but what about the outward movement of carbon dioxide? Return to page 12, frame 8, and review the material; then try the question again.

16C (from page 13, frame 10)
Correct. The right lung contains 10 segments and the left lung has only 9 segments. Please continue on page 14, frame 11.

16D (from page 12, frame 9)
Wrong. The heart occupies the pericardial area. Turn to page 13, frame 10; you will see that the lungs are situated in the pleural cavity.

16a (from page 10, frame 6)
Correct. Terminal bronchioles lead directly to respiratory bronchioles. Please continue on page 11, frame 7.

16b (from page 12, frame 8)
Correct. Oxygen diffuses into the blood in the pulmonary capillaries, and carbon dioxide diffuses out of blood into the alveoli until an equilibrium is reached. Please continue on page 12, frame 9.

16c (from page 12, frame 9)
Correct. Turn to page 13, frame 10 to see how the lungs are positioned in the pleural cavity.

16d (from page 15, frame 12)
Wrong. The diaphragm has a domed shape at rest and becomes flat when the muscle contracts during inspiration. Please continue on page 18, frame 13.

17A (from page 5, frame 2)
Wrong. The trachea serves simply as an airway. Although some of the air is left in the trachea, the amount is small. Return to page 5, frame 2, and select another answer.

17B (from page 6, frame 4)
Wrong. The exchange of gases does not take place in the bronchial tree. The alveoli and respiratory bronchioles, the functional units of the lungs, are the principal structures in which the exchange of gases takes place. Return to page 6, frame 4, and review the material; then select another answer.

17C (from page 10, frame 6)
Wrong. The airways divide several times before terminating at the alveolar atrium. Return to page 10, frame 6, and review the material; then try the question again.

17D (from page 11, frame 7)
Careful! The purpose of the exchange of gases is to provide a continual supply of oxygen to the blood and to eliminate excess carbon dioxide from the blood. The answer you selected says just the opposite. The diagram on page 11 shows that the blood going to the lungs carries an increased amount of carbon dioxide (CO_2) to be excreted into the alveoli and a decreased amount of oxygen. Additional oxygen then diffuses from the alveoli into the pulmonary capillaries and eventually is delivered to the cells via the arteries. Return to page 11 and study Figure 1-3.

17a (from page 11, frame 7)
Correct. Oxygen diffuses from the alveoli into the capillaries. Carbon dioxide moves into the alveoli from the capillaries. Please continue on page 12, frame 8.

17b (from page 12, frame 8)
Wrong. This would account for carbon dioxide diffusing into the alveoli, but what about the diffusion of oxygen? Return to page 12, frame 8, and try again.

17c (from page 13, frame 10)
Wrong. Remember the diagram is facing you. It is the *right* lung that has 10 segments. The left lung has only nine segments. Please continue on page 12, frame 9.

17d (from page 12, frame 9)
Wrong. The mediastinal area is the space *between* the lungs that is occupied by the trachea, esophagus, pericardial sac, and other structures. Turn to page 13, frame 10, and you will see that the lungs occupy the pleural area.

FRAME 13. INTERCOSTAL MUSCLES

The external and internal intercostal muscles occupy the spaces between the ribs (Fig. 1–7). The fibers of these two sets of muscles are aligned almost at right angles to each other, from the bottom of one rib to the top of the rib below it. Contraction of these muscles during inhalation often elevates the ribs and thus increases the thoracic volume.

The central part of the diaphragm is made of a tough membrane called the central tendon. Into this membrane are inserted the muscles of the diaphragm. These fibers arise from the lumbar vertebrae as two stout bundles called the crura (singular, crus) (Fig. 1–8). The right crus arises from the upper three or four lumbar vertebrae, and the left from the upper two or three. Anteriorly, the diaphragm's muscle fibers arise from the pointed lower part of the sternum (the xiphoid process) and the lower six ribs.

(Q) The muscle(s) primarily involved in inspiration are

a. the diaphragm. 21 B
b. the external intercostal muscles. 21 a
c. both of the above. 21 d

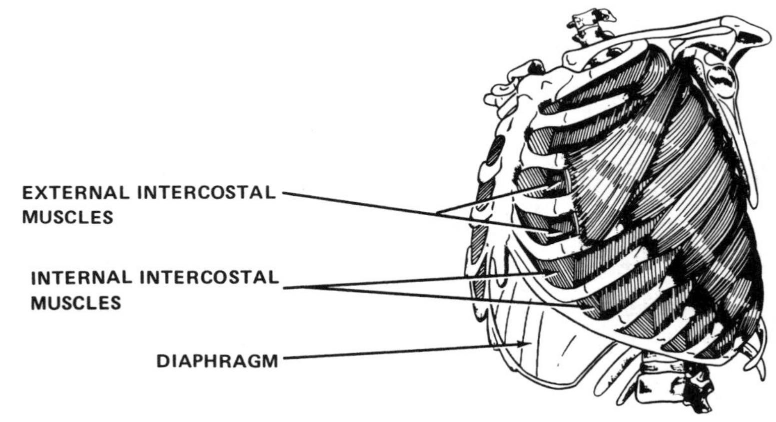

Figure 1–7

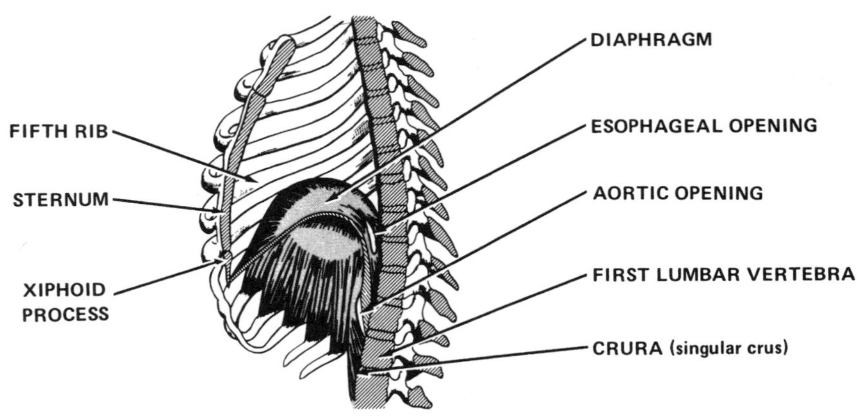

Figure 1–8

FRAME 14. THE RESPIRATORY MUSCULATURE

Contraction of the external intercostals elevates the ribs and along with contraction of the diaphragm initiates inspiration by causing the thoracic cavity to become elongated and to increase in diameter, thus drawing air into the lungs. Other accessory inspiratory muscles, such as the scalenus, help to elevate and fix the sternum and upper ribs at high levels of ventilation. When the muscles relax, the size of the thoracic cavity decreases, forcing air out of the lungs. During quiet breathing, expiration occurs from passive recoil of the lungs. Active exhalation occurs when the internal intercostal muscles depress the ribs downward. Abdominal muscles (rectus abdominis, external oblique, and transversus abdominis) assist active exhalation by depressing lower ribs and compressing abdominal contents, which helps the diaphragm to ascend (See Fig. 1–9).

The thoracic cavity is a closed unit that is sealed from the outside except for a small opening (the trachea). Inhalation takes place in accordance with the physical principle that enlargement of a chamber with a subsequent drop in pressure will draw in air from the outside through the opening. The air filling the enlarged space then equalizes the pressures inside and outside the chamber.

(Q) When the thoracic cavity becomes elongated and increases in diameter, the volume capacity increases during inhalation, and pressure inside the lungs

a. increases. 21 C

b. decreases. 21 b

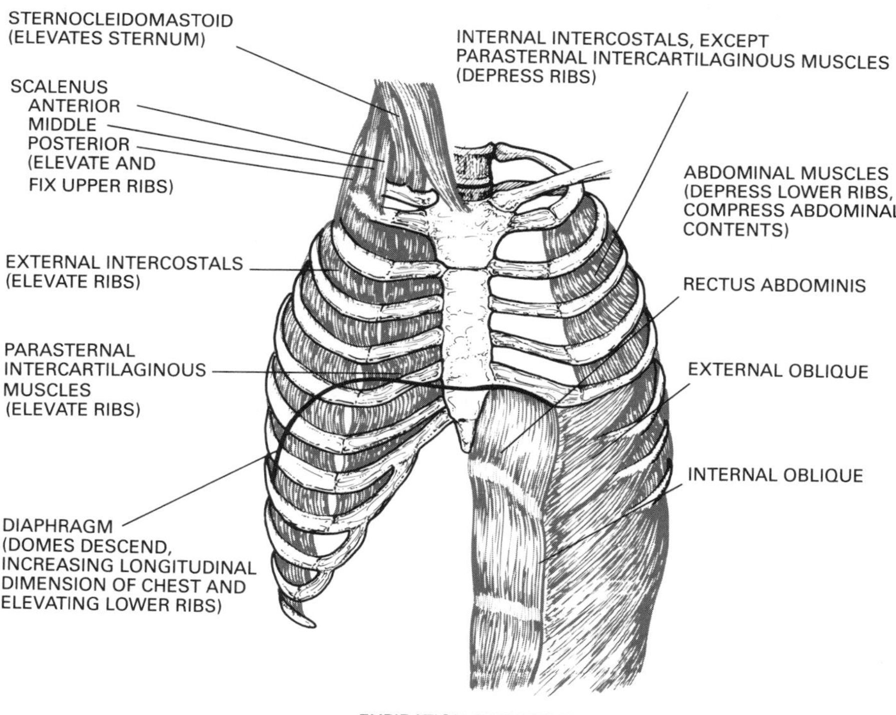

Figure 1–9

ANSWERS TO FRAMES

20A (from page 23, frame 16)

1. Nose
2. Pharynx
3. Epiglottis
4. Larynx
5. Trachea
6. Right and left main stem bronchi
7. Bronchioles
8. Alveolar ducts
9. Alveoli
10. Lung

The plurals of bronchus, bronchiole, and alveolus are bronchi, bronchioles, and alveoli. If you missed any of the answers listed above, return to page 23, frame 16, and try it again. If you got them all correct, please continue on page 24, frame 17.

20B (from page 24, frame 17)

1. Venous blood carrying high levels of CO_2 enters the *right atrium* of the heart. From there, it is pumped into the *right* ventricle and on to the *lungs* via the pulmonary artery.
2. Oxygenated blood flows via the pulmonary veins from the lungs into the left *atrium* of the heart. From there it is pumped into the left *ventricle,* then into the aorta for delivery to the tissues.

If you didn't fill in the blanks correctly, return to page 24, frame 17, and try again. Otherwise, please continue on page 25, frame 18.

21A (from page 15, frame 12)
Correct. The diaphragm separates the thoracic cavity from the abdominal cavity and is dome-shaped at rest. It becomes flat when contracting during inspiration. Please continue on page 18, frame 13.

21B (from page 18, frame 13)
True, but it works in cooperation with other muscles. Return to page 18, frame 13, and try again.

21C (from page 19, frame 14)
Wrong. If you review Figure 1–9, you will notice that when the muscles contract, the diaphragm is pulled down. What does this do to the pressure inside the lungs? Return to page 19, frame 14, and study Figure 1–9; then select another answer.

21D (from page 22, frame 15)
Wrong. The cycle of inhalation and exhalation takes place about 12 to 20 times per minute in the normal healthy adult at rest. The number of breaths per minute may be higher under certain emotional and metabolic conditions. Please continue on page 23, frame 16.

21a (from page 18, frame 13)
True, but they work in cooperation with other muscles. Return to page 18, frame 13, and try again.

21b (from page 19, frame 14)
Correct. When the thoracic cavity's volume capacity is increased, the pressure inside the lungs decreases. In addition, the thoracic cage moves up and forward, further increasing the volume of the thoracic cage. Thus, routine, moment-to-moment breathing is caused by the phased contraction and relaxation of the diaphragm and the external intercostal muscles. Please continue on page 22, frame 15.

21c (from page 22, frame 15)
Correct. In a healthy adult at rest, breathing occurs 12 to 20 times per minute. Please continue on page 23, frame 16.

21d (from page 18, frame 13)
Correct. Primarily the diaphragm and external intercostal muscles are involved in inspiration. Please continue on page 19, frame 14.

FRAME 15. RESPIRATORY RATE

When the volume of the thoracic cavity is increased by the contraction of the diaphragm and external intercostal muscles, the chest wall is raised and air is drawn into the lungs (inhalation). The chest wall is returned to its original position by the relaxation of the respiratory muscles and air is expelled (exhalation). A healthy adult at rest breathes at a rate of 12 to 20 times per minute. The number of inhalations per minute (respiratory rate) is increased by emotional excitement, exercise, fever, hyperthyroidism, and diseases or drugs that increase the general rate of metabolism. The result is greater ventilation (which may result in hyperventilation), which increases the amount of oxygen delivered to the lungs and the amount of carbon dioxide eliminated from the body. Conversely, with some illnesses and depressant drugs the amount of breathing decreases, causing hypoventilation. Hypoventilation results in insufficient carbon dioxide being removed; without oxygen therapy inadequate oxygen enters the alveolar space.

Other respiratory muscles not actively used for quiet breathing are referred to as accessory muscles and include the scalene, sternocleidomastoid, trapezius, and pectoralis muscles. The function of these accessory muscles is to stabilize and elevate the chest wall so that the diameter is increased, thus improving the efficiency of diaphragmatic excursion when higher levels of ventilation are needed. Abdominal muscles play an important role in active exhalation by contracting and depressing the lower ribs, flexing the trunk, and forcing the diaphragm up by increasing the intra-abdominal pressure. These muscles include the external oblique, internal oblique, and rectus abdominis muscles (Fig. 1–10).

(Q) In a healthy adult at rest, breathing occurs at a rate of
   a. 15 to 20/min. 21 D
   b. 11 to 14/min. 21 c

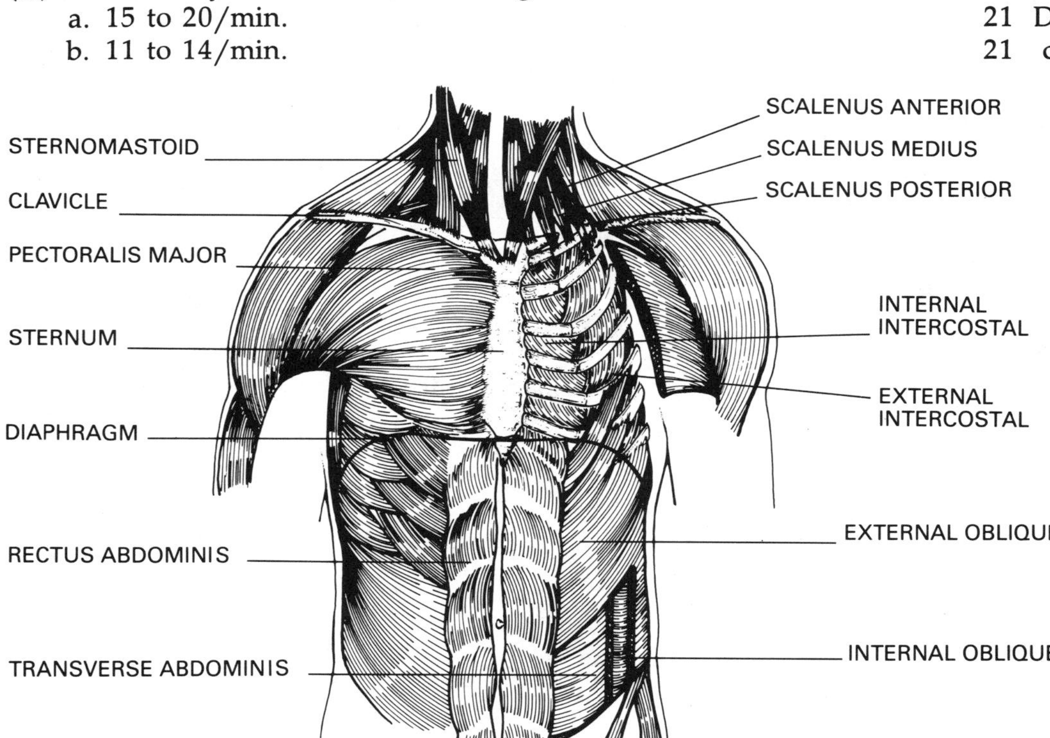

Figure 1–10

FRAME 16. COMPONENTS OF THE RESPIRATORY SYSTEM

On a separate piece of paper, see how well you can identify the components of the respiratory system numbered from 1 to 10 in Figure 1–11 below. When you have finished, turn to page 20A and compare your answers.

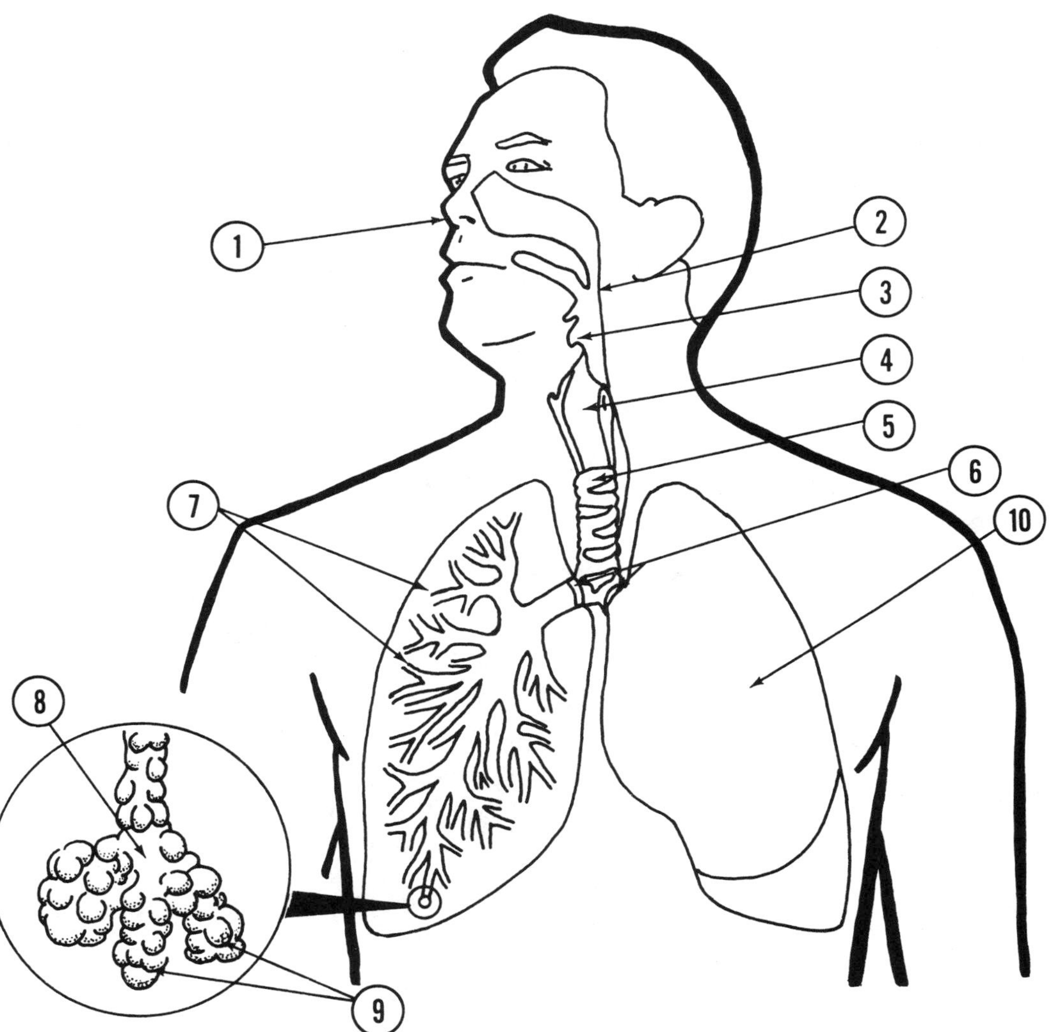

Figure 1–11

FRAME 17. PULMONARY CIRCULATION

Carbon dioxide and oxygen (respiratory gases) are transported to and from the lungs by the circulatory system, which consists of the heart and blood vessels. The systemic veins carry the blood to the heart from the various parts of the body. The systemic arteries carry the freshly oxygenated blood to the body tissues.

In Figure 1–12, you can trace the flow of venous blood carrying elevated levels of carbon dioxide (CO_2) to the lungs, and the flow of arterialized (oxygenated) blood (O_2) from the lungs to the heart and to the tissues. On a separate piece of paper fill in the blanks below.

1. Venous blood carrying high levels of CO_2 enters the ______________ of the heart. From there, it is pumped into the ______________ ventricle and on to the ______________ via the pulmonary artery.
2. Oxygenated blood flows via the pulmonary veins from the lungs into the left ______________ of the heart. From there it is pumped in to the left ______________, then into the aorta for delivery to the tissues.

When you have filled in the blanks turn to page 20B and check your answers.

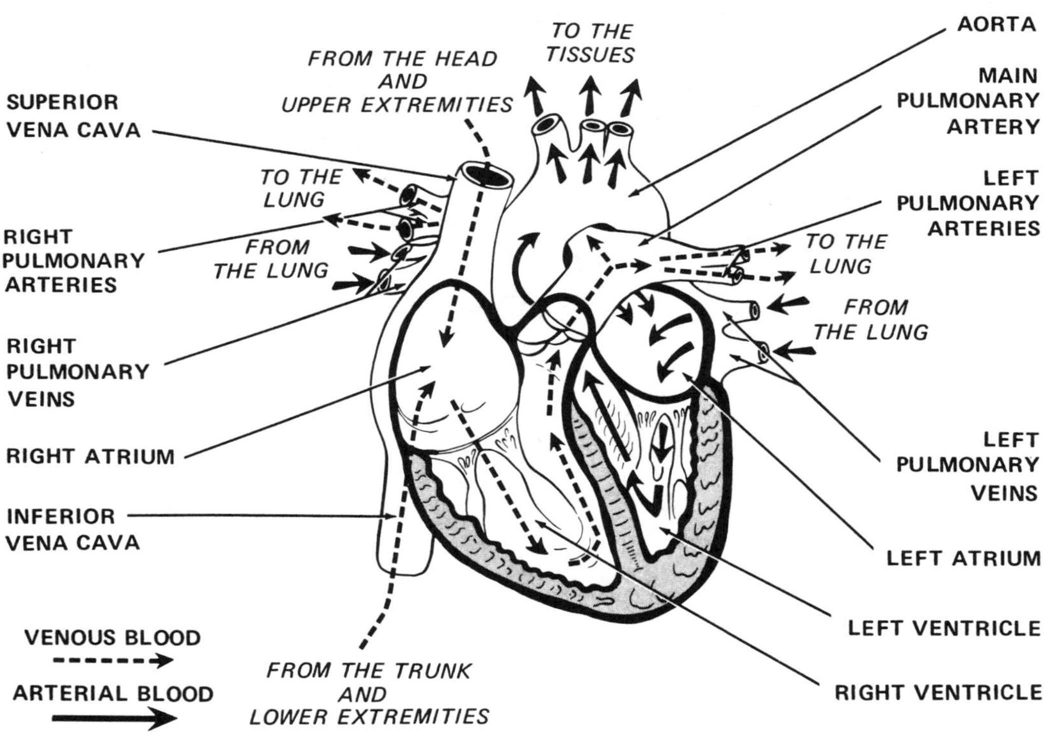

Figure 1–12

FRAME 18. EXTERNAL AND INTERNAL RESPIRATION

There are two kinds of respiration, external and internal. External respiration is the diffusion of carbon dioxide from the pulmonary capillaries into the alveoli, concurrent with the diffusion of oxygen from the alveoli into pulmonary capillary blood. Internal respiration is the diffusion of oxygen from tissue capillaries to the cells, concurrent with outward diffusion of hydrogen ions and carbon dioxide from cells to the tissue capillaries. See Figure 1–13.

(Q) External respiration takes place in the

a. pulmonary capillaries. 29 D
b. tissue capillaries. 33 B
c. alveoli and pulmonary capillaries. 29 A

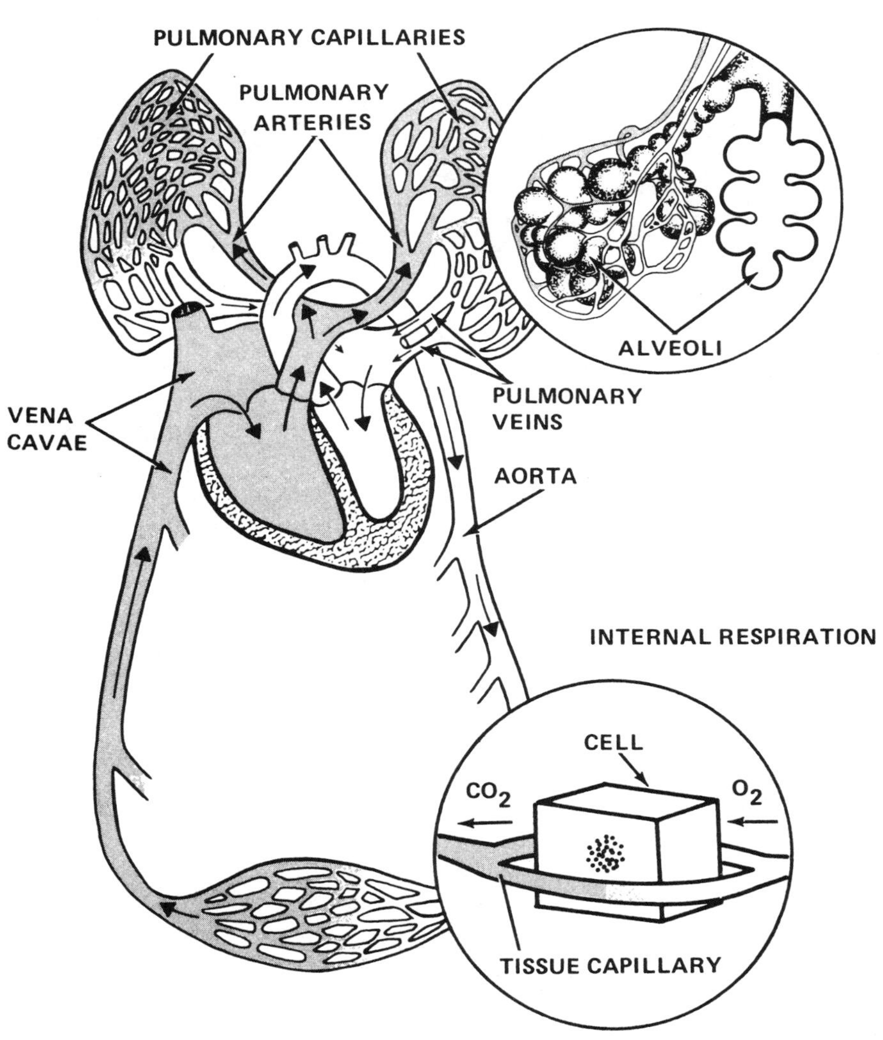

Figure 1–13

FRAME 19. ANATOMY OF THE PULMONARY CIRCULATION

See how well you can identify the structures involved in pulmonary circulation. In Figure 1–14 (below), which numbers identify the following structures? List the structures and your answers on a separate piece of paper. When you have finished, compare your answers to those on page 28A.

Right atrium	______	Left atrium	______
Right ventricle	______	Left ventricle	______
Right pulmonary vein	______	Capillaries	______
Right pulmonary artery	______	Alveolus	______
Inferior vena cava	______	Left pulmonary artery	______
Superior vena cava	______	Left pulmonary vein	______

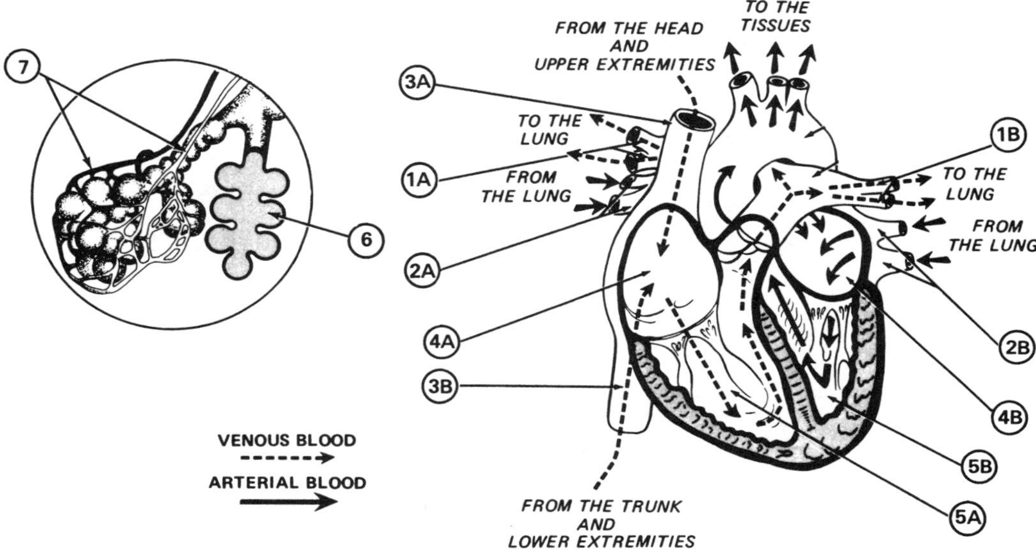

Figure 1–14

FRAME 20. THE HEART

The heart pumps blood to the pulmonary and systemic circulatory systems. The right side of the heart is considered to be a low-pressure pump and the left side a high-pressure pump because of the differences in blood pressure between pulmonary and systemic circulation.

(Q) The heart consists of how many chambers?

a. two chambers 29 C

b. four chambers 33 A

FRAME 21. THE CARDIOVASCULAR SYSTEM

Figure 1-15 shows the relation of arteries, veins, and capillaries in the circulatory system. The light areas represent blood containing greater amounts of oxygen than venous blood. The arteries deliver this blood to the tissues. The dark areas represent blood carrying increased amounts of carbon dioxide and decreased amounts of oxygen.

(Q) Which statement about blood returning from the tissues is correct?

a. Venous blood goes directly to the lungs, where the gases are exchanged, and the oxygenated blood goes back to the heart to be pumped into the arteries. 29 E

b. Venous blood goes to the right heart, where it is pumped into the lungs for gaseous exchange. From the lungs it goes into the arteries for distribution throughout the body. 33 C

c. Venous blood goes to the right heart, where it is pumped into the lungs for gas exchange. From the lungs the oxygenated blood goes back to the left heart, where it is pumped into the arteries. 29 B

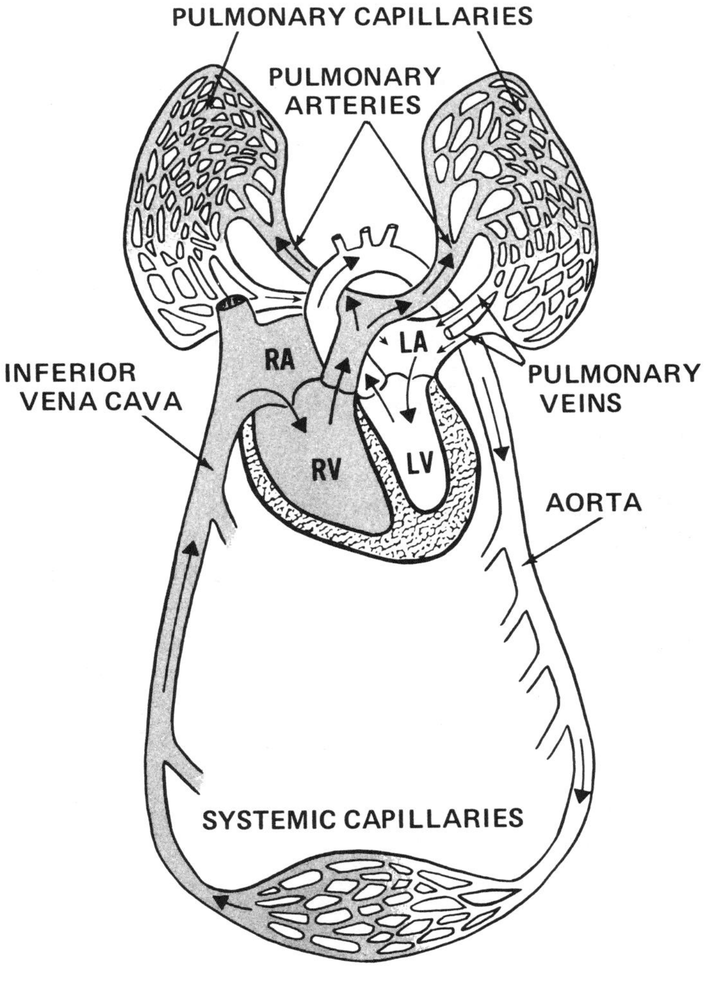

Figure 1-15

28A (from page 26, frame 19)
Answers

Right atrium—4A
Right ventricle—5A
Right pulmonary vein—2A
Right pulmonary artery—1A
Inferior vena cava—3B
Superior vena cava—3A
Left atrium—4B
Left ventricle—5B
Capillaries—7
Alveolus—6
Left pulmonary artery—1B
Left pulmonary vein—2B

If you missed any, return to page 26, frame 19, and try it again. If you identified all of these correctly, please continue on page 26, frame 20.

28B (from page 30, frame 22)
Wrong. Approximately 150 mL of the inspired air remains in the dead space (airways). The rest of it enters the alveoli for gaseous exchange. Return to page 30, frame 22, and try again.

28C (from page 31, frame 23)
Wrong. The volume of air per minute (in liters) that ventilates the physiologic dead space (anatomic and alveolar dead space) is called dead-space ventilation. In dead-space ventilation, the areas are aerated, but rapid gas exchange does not take place. Total ventilation includes this ventilation of dead space, as well as ventilation of the functioning alveoli. Return to page 31, frame 23, and select another answer.

28D (from page 31, frame 23)
Correct. Total ventilation means the volume of air moved into and out of the entire respiratory tract. This includes dead-space ventilation (both anatomical and alveolar dead space) and alveolar ventilation of the functional alveoli. The average total (minute) ventilation of a young healthy male is about 6 L/min (about 500 mL, 12/min). If breathing is shallow, the volume of air inhaled (tidal volume) is small. There may be just enough tidal volume to ventilate the dead space, with very little getting through to the alveoli. Please continue on page 31, frame 24.

28E (from page 39, frame 31)

1. $P\bar{v}O_2$
2. $S\bar{v}O_2$
3. TLC

Please continue on page 42, frame 32.

29A (from page 25, frame 18)
Correct. External respiration takes place only between functioning alveoli and pulmonary capillaries. The capillaries surrounding alveoli are small, thin-walled blood vessels that connect arterioles to venules. The gases are exchanged between pulmonary capillaries and the alveoli. The *arterialized* blood (blood containing a greater amount of oxygen) then flows from the pulmonary capillaries into the pulmonary venules and on through into the pulmonary veins, until it reaches the left atrium of the heart.

The lungs themselves play a passive role in the exchange of gases. The diffusion of oxygen from the alveoli is caused by the unequal pressures of oxygen and carbon dioxide on either side of the semipermeable membranes separating the alveoli and the capillaries. Since oxygen exerts a greater pressure in the alveoli than in the blood, O_2 diffuses into the bloodstream. Since the pressure of carbon dioxide is greater in the blood than in the alveoli, CO_2 diffuses out of the blood into the alveoli. From there, it is expelled from the body into the atmosphere. Please continue on page 26, frame 19.

29B (from page 27, frame 21)
Correct. Venous blood from the head and upper extremity enters the right heart via the superior vena cava. From the trunk and lower extremity, venous blood enters the right heart via the inferior vena cava. The blood is then pumped to the lungs for gas exchange. The oxygenated blood is returned to the left heart, from which it is pumped into the arteries for distribution to the body. Please continue on page 30, frame 22.

29C (from page 26, frame 20)
Wrong. The right heart pumps the venous blood to the lungs to be oxygenated, and the left heart pumps the oxygenated blood to the tissues. Each "pump" has two chambers—an atrium and a ventricle. Return to page 26, frame 20, and study Figure 1-14; then try the question again.

29D (from page 25, frame 18)
Not quite. The pulmonary capillaries are the small, thin-walled vessels that envelop the alveoli in the lungs. Blood travels from the pulmonary arteries into the pulmonary arterioles and on to the pulmonary capillaries, then through the pulmonary venules into the pulmonary veins. Along this route, the carbon dioxide from the blood is exchanged for oxygen. Where does this exchange between capillary blood and alveolar air take place? Return to page 25, frame 18, and try again.

29E (from page 27, frame 21)
Careful! You've bypassed the heart. Venous blood from the head and upper extremities enters the right heart through the inferior vena cava. From there, it is pumped into the lungs for gas exchange. Return to page 27, frame 21, and select another answer.

FRAME 22. NORMAL ALVEOLAR VENTILATION

In a normal inhalation, you breathe in about 500 mL of air. This amount is called the *tidal volume.* Only about two thirds of this amount, however, reaches the area of gas exchange — the alveoli. The rest remains in the airways, where gas exchange does not take place. See Figure 1–16.

(Q) During normal ventilation, approximately how much air enters the alveoli from the atmosphere?

a. 350 mL — 33 D
b. 150 mL — 28 B
c. 500 mL — 32 A

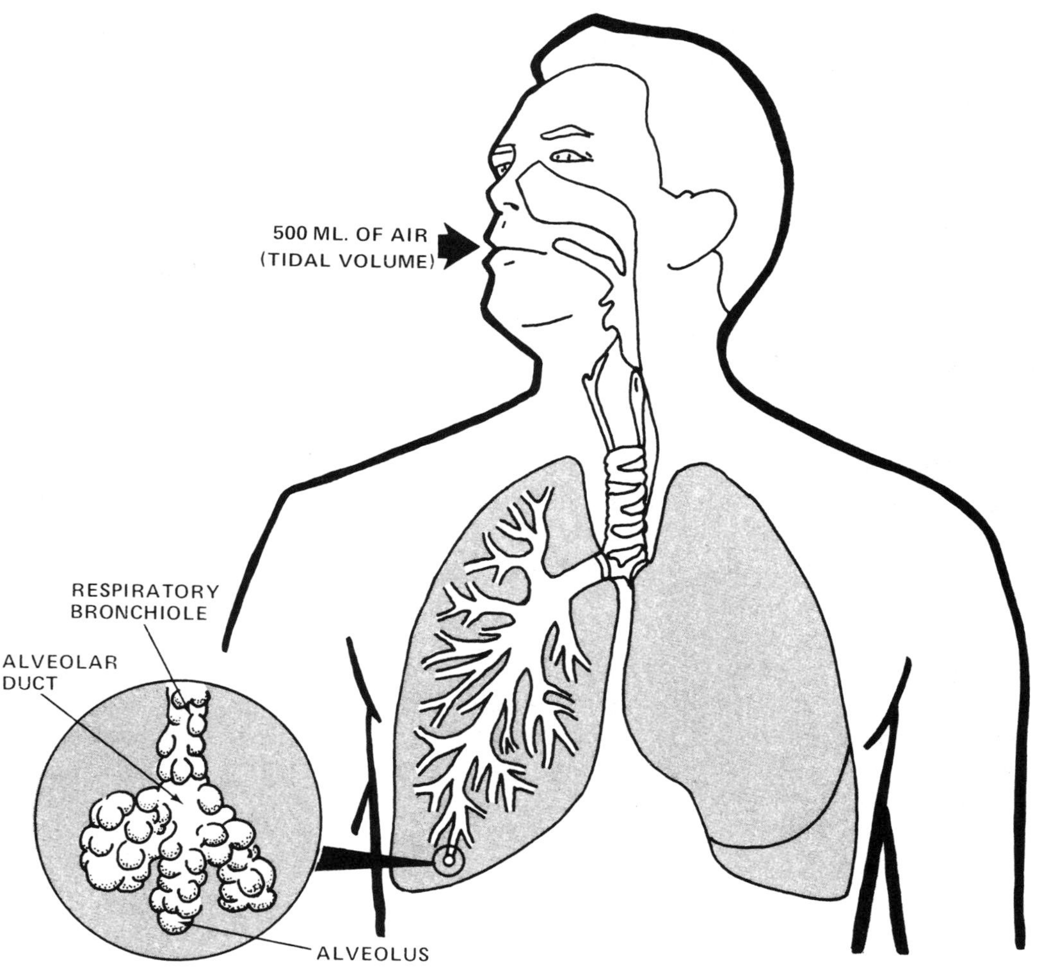

Figure 1–16

FRAME 23. PHYSIOLOGIC DEAD SPACE

The fresh air that enters the alveoli is mixed with a volume of gas already filling the millions of alveoli. When you breathe out, you first exhale the air from the *anatomic dead space,* which is followed by a larger amount of air from the alveoli. This causes the anatomic dead space to be filled with mixed alveolar gas, which is drawn back into the lungs on the next breath, followed by fresh air. If you were to continue rebreathing the air in the dead space by breathing through a long tube, the air entering the alveoli would soon lose most of its oxygen and accumulate a dangerously high level of carbon dioxide, with fatal consequences.

The dead space from the mouth and nose to the terminal bronchiole is called the anatomic dead space. However, dead space also may occur in the alveoli themselves. Alveoli that are ventilated but cannot function properly in the exchange of gases are considered alveolar dead space. The sum of the *anatomic* and *alveolar dead space* is referred to as *physiologic dead space.*

(Q) Minute volume includes which of the following?
- a. dead space ventilation — 28 C
- b. alveolar ventilation — 33 a
- c. both of the above — 28 D

FRAME 24. ABNORMAL VENTILATION

Normal ventilation is that amount of ventilation per minute that provides adequate alveolar ventilation at a normal rate and with a minimum of effort. Hypoventilation is a condition in which not enough fresh air is breathed into and out of the alveoli (underbreathing). It results in a decreased amount of oxygen intake and an accumulation of CO_2. Hypoventilation may occur with a reduction in tidal volume (amount of inhaled gas per breath), reduction in respiratory rate, or an increase in dead space. By contrast, hyperventilation is a condition in which too much fresh air is being moved into and out of the alveoli (overbreathing). Hyperventilation results in increased carbon dioxide excretion and increased oxygen intake. The only way to determine if a patient has a normal alveolar ventilation is to analyze an arterial blood sample. In normal individuals an arterial CO_2 tension *above* 40 mm Hg would indicate hypoventilation and an arterial CO_2 *below* 40 mm Hg would indicate hyperventilation.

(Q) A reduction in the breathing rate and/or tidal volume may cause
- a. hyperventilation. — 33 b
- b. hypoventilation. — 32 B

32A (from page 30, frame 22)
Wrong. 500 mL is the tidal volume—the total amount inhaled. But all of this does not reach the alveoli for gas exchange. Some of it remains in the dead space (nose, mouth, pharynx, trachea, bronchi, bronchioles), where rapid exchange of gases does not take place. Return to page 30, frame 22, and try again.

32B (from page 31, frame 24)
Correct. The care of patients who are hypoventilating (where not enough oxygen is being supplied or not enough carbon dioxide removed) is one of the most important responsibilities of respiratory care practitioners. Sometimes, certain respiratory care procedures may cause hyperventilation. Normal body functions are disrupted if the carbon dioxide is too low. Then the breathing rate must be slowed or the tidal volume decreased to prevent excessive elimination of carbon dioxide from the body. A less common problem is treatment of hyperventilation caused by severe pain or lung disease. Please continue on page 34, frame 25.

32C (from page 50, frame 38)
Correct. Although the oxygen molecules diffuse into the plasma and are carried in solution, most of them are transported in chemical combination with hemoglobin, the pigment of the erythrocytes (red blood cells). In anemia the hemoglobin content is decreased, and less oxygen can be carried to the cells because the means of transport has been decreased. Please continue on page 51, frame 39.

32D (from page 52, frame 40)
Correct. The reduced alveolar oxygen tension that causes hypoxia can result from an insufficient supply of oxygen in the inspired air (as at high altitudes) or inadequate alveolar ventilation of some other origin. Please continue on page 53, frame 41.

32E (from page 55, frame 43)
Wrong. The oxygen molecule increases or decreases its affinity for hemoglobin when the curve shifts. In this example the curve has shifted to the right and the amount of usable oxygen will change. Return to page 55, frame 43, and try again.

33A (from page 26, frame 20)
Correct. We may consider the heart as having two "pumps." The right heart pumps the venous blood to the lungs to be oxygenated and the left heart pumps the oxygenated blood to the tissues. Each pump has two chambers—an atrium and a ventricle. The heart thus consists of four chambers—the right atrium, right ventricle, left atrium, and left ventricle. Please continue on page 27, frame 21.

33B (from page 25, frame 18)
External respiration does not take place in the tissue capillaries. Return to page 25, frame 18, and select another answer.

33C (from page 27, frame 21)
Careful! You've bypassed the heart. Oxygenated blood does not flow directly from the lungs to the body tissues. It must be pumped by the heart into the arteries. Return to page 27, frame 21, and try again.

33D (from page 30, frame 22)
Correct. Keep in mind that all of the air that enters the respiratory system does not reach the alveoli. About one third of it remains in the dead space (airways, where rapid gas exchange does not take place). Two thirds of the tidal volume is available for the exchange of gases with capillary blood. Please continue on page 31, frame 23.

33a (from page 31, frame 23)
Wrong. The volume of air per minute (in liters) that ventilates all the functioning alveoli (where rapid gas exchange takes place) is called alveolar ventilation. But remember that the dead space is also ventilated, even though rapid gas exchange does not take place in those areas. Return to page 31, frame 23, and select another answer.

33b (from page 31, frame 24)
Wrong. Hyperventilation is a condition that may be caused by a fast breathing rate and/or a large tidal volume. Return to page 31, frame 24, and try again.

33c (from page 35, frame 26)
Wrong. 6000 mL is the *total lung capacity*—the amount of gas you would have in your lungs after maximal inspiration. Return to page 35, frame 26, and study Figures 1-17 and 1-18; then select another answer.

33d (from page 36, frame 27)
Wrong. The ERV is that volume of air that *can still be exhaled* from the resting expiratory level. We're talking about the RV, the amount of air left in the lungs *after a maximal expiration*. Return to page 36, frame 27, and select another answer.

FRAME 25. THE LANGUAGE OF RESPIRATORY PHYSIOLOGY

Before lung volumes and capacities can be discussed, you should become familiar with some of the language and symbols used by respiratory physiologists to define lung capacities and volumes, gas pressures, and symbols used to describe the physiology of breathing. The effect of gases is frequently considered in terms of their partial pressures. Dalton's law of partial pressure demonstrates that the total pressure of a gas mixture is equal to the sum of the partial pressures of the constituent gases. The partial pressure generated by each gas in a mixture is the same as the pressure it would exert if it occupied the entire volume alone. We will discuss the partial pressures of carbon dioxide and oxygen in the blood subsequently. The following symbols are examples of those used by respiratory care practitioners.

For Gases

Selected Primary Symbols

V = Gas volume
P = Gas pressure
F = Fractional concentration in dry-gas phase
f = Respiratory rate

Selected Secondary Symbols

I = Inspired gas
E = Expired gas
A = Alveolar gas
T = Tidal gas
D = Dead space

For Blood

Selected Primary Symbols

S = Percent saturation of Hb with O_2 or CO
C = Concentration in blood phase

Selected Secondary Symbols

a = Arterial blood
v = Venous blood
c = Capillary blood

Examples

V_T = Tidal volume
$Paco_2$ = Partial pressure of CO_2 in arterial blood
$P\bar{v}o_2$ = Partial pressure of O_2 in mixed venous blood
$S\bar{v}o_2$ = Percent saturation of Hb with O_2 in mixed venous blood

For Lung Volumes

TLC = Total lung capacity, volume of gas in the lungs at the end of a maximal inspiration
VC = Vital capacity, maximal volume that can be expired after maximal inspiration
RV = Residual volume, volume of gas in the lungs at end of maximal expiration

Please turn to page 35, frame 26.

FRAME 26. NORMAL LUNG VOLUMES AND CAPACITIES

In a young healthy male, the total amount of gas contained in the lungs after a maximal inspiration is called the total lung capacity (TLC) (Fig. 1–17). It is normally about 6000 mL.

(Q) The amount of air normally breathed in and out (tidal volume) is ideally about

a. 6000 mL. 33 c

b. 500 mL. 41 A

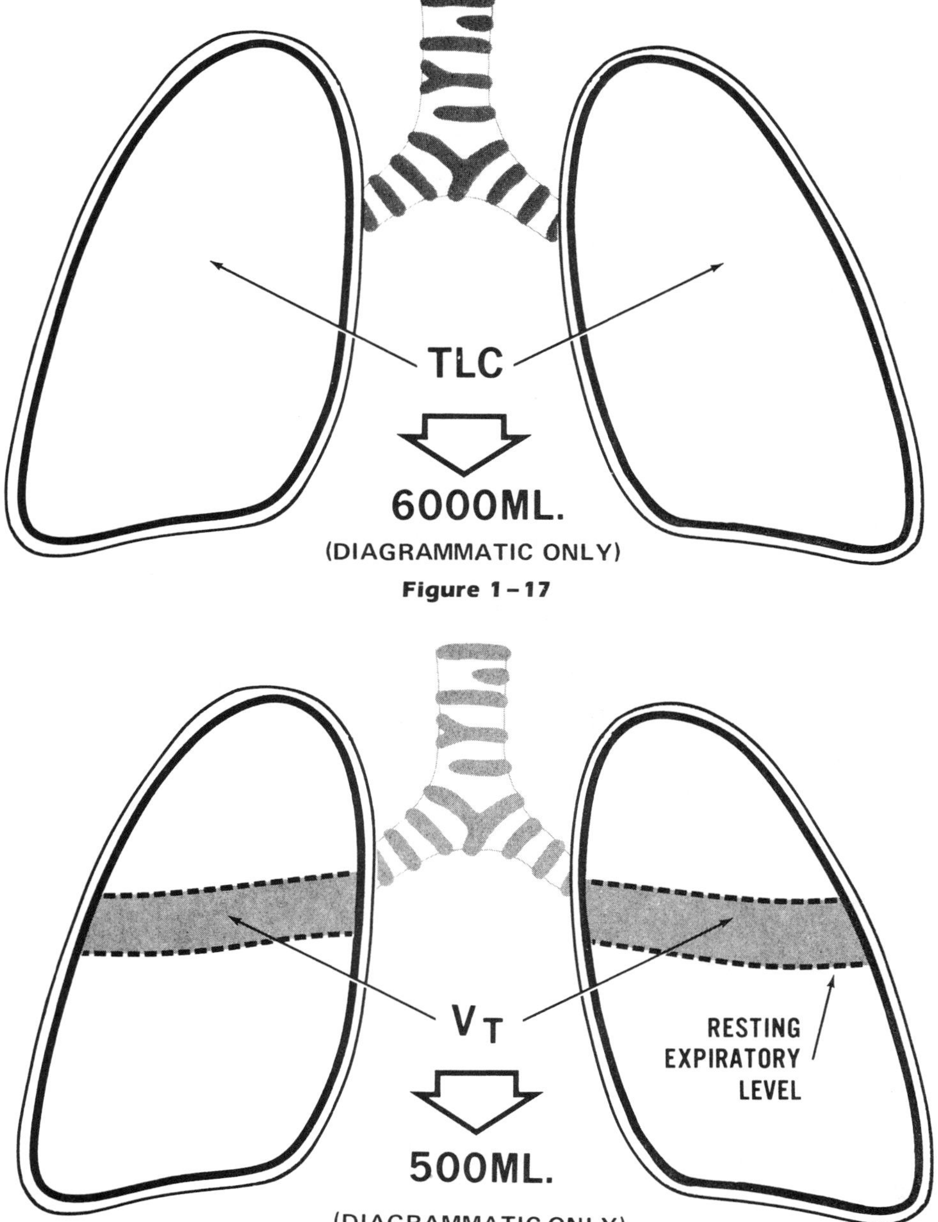

Figure 1–17

Figure 1–18

FRAME 27. EXPIRATORY RESERVE AND RESIDUAL VOLUMES

If you breathe in normally and exhale normally (tidal volume, or V_T), you have reached the *resting expiratory level* (Fig. 1–18). If you try, you will find that you can continue to exhale an additional amount of air. This additional amount is called the *expiratory reserve volume* (ERV), as shown in Figure 1–19. At this point, you have made a maximal expiration. However, there is still some air remaining in your lungs. This is called the *residual volume* (RV).

(Q) The amount of air left in the lungs after a maximal exhalation is called the

a. expiratory reserve volume. 33 d

b. residual volume. 41 B

EXPIRATORY RESERVE AND RESIDUAL VOLUMES

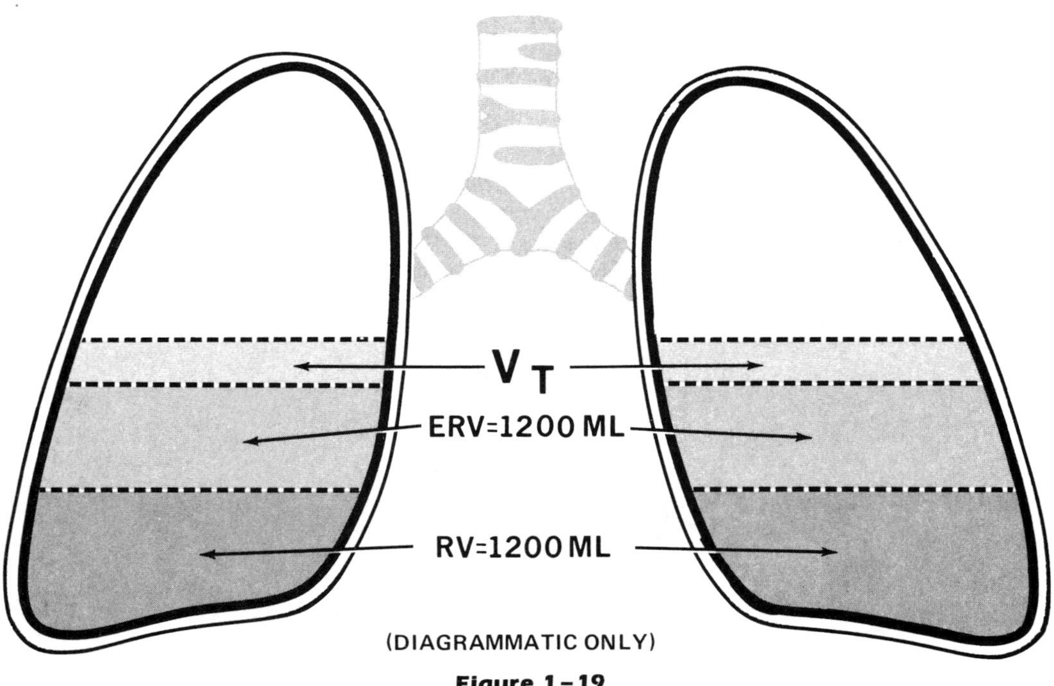

Figure 1–19

FRAME 28. FUNCTIONAL RESIDUAL CAPACITY

As you can see in Figure 1–20, the RV of gas in the lungs is about 1200 mL and the ERV about 1200 mL. The total of these two (RV + ERV) equals the volume of gas in the lungs after a normal exhalation. This volume is called the functional residual capacity (FRC).

(Q) The normal value for the functional residual capacity in a healthy young male should be about

a. 3600 mL. 41 C

b. 2400 mL. 41 a

LUNG VOLUMES

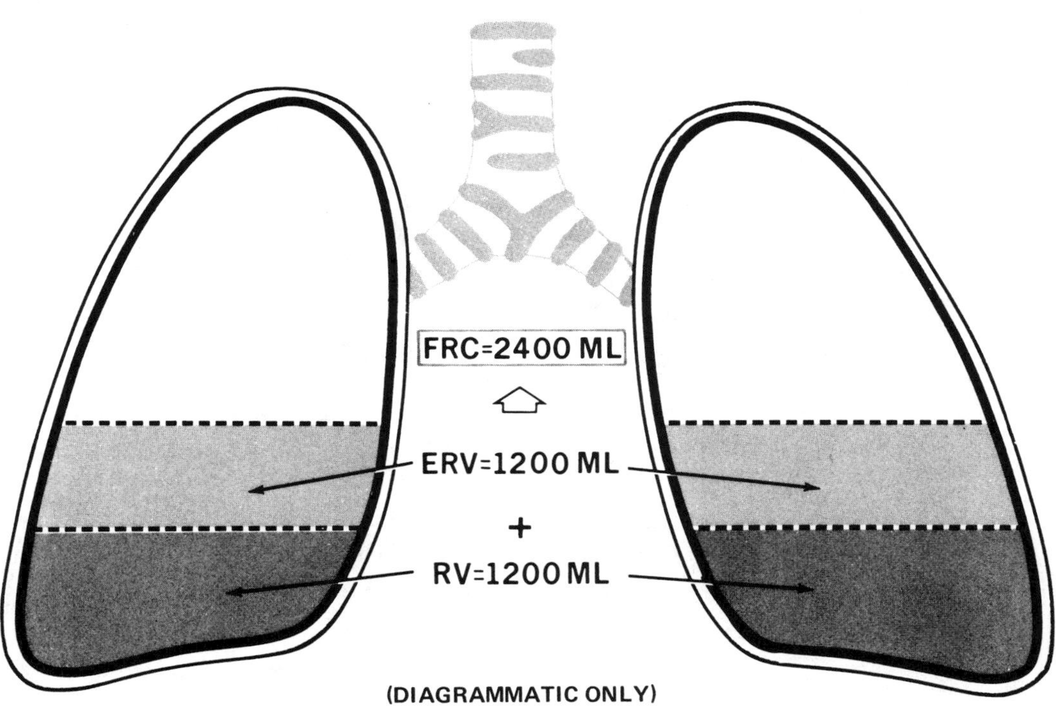

(DIAGRAMMATIC ONLY)

Figure 1–20

FRAME 29. VITAL CAPACITY

The maximum amount of air that can be inhaled from the resting expiratory level is called the inspiratory capacity (IC). The vital capacity of the lung (VC) is the maximal volume that can be exhaled after a maximal inspiration. Of the 6000 mL TLC, 1200 mL will remain in the lung as residual volume (Fig. 1–21). The rest can be exhaled. This includes the IC and the ERV.

(Q) The VC includes

a. RV + ERV. 41 D

b. IC + FRC. 41 b

c. ERV + IC. 40 D

LUNG VOLUMES

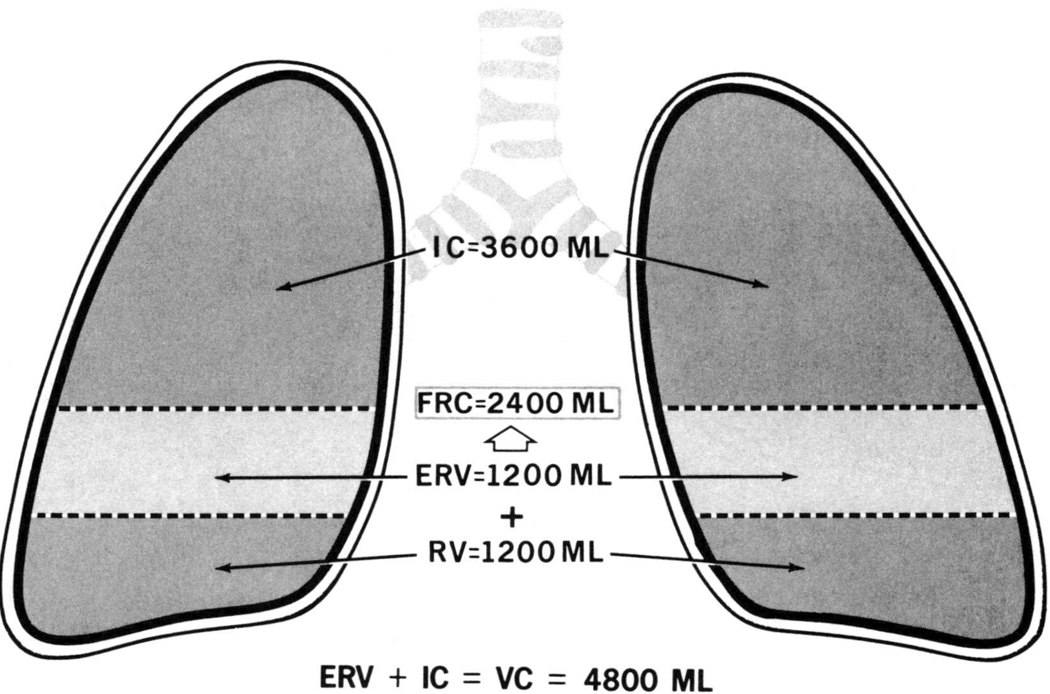

(DIAGRAMMATIC ONLY)

Figure 1–21

FRAME 30. INSPIRATORY CAPACITY

(Q) As illustrated in Figure 1–22, the normal value for the IC in a healthy young male is about

a. 3600 mL. 40 A
b. 3100 mL. 40 a
c. 500 mL. 49 A

LUNG VOLUMES

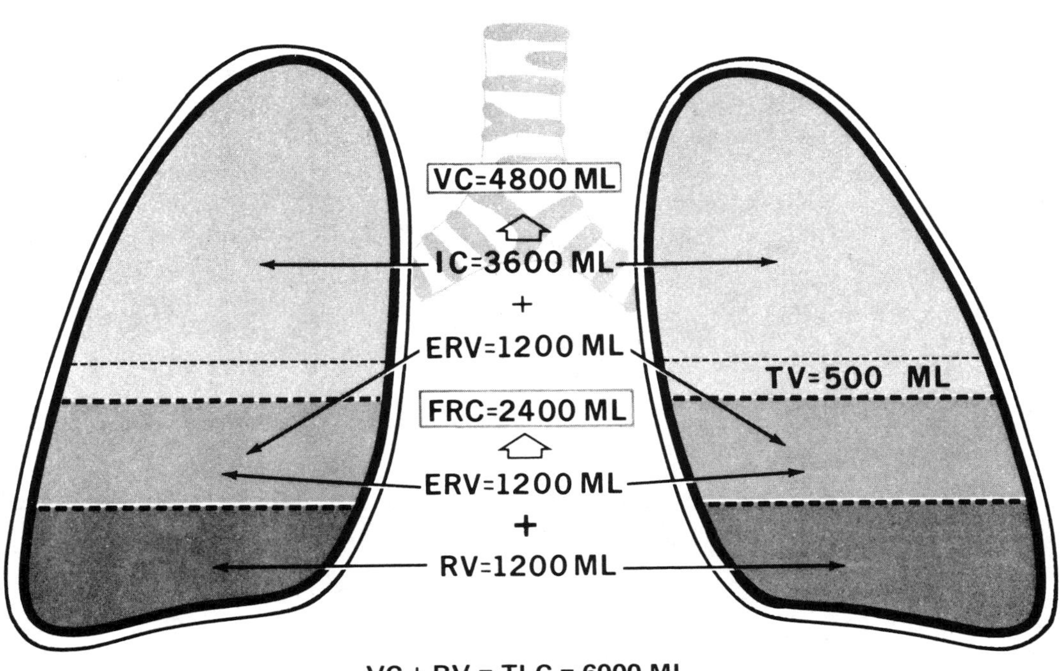

VC + RV = TLC = 6000 ML

(DIAGRAMMATIC ONLY)

Figure 1–22

FRAME 31. PRIMARY AND SECONDARY PHYSIOLOGY SYMBOLS

The symbols reviewed on page 34 will be used in discussing lung volumes and partial pressures of gases in the blood.

(Q) On a separate piece of paper, write down the symbols used for the following:

1. partial pressure of oxygen (O_2) in mixed venous blood
2. saturation of hemoglobin (Hb) with O_2 in mixed venous blood
3. volume of gas in the lungs at the end of a maximal inspiration

Turn to page 28E and compare your answers.

40A (from page 39, frame 30)
Correct. After you inhale normally, there still remains in the lungs an inspiratory reserve volume (which still can be inhaled). The tidal volume (VT) and the inspiratory reserve volume (IRV) constitute the inspiratory capacity (IC), which should be about 3600 mL in a healthy young male. Please continue on page 39, frame 31.

40B (from page 43, frame 33)
Almost. But there is another part of the brain also involved. Return to page 43, frame 33, and select another answer.

40C (from page 47, frame 37)
Wrong. Partial pressure of carbon dioxide in arterial blood would be symbolized as $Paco_2$. Return to page 47, frame 37, and try again.

40D (from page 38, frame 29)
Correct. The VC is the maximal volume that can be exhaled after maximal inhalation. If 3600 mL is the IC (the volume that can be inspired from the resting expiratory level), then all of this plus the ERV of 1200 mL can be exhaled. The total of these two volumes—ERV and IC—is 4800 mL, the normal vital capacity. Please continue on page 39, frame 30.

40a (from page 39, frame 30)
Not quite enough. The inspiratory capacity includes the tidal volume and inspiratory reserve volume. Return to page 39, frame 30, and try again.

40b (from page 46, frame 36)
Wrong. If this were true, the oxygen would diffuse from the venous blood into the alveoli. Return to page 46, frame 36, and study Figure 1-26; then try again.

40c (from page 51, frame 39)
True, but certainly emergency action is required in severe hypoxia. Return to page 51, frame 39, and select another answer.

40d (from page 53, frame 41)
Wrong. Histotoxic substances are chemicals or drugs that cause hypoxia by interfering with the oxidative-enzyme mechanism of the cell. When you apply a tourniquet, what happens to the blood flow? Return to page 53, frame 41, and review the causes of hypoxia; then try again.

41A (from page 35, frame 26)
Correct. The normal tidal volume (VT) for a young healthy male at rest is about 500 mL. Please continue on page 36, frame 27.

41B (from page 36, frame 27)
Correct. The residual volume is the amount of air left in the lungs after a maximal exhalation. Please continue on page 37, frame 28.

41C (from page 37, frame 28)
Wrong. The residual volume (1200 mL) and the expiratory reserve volume (1200 mL) constitute the *functional residual capacity* (FRC) which has a normal value of 2400 mL. Please continue on page 38, frame 29.

41D (from page 38, frame 29)
Wrong. The residual volume is not exhaled. It is the amount that remains in the lungs after a maximal expiration. The vital capacity includes only the air that can be exhaled after maximal inspiration. Return to page 38, frame 29, and try again.

41E (from page 55, frame 43)
Wrong. The oxygen molecule increases its affinity for hemoglobin when the curve shifts to the left. As blood flows through systemic capillaries, the curve shifts right. Return to page 55, frame 43, and try again.

41a (from page 37, frame 28)
Correct. The FRC has a normal value of 2400 mL. Please continue on page 38, frame 29.

41b (from page 38, frame 29)
Wrong. The vital capacity is the maximal volume that can be exhaled after a maximal inspiration. The functional residual capacity contains the residual volume, which cannot be exhaled. Return to page 38, frame 29, and try the question again.

41c (from page 42, frame 32)
Wrong. This is the amount that occupies the anatomic dead space. About 350 mL actually reach the alveoli to take part in gas exchange. The alveolar minute ventilation can be calculated by multiplying 350 × respiratory rate (e.g., $350 \times 12 = 4.2$ L/min). Please continue on page 43, frame 33.

41d (from page 46, frame 36)
Correct. Because the partial pressure of oxygen is higher in the alveoli than in the venous blood, the oxygen diffuses across the thin alveolar capillary membranes into the pulmonary capillaries. Conversely, because the partial pressure of carbon dioxide is greater in the venous blood than in the alveoli, carbon dioxide diffuses across the membranes into the alveoli. Please continue on page 47, frame 37.

FRAME 32. DEAD-SPACE VENTILATION

Ideally, the tidal volume (the amount taken in during a normal inspiration) is about 500 mL. However, 150 mL of the tidal volume is dead-space ventilation (Fig. 1–23), which never reaches the alveoli.

(Q) Of the 500 mL of air inspired, how much of it actually reaches the alveoli for the exchange of gases?
   a. 150 mL 41 c
   b. 350 mL 49 a

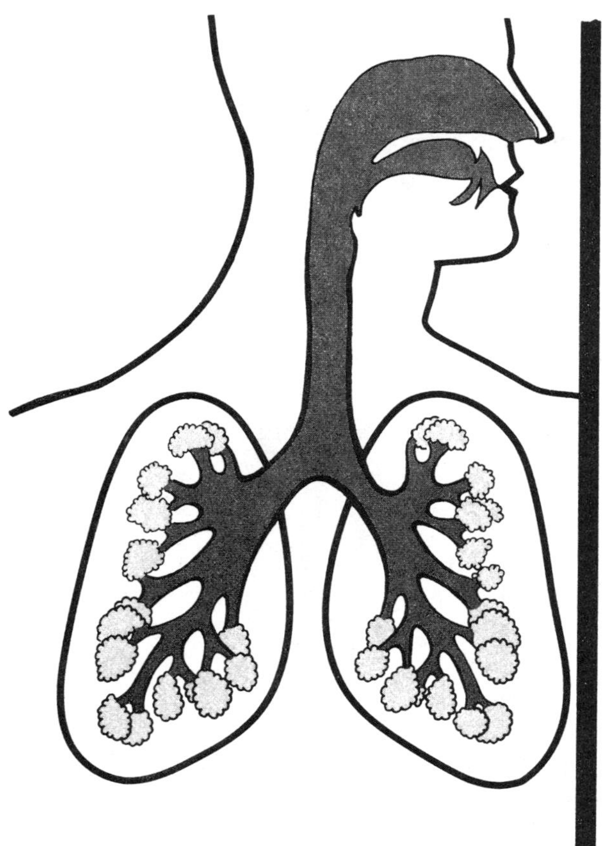

VENTILATION

TV = 500ml

■ DEAD SPACE VENTILATION 150ml PER BREATH

□ ALVEOLAR VENTILATION 350ml PER BREATH

Figure 1–23

FRAME 33. REGULATION OF VENTILATION

Ventilation is caused by the alternate contraction and relaxation of the diaphragm and the external intercostal muscles. But what initiates the actions of these muscles? When certain parts of the brainstem—the medulla oblongata and the pons (Fig. 1–24)—are stimulated, they direct the respiratory muscles to contract and relax in a regulated pattern.

(Q) The cerebral cortex also plays a part in voluntary control (such as holding your breath), but what controls the regular automatic pattern of ventilation?

a. the pons 49 b
b. the medulla 40 B
c. both of the above 49 B

FUNCTION AND LOCATION OF RESPIRATORY CENTERS

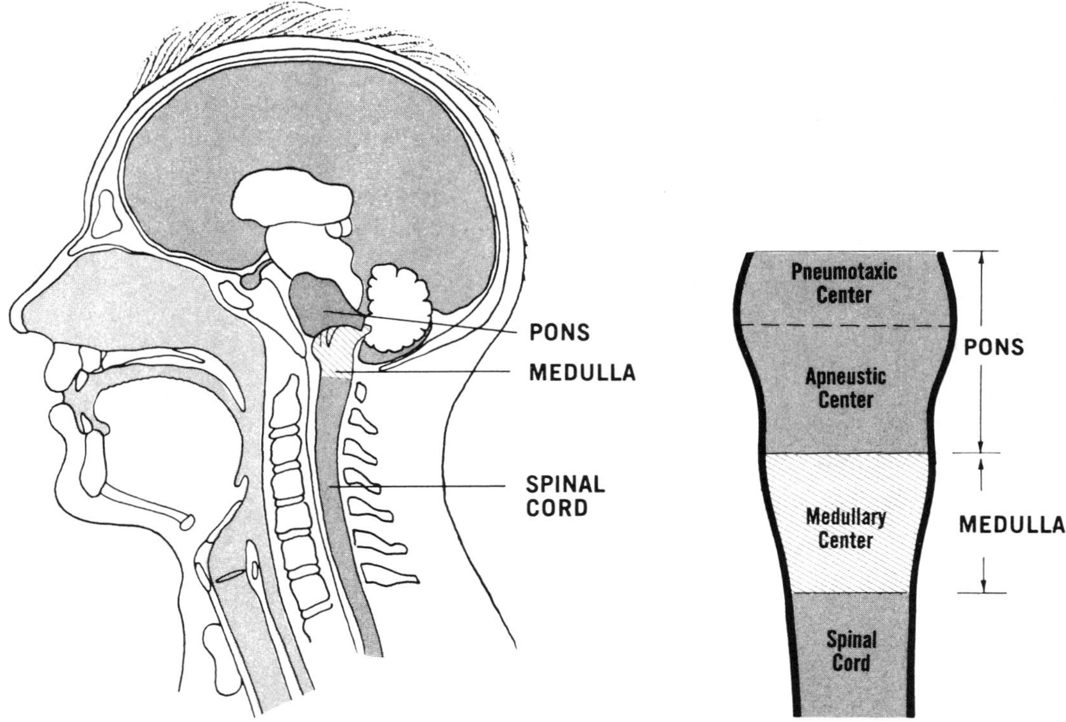

Figure 1–24

FRAME 34. NERVE IMPULSES

Nerve impulses are sent from the respiratory centers in the brain to the spinal cord. From the upper spinal cord, the phrenic nerves send impulses to the diaphragm. Lower in the spinal cord, the intercostal nerves send impulses to the intercostal muscles. The alternate contraction and relaxation of the diaphragm and the external intercostal muscles provide the major power for quiet breathing.

Sudden death can be caused by the various factors that interfere with nerve impulses from the brain reaching the spinal cord and respiratory muscles. Depression due to drug overdose, damage to the base of the skull (resulting in damage to the brainstem), or damage to the spinal cord can all result in cessation of breathing.

Severe factors affect the rate of impulses from the brain to the respiratory musculature. Some are the level of physical activity, the chemical composition of the blood and spinal fluid supplying and surrounding the respiratory centers in the brain, nerve impulses received by the respiratory centers from the rest of the body, or a combination of these factors.

The rate and depth of breathing determine how much air will reach the alveoli, allowing oxygen and carbon dioxide to diffuse across the alveolar capillary membranes. During exercise, emotional stress, and illness, different types of breathing can be observed. Several different patterns are described below and illustrated on page 45.

1. Abnormal increase in the depth and the rate of respiratory movements
2. Abnormal slowness in the rate of breathing
3. Cessation of breathing
4. Abnormally fast rate of breathing
5. A condition seen especially during a coma resulting from damage to the nervous centers, characterized by a rhythmic increase, then decrease, in the tidal volume, followed by periods of apnea (no breathing)
6. Abnormal decrease in the depth of respiratory movements

Turn to page 45, frame 35, and review Figure 1–25, which shows the different types of breathing you may encounter.

FRAME 35. BREATHING PATTERNS

The illustration of eupnea (Fig. 1–25) shows the normal rate and depth of breathing. As the patient inhales, gas is removed from the spirometer bell and the stylus moves upward on the graph paper. During exhalation, the patient's exhaled air flows into the bell and the stylus moves downward. The other breathing patterns are abnormal types brought on by emotional or physiological disturbances. From Figure 1–25 above and the descriptions on page 44, frame 34, see how many of these abnormal patterns you can define. Write your answers on a separate piece of paper.

When you have defined the six abnormal patterns of breathing, turn to page 48A to see how well you have done.

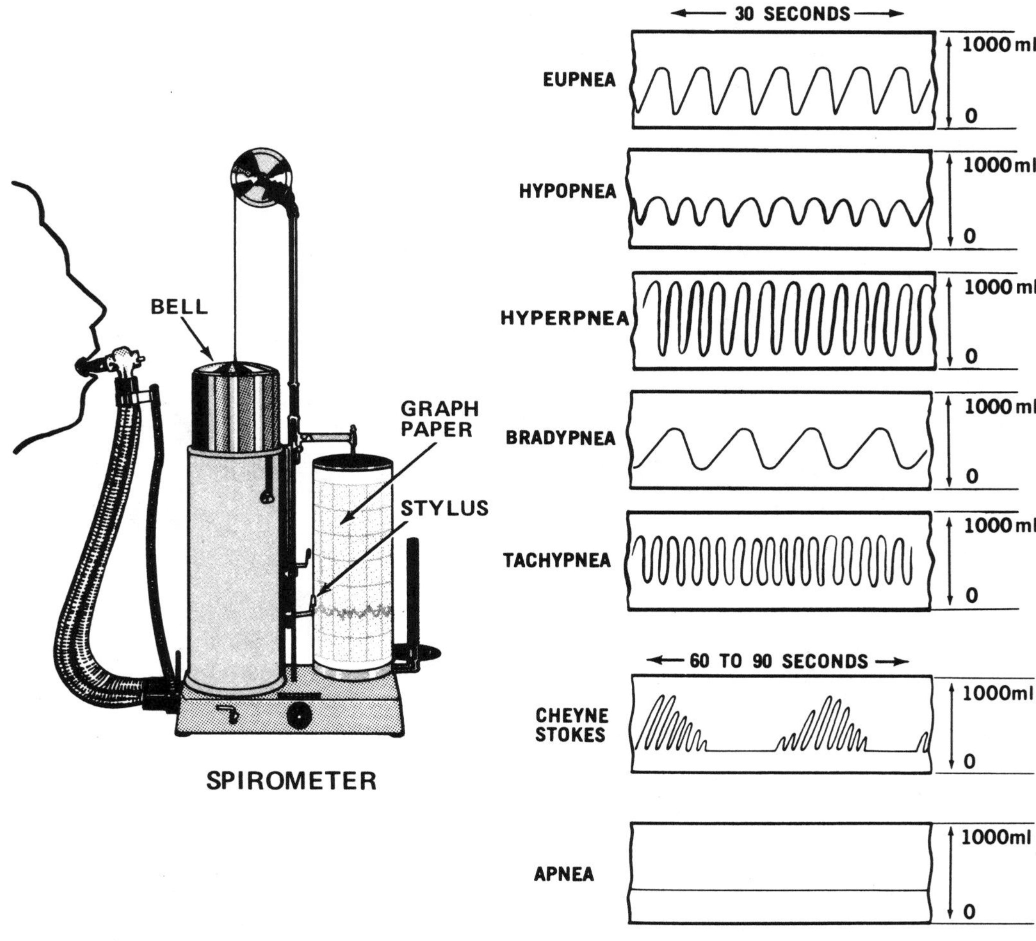

Figure 1–25

FRAME 36. OXYGEN UPTAKE

You can see how different types and rates of breathing can affect the amount of oxygen reaching the alveoli for gas exchange. Hypoventilation (underbreathing) is a reduction in alveolar ventilation. During hypoventilation, the amount of carbon dioxide in the body increases above normal. Hyperventilation (overbreathing) results in an increase in alveolar ventilation, which causes the amount of carbon dioxide in the body to decrease below normal. Keep in mind that there is always a certain partial pressure of carbon dioxide and oxygen in blood, usually maintained by a normal breathing pattern. Hypoventilation or hyperventilation disturbs this balance. Gas exchange in the lungs takes place because of the differences in partial pressure of oxygen and carbon dioxide between the blood and the alveoli (Fig. 1–26).

(Q) Which of the following statements is correct?

a. The partial pressure of oxygen is higher in the alveolus than in the venous blood. 41 d

b. The partial pressure of oxygen is higher in the venous blood than in the alveolus. 40 b

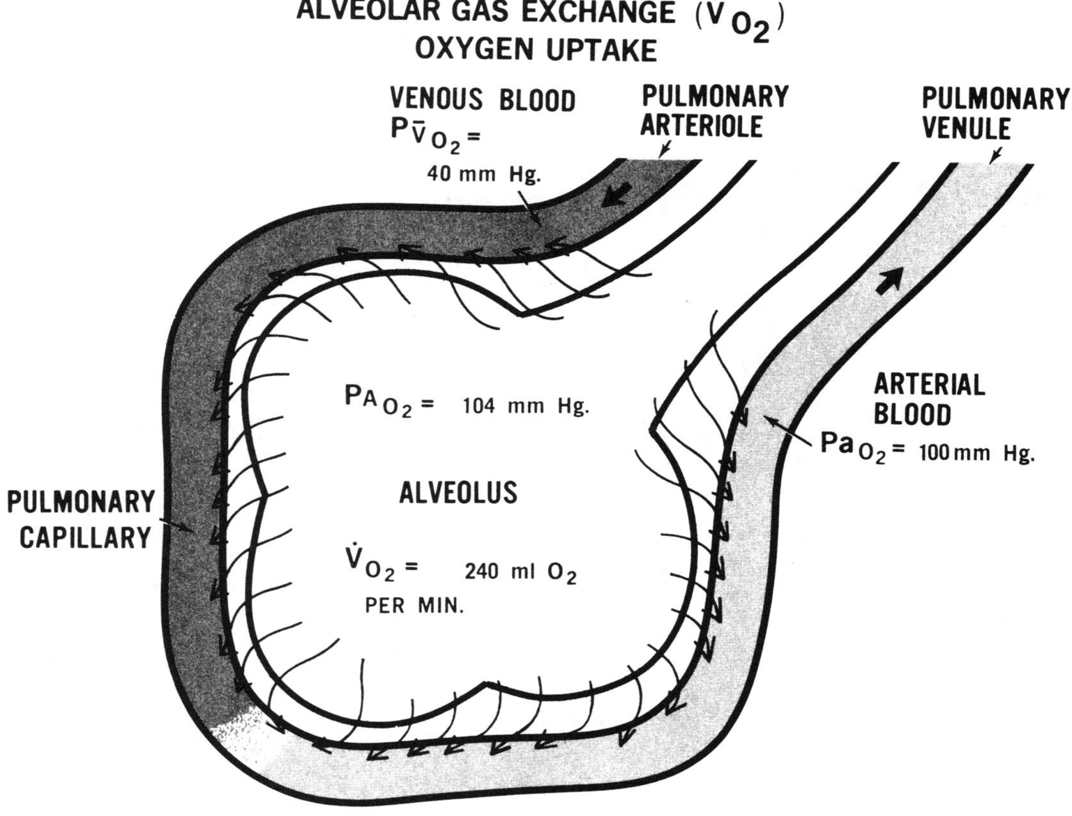

Figure 1–26

FRAME 37. CARBON DIOXIDE OUTPUT

Carbon dioxide leaves the pulmonary capillary blood until the CO_2 pressure in the blood comes into equilibrium with the CO_2 tension in the alveoli (Fig. 1–27).

(Q) The symbol $P\bar{v}CO_2$ refers to the partial pressure of

a. carbon dioxide in mixed venous blood. 49 c
b. carbon dioxide in arterial blood. 40 C
c. oxygen in arterial blood. 49 C

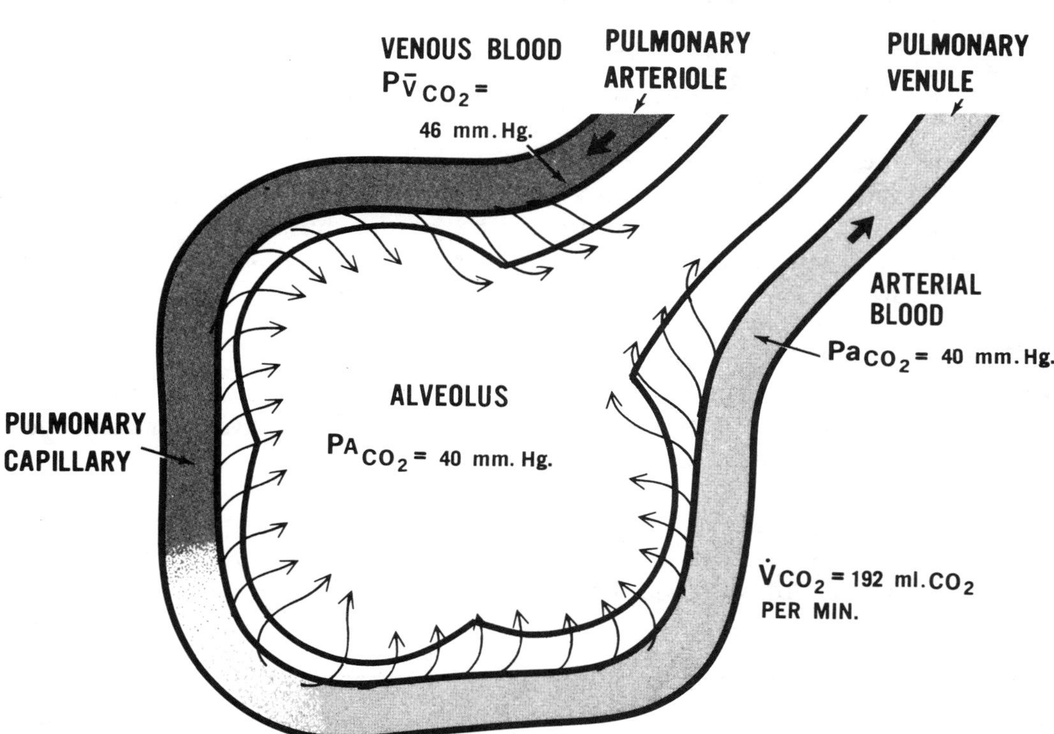

Figure 1–27

48A (from page 45, frame 35)

1. *Hyperpnea:* Abnormal increase in depth and rate of tidal volumes
2. *Bradypnea:* Abnormal slowness in the rate of breathing
3. *Apnea:* cessation of breathing
4. *Tachypnea:* Abnormally fast rate of breathing
5. *Cheyne-Stokes breathing:* A condition seen especially during a coma resulting from damage to the nervous centers, characterized by the rhythmic increase, then decreases in the tidal volume, followed by periods of apnea (no breathing)
6. *Hypopnea:* Abnormal decrease in the depth of tidal volumes

Please continue on page 46, frame 36.

48B (from page 50, frame 38)
Wrong. Plasma is the fluid portion of the blood in which the red cells are suspended. Some oxygen molecules diffuse into the plasma, but *most* of the oxygen is transported in chemical combination with hemoglobin in the erythrocytes (red blood cells). Return to page 50, frame 38, and try again.

48C (from page 52, frame 40)
Wrong. We are talking about hypoxia caused not by dysfunction of the respiratory system, but by a lack of oxygen in the atmosphere, such as occurs at high altitudes. Return to page 52, frame 40, and try again.

48D (from page 53, frame 41)
Correct. Blue-colored skin or cyanosis (si-a-*no*-sis) is caused by the tourniquet interfering with the flow of blood through the capillaries. Please continue on page 54, frame 42.

48a (from page 52, frame 40)
Wrong. Hemoglobin deficiency is a physiological disturbance. The hypoxia is caused by a lack of oxygen in the atmosphere, such as occurs at high altitudes. Return to page 52, frame 40, and review; then try again.

48b (from page 51, frame 39)
Yes, but even moderate hypoxemia can lead to cardiac arrest if neglected. This is not the best answer. Return to page 51, frame 39, and select another answer.

49A (from page 39, frame 30)
Wrong. 500 mL is the tidal volume—the amount taken in with a normal inhalation. The inspiratory capacity consists of the tidal volume plus the inspiratory reserve volume. Return to page 39, frame 30, and try again.

49B (from page 43, frame 33)
Correct. Both the pons and the medulla oblongata contain the respiratory centers, which regulate the patterns of ventilation. Peripheral chemoreceptors located in the bifurcation of the carotid arteries also stimulate breathing by sending impulses to the respiratory centers via afferent nerves when the $Pa{O_2}$ drops below 60 mm Hg or $Pa{CO_2}$ increases by 10 mm Hg. Please continue on page 44, frame 34.

49C (from page 47, frame 37)
Wrong. The symbol for oxygen is O_2. We're talking about carbon dioxide. Return to page 47, frame 37, and try again.

49D (from page 55, frame 43)
Correct. The oxygen molecule becomes less tightly bound to hemoglobin when the curve shifts to the right. There will be more oxygen released from hemoglobin and available to diffuse into the surrounding tissue and cells. Please continue on page 56 and complete the chapter exercises.

49a (from page 42, frame 32)
Correct. About two thirds of the tidal volume reaches the alveoli for gas exchange. The rest remains in the anatomic dead space. The alveolar minute ventilation can be calculated by multiplying 350 $\times$ the respiratory rate (e.g., $350 \times 12 = 4.2$ L/min). Please continue on page 43, frame 33.

49b (from page 43, frame 33)
Wrong. Another part of the brain is also involved. Return to page 43, frame 33, and select another answer.

49c (from page 47, frame 37)
Correct. P = partial pressure, $\bar{v}$ = mixed venous blood, CO_2 = carbon dioxide. The partial pressure of carbon dioxide in mixed venous blood coming from the systemic veins is about 46 mm Hg. Because the carbon dioxide tension is higher in mixed venous blood than in alveolar gas, carbon dioxide diffuses into the alveoli. By the same mechanism, the tension of oxygen in the alveoli is higher than the 40 mm Hg partial pressure found in the venous blood, and thus oxygen diffuses across the alveolar capillary membrane into the pulmonary capillaries. The blood from the pulmonary capillaries is returned to the left atrium of the heart. Please continue on page 50, frame 38.

49d (from page 51, frame 39)
Correct. Emergency action is certainly required in severe hypoxemia, but oxygen therapy also is needed at the first signs of moderate hypoxemia. It is not wise to wait until the signs of severe of hypoxemia are present before oxygen is administered. Please continue on page 52, frame 40.

FRAME 38. NORMAL BLOOD GAS VALUES

A small amount of oxygen is transported in simple solution in the plasma; a much larger amount of oxygen is transported in chemical combination with the hemoglobin in red cells. This combination, called oxyhemoglobin, is about 97% saturated with oxygen in arterial blood found in the systemic circulation (Fig. 1–28). The hemoglobin in venous blood is only about 75% saturated with oxygen. In the systemic circulation, oxygen is distributed to the tissues, which results in a lower oxygen saturation in venous blood.

(Q) Which part of the blood carries more oxygen?

- a. plasma — 48 B
- b. red cells — 32 C

BLOOD GAS VALUES

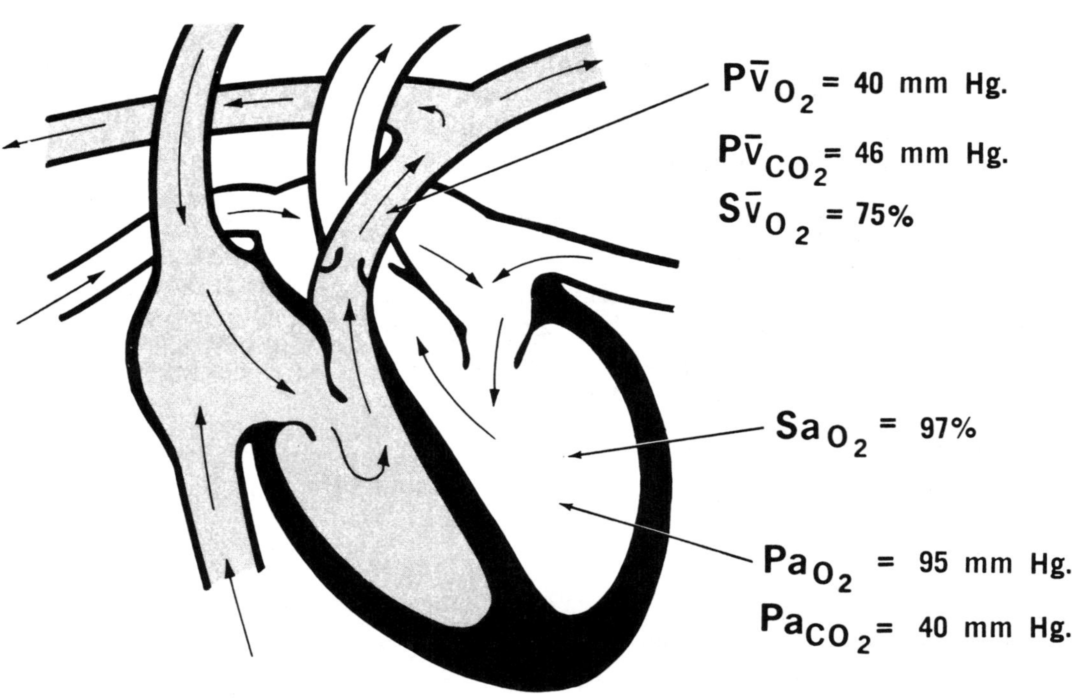

Figure 1–28

FRAME 39. OXYGEN TRANSPORT

One gram of hemoglobin (Hb) will chemically combine with 1.34 mL of oxygen. If the hemoglobin carried by red cells is 100% saturated, it will carry 20.1 mL of oxygen for each 100 mL aliquot of blood (if the aliquot has 15 g of hemoglobin). The maximum amount of O_2 that can be carried by hemoglobin when 100% saturated is determined by multiplying the amount of oxygen carried by 1 gram by the number of grams of hemoglobin in the sample (15 g $\times$ 1.34 mL/g $\times$ 100% = 20.1 mL of oxygen).

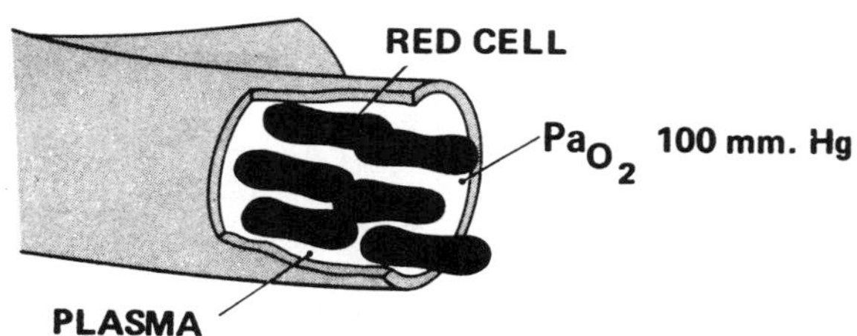

Figure 1–29

Figure 1–29 illustrates how plasma (the liquid part of blood) will carry 0.003 mL of oxygen for every millimeter of oxygen tension (pressure) in the blood; 100 mL of plasma with an oxygen tension of 100 mm Hg (Pao_2) carries 0.30 mL of oxygen (100 mm Hg $\times$ 0.003 mL O_2/mm Hg = 0.30 mL O_2).

Evaluation of oxygen transport in blood must consider arterial oxygen tension, arterial oxygen content, and the volume and distribution of cardiac output (amount of blood pumped by the heart per minute). Abnormalities in the balance between perfusion of alveoli and ventilation in the lung have been established as the most important cause of decreased arterial oxygen tension. The arterial oxygen content depends upon the hemoglobin concentration (normal 16 g/100 mL for men, and 14 g/100 mL for women), the arterial O_2 tension, and, to a smaller extent, on the position of the oxyhemoglobin dissociation curve (see frame 43). For tissues to utilize oxygen, cellular metabolism and the permeability of capillaries and cell membranes must be normal.

Normal respiration requires (1) an adequate concentration of oxygen in the alveoli, (2) adequate alveolar capillary diffusion, (3) adequate systemic circulation, (4) a sufficient amount of hemoglobin to transport the oxygen to the tissues at a rate capable of filling tissue needs, and (5) the ability of the body cells to utilize the oxygen delivered. Any unfavorable variation in these processes, beyond the ability of the body to compensate for the change, will result in hypoxia. Moderate hypoxemia (insufficient oxygen in blood, e.g., Pao_2 of 40 to 60 mm Hg) is accompanied by restlessness, tachycardia (heart rate above 100 beats per minute), and eventually the possibility of cyanosis (blue color of the skin and mucous membranes). Severe hypoxemia ($Pao_2 < 40$ mm Hg) results in unconsciousness, apnea (cessation of breathing), bradycardia (heart rate below 60 beats per minute), and eventually asystole (absence of a heart beat).

(Q) In which type of hypoxemia would oxygen therapy be recommended?

a. moderate hypoxemia 40 c
b. severe hypoxemia 48 b
c. both moderate and severe hypoxemia 49 d

FRAME 40. CAUSES OF HYPOXIA

There are several different causes of hypoxia. It can result from reduced alveolar oxygen tension (partial pressure), impaired alveolar capillary diffusion, hemoglobin deficiency, circulatory failure, or histotoxic problems (inability of cells to utilize the oxygen).

Reduced Alveolar Oxygen Tension The ability of the blood to carry O_2 may be normal, but there is incomplete oxygenation of the arterial blood when alveolar oxygen tension is reduced. The cause may be insufficient O_2 in the inspired air, such as at high altitudes, or inadequate ventilation of the alveoli due to insufficient depth or rate of breathing, obstructive lesions of the airways, or diseases such as asthma and emphysema.

Impaired Alveolar Capillary Diffusion Impaired diffusion results in fewer oxygen molecules that are able to penetrate the alveolar capillary membranes, even with normal alveolar oxygen tension. This condition may be caused by pathologic changes in any of the structures of the alveolar capillary membranes or widening of the interstitial space in between.

Hemoglobin Deficiency Hemoglobin deficiency results from a decrease in the amount of functional hemoglobin with or without a decrease in the number of red cells. The result is a decrease in the oxygen-carrying capacity of the blood. Of course, this capacity can also be affected by toxic agents that prevent the red blood cells from carrying the normal amount of oxygen. For example, hemoglobin has a greater affinity for carbon monoxide than it does for oxygen. If both gases are present in the atmosphere, the hemoglobin will reject the oxygen and combine with carbon monoxide.

(Q) Without means for supplying additional oxygen, mountain climbers at high altitudes would suffer from hypoxia because of

a. reduced alveolar ventilation. 48 C
b. reduced alveolar oxygen tension. 32 D
c. hemoglobin deficiency. 48 a

FRAME 41. CIRCULATORY, ANEMIC, AND HISTOTOXIC HYPOXIA

Circulatory Hypoxia In circulatory hypoxia the oxygen content and the oxygen-carrying capacity of blood may be normal, but the blood flow through the capillaries is slowed to such a degree that the blood cannot be delivered to the tissues at an adequate rate to meet tissue demands. Hypoxemia caused by circulatory failure may be localized or general. General hypoxemia may be associated with congestive heart failure, shock, inpaired venous return, or obstruction to the arterial or venous blood flow by injury, or increased oxygen demand caused by fever or tissue trauma.

Histotoxic Hypoxia Even if there is sufficient oxygen intake through the respiratory system, *histotoxic* (tissue-poisoning) substances can prevent cells from utilizing the oxygen they receive. Histotoxic substances, such as cyanide, impair the oxidative-enzyme mechanism of the cell, thus interfering with metabolism.

Anemic Hypoxia Inadequate amounts of hemoglobin will seriously affect oxygen-carrying capacity and result in hypoxia. Each gram of hemoglobin, when 100% saturated, has the capability of carrying 1.34 mL of oxygen compared with the 0.3 mL of oxygen that dissolves in 100 mL of blood with a Pa_{O_2} of 100 mm Hg.

(Q) When a tourniquet is applied, the skin beyond the tourniquet will become blue because of

a. histotoxic substances. 40 d

b. circulatory failure. 48 D

FRAME 42. CLINICAL SIGNS OF HYPOXEMIA

The effects produced by hypoxemia will depend upon the type and degree of dysfunction, how rapidly it develops, how long it lasts, and how well the cells were functioning before its onset. The brain, heart, and retina are particularly sensitive to lack of oxygen.

It is important, therefore, that physicians and respiratory care practitioners be sensitive to the possibility of hypoxemia, since the early clinical signs of mild hypoxemia are usually hard to detect. Oxygen therapy should be started before moderate or severe hypoxemia develops. It is dangerous to wait until the patient has severe dyspnea (difficult or labored breathing) or cyanosis. Concern about hypoxemia can be confirmed by analysis of arterial blood. Blood gas analysis can determine if the oxygen saturation of hemoglobin (Sa_{O_2}), hemoglobin concentration (Hb), oxygen content (Ca_{O_2}), and oxygen tension (Pa_{O_2}) are normal.

(Q) On a separate piece of paper write down the clinical signs of
1. moderate hypoxemia.
2. severe hypoxemia.

When you have finished, turn to page 8a and compare your answers.

FRAME 43. THE OXYHEMOGLOBIN DISSOCIATION CURVE

The shape of the oxyhemoglobin dissociation curve represents the proportion of hemoglobin molecules saturated with oxygen at a given partial pressure of oxygen (Fig. 1–30A). It is important to notice that a drop in Pao_2 from 70 to 40 mm Hg will result in a huge and dangerous drop in oxygen saturation of hemoglobin from 90% to 72%. However, a drop in Pao_2 from 100 to 70 mm Hg results in only a small drop in saturation from 97% to 93%. This also means that an increase in Pao_2 above 70 mm Hg will result in only a small increase in the oxygen carried by the blood. However, to protect the patient from sudden falls in oxygen saturation, the Pao_2 should be raised to 100 mm Hg so that a subsequent sudden decrease in oxygen tension will result in only a small decrease in the oxygen carried by hemoglobin. The oxyhemoglobin curve shifts left or right with changes in the pH, Pco_2, 2,3-diphosphoglycerate, and temperature of the blood (Fig. 1–30B). A shift to the left means oxygen will be more strongly bound to hemoglobin, and a higher saturation of hemoglobin will occur at a given oxygen tension. When the curve shifts to the right, oxygen is bound less strongly to hemoglobin and is less saturated at a given oxygen tension.

(Q) As blood flows through the capillaries of the systemic circulation, the pH falls and the Pco_2 of the blood increases, causing the oxyhemoglobin dissociation curve to shift toward the right. This means that

a. more oxygen is available. 49 D
b. less oxygen is available. 41 E
c. there is no change in usable oxygen. 32 E

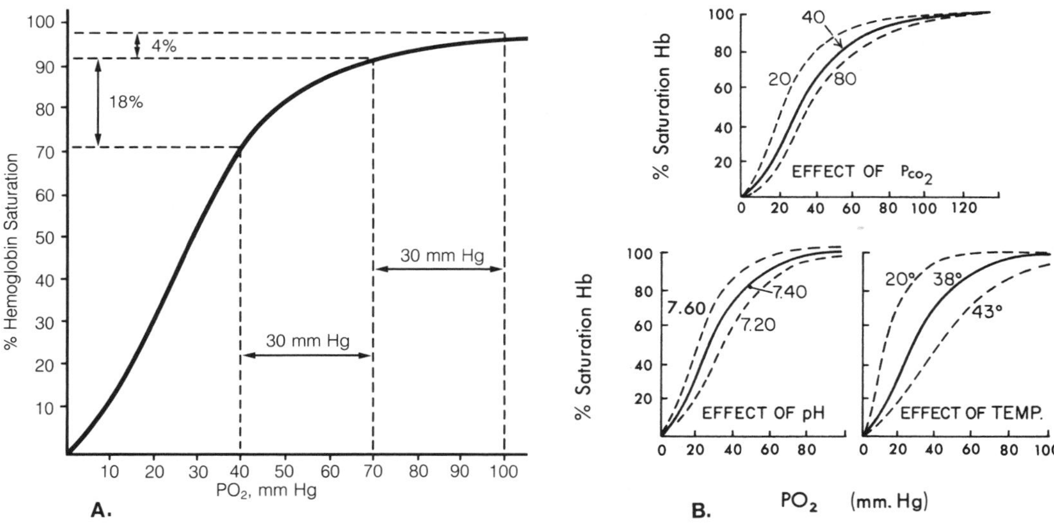

Figure 1–30A The effect of the steep portion of the oxyhemoglobin dissociation curve on equal changes in the PaO_2 and resultant percent hemoglobin saturation. (Source: Barnes, TA: Respiratory Care Practice. Year Book Medical Publishers, Chicago, 1988. Used with permission.) **B** Changes in the reaction between oxygen and hemoglobin are represented by changes in the position of the oxyhemoglobin dissociation curve. (Source: Cherniak, RM and Cherniak, L: Respiration in Health and Disease, ed 3. WB Saunders, Philadelphia, 1983. Used with permission.)

EXERCISES

1. If the ratio of dead space to tidal volume (VD/VT) is 0.60 for a patient with emphysema, calculate the alveolar ventilation per minute ($\dot{V}A$) if the tidal volume is 500 mL and the respiratory rate is 15/min.
2. List all the symbols used to describe the amount of oxygen and carbon dioxide found in arterial blood.
3. Calculate the inspiratory reserve volume, given the following: expiratory reserve volume of 1200 mL, tidal volume of 450 mL, and vital capacity of 4800 mL.
4. Using 10 × 10 squares/inch graph paper draw the oxyhemoglobin dissociation curve; label the vertical axis Sao_2 and horizontal axis Pao_2, and make sure the curve is not shifted left or right. When the curve is drawn, determine the Pao_2 that corresponds to a Sao_2 of 50% (this value is called P_{50}).
5. List three clinical signs of moderate hypoxemia and three clinical signs of severe hypoxemia.
6. Name all the airways, starting at the nose and mouth and finishing at the alveoli.
7. Name all the blood vessels, heart chambers, and valves, starting with the vena cava and finishing at the aorta.
8. List the normal blood gas values (Po_2, Pco_2, So_2, Co_2) for the pulmonary artery and pulmonary vein.
9. Describe the relative contributions of hemoglobin and plasma in transporting oxygen to the tissues.
10. Describe how the accessory muscles help generate a larger tidal volume at high levels of ventilation.

POSTTEST

This test is designed to evaluate what you learned from completing Chapter 1. Check your answers on page 59 and review the topics where your answer is incorrect.

1. Which of the following is an end product of internal respiration?
   A. oxygen
   B. carbon dioxide
   C. glucose
   D. hydrogen ions
   E. both *B* and *D*
2. Which of the following combinations of tidal volume and respiratory rate will provide the highest alveolar ventilation?
   A. 1000 mL × 10/min
   B. 800 mL × 12/min
   C. 700 mL × 14/min
   D. 500 mL × 20/min
   E. 400 mL × 25/min
3. The smallest airway that is part of the anatomical dead space is the
   A. lobar bronchus.
   B. segmental bronchus.
   C. terminal bronchiole.
   D. respiratory bronchiole.
   E. alveolar duct.
4. How many lobes and lung segments does the right lung have?
   A. 2 lobes, 9 segments
   B. 2 lobes, 10 segments
   C. 3 lobes, 9 segments
   D. 3 lobes, 10 segments
   E. 4 lobes, 12 segments
5. All of the following muscles participate in active exhalation *except*
   A. rectus abdominis.
   B. scalenus anterior.
   C. external oblique.
   D. transversus abdominis.
   E. internal intercostals.
6. Exhalation occurs during quiet breathing as a result of
   A. contraction of the diaphragm.
   B. contraction of internal intercostals.
   C. relaxation of internal intercostals.
   D. elastic recoil of the lungs.
   E. elastic recoil of the diaphragm.
7. During normal breathing which of the following muscles increase tidal volume by elevating and fixing the sternum and ribs?
   A. scalenus
   B. external intercostals
   C. internal intercostals
   D. external oblique
   E. parasternal intercartilaginous

8. Which of the following statements about the pulmonary circulation are true?
   I. It is a low pressure system.
   II. It returns blood to the right ventricle.
   III. The pulmonary artery carries venous blood.
   IV. Pulmonary veins carry arterial blood.
   A. I only
   B. II only
   C. I, II only
   D. I, III, IV only
   E. II, III, IV only

9. The systemic circulation is responsible for
   A. external respiration.
   B. oxygen transport.
   C. oxygen uptake.
   D. CO_2 excretion.
   E. both *A* and *C*.

10. Which of the following has the lowest systolic blood pressure?
   A. aorta
   B. left ventricle
   C. left atrium
   D. right ventricle
   E. pulmonary artery

11. The anatomical dead space for a young healthy male weighing 150 lb with a tidal volume of 450 mL is
   A. 50 mL.
   B. 100 mL.
   C. 150 mL.
   D. 300 mL.
   E. 450 mL.

12. Adequate ventilation is best determined by measuring
   A. tidal volume.
   B. minute volume.
   C. arterial oxygen tension.
   D. arterial CO_2 tension.
   E. venous oxygen tension.

13. The symbol Cao_2 can be defined as
   A. partial pressure of oxygen in arterial blood.
   B. saturation of hemoglobin with oxygen in arterial blood.
   C. amount of oxygen in 100 mL of arterial blood.
   D. amount of CO_2 in arterial blood.
   E. none of the above.

14. The vital capacity comprises the
   A. RV and IC.
   B. ERV, V_T, IRV.
   C. FRC and IC.
   D. ERV and IRV.
   E. RV and IC.

15. Peripheral chemoreceptors increase ventilation in response to a Pao_2 of
   A. 55 mm Hg.
   B. 65 mm Hg.
   C. 80 mm Hg.
   D. 100 mm Hg.
   E. all of the above.
16. A breathing pattern with a normal respiratory rate and an above-normal tidal volume is best described as
   A. tachypnea.
   B. bradypnea.
   C. hypopnea.
   D. hyperpnea.
   E. eupnea.
17. Normally oxygen diffuses out of alveoli into the pulmonary capillaries across a pressure gradient of
   A. 6 mm Hg.
   B. 40 mm Hg.
   C. 60 mm Hg.
   D. 80 mm Hg.
   E. 100 mm Hg.
18. The maximum amount of oxygen that 15 g of hemoglobin can carry is
   A. 0.03 mL.
   B. 14.50 mL.
   C. 19.50 mL.
   D. 20.10 mL.
   E. 23.20 mL.
19. Moderate hypoxemia will occur when the arterial oxygen tension is
   A. 50 mm Hg.
   B. 70 mm Hg.
   C. 90 mm Hg.
   D. 100 mm Hg.
   E. 110 mm Hg.
20. Which of the following is *not* true about the oxyhemoglobin dissociation curve?
   A. It shifts right with fever.
   B. It shifts left with a pH of 7.50.
   C. It shifts right with Pco_2 of 30 mm Hg.
   D. It shifts left with hypothermia.
   E. It shifts right in venous blood.

ANSWERS TO POSTTEST

1. E (F18)
2. A (F32)
3. C (F23)
4. D (F10)
5. B (F14)
6. D (F14)
7. B (F14)
8. D (F17)
9. B (F21)
10. C (F20)
11. C (F22)
12. D (F24)
13. C (F25)
14. B (F29)
15. A (F33)
16. D (F35)
17. C (F36)
18. D (F40)
19. A (F43)
20. C (F43)

BIBLIOGRAPHY

Barnes, TA: Respiratory Care Practice. Year Book Medical Publishers, Chicago, 1988.

Bates, B: A Guide to Physical Examination and History Taking, ed 4. JB Lippincott, Philadelphia, 1987.

Finucane, BT and Santora, AH: Principles of Airway Management. FA Davis, Philadelphia, 1988.

Forster, RE, Fisher, AB, DuBois, AB, and Briscoe, WA: The Lung—Physiologic Basis of Pulmonary Function Tests, ed 3. Year Book Medical Publishers, Chicago, 1986.

Lane, EE and Walker, JF: Clinical Arterial Blood Gas Analysis. CV Mosby, St. Louis, 1987.

Murray, JF: The Normal Lung, ed 2. WB Saunders, Philadelphia, 1986.

Netter, FH. The Ciba Collection of Medical Illustrations, Vol 7, Respiratory System. CIBA Pharmaceutical Co, Summit, NJ, 1979.

Shapiro, BA, Harrison, RA, Cane, RD, Templin, RK, and Walton, JR: Clinical Application of Blood Gases, ed 4. Year Book Medical Publishers, Chicago, 1988.

Slonim, NB and Hamilton, LH: Respiratory Physiology, ed 5. CV Mosby, St. Louis, 1988.

West, JB: Pulmonary Pathophysiology, ed 3. Williams & Wilkins, Baltimore, 1987.

2

Acid-Base Physiology

PRETEST

This pretest is designed to measure what you already know about acid-base physiology. Check your answers on page 64 and then continue on page 65, frame 44.

1. If the rate of CO_2 production suddenly increases and the rate of CO_2 excretion remains *unchanged*
   A. plasma Pco_2 will decrease.
   B. plasma Pco_2 will increase.
   C. plasma pH will remain unchanged.
   D. plasma HCO_3^- will increase.
   E. both *B* and *C*.

2. Most carbon dioxide is transported to the lungs in the form of
   A. plasma Pco_2.
   B. plasma bicarbonate.
   C. carbonic acid.
   D. carbonate.
   E. phosphate.

3. Which of the following buffers stabilize the pH of whole blood?
   A. hemoglobin and oxyhemoglobin
   B. plasma bicarbonate
   C. erythrocytes
   D. plasma proteins
   E. all of the above

4. The range of normal pH is
   A. 7.20 to 7.30.
   B. 7.25 to 7.35.
   C. 7.30 to 7.40.
   D. 7.35 to 7.45.
   E. 7.40 to 7.50.

5. The pH_a refers to the concentration of
   A. buffers in arterial blood.
   B. hemoglobin in arterial blood.
   C. hydrogen ions in arterial blood.
   D. bases in body fluids.
   E. organic salts in body fluids.

6. The normal range of arterial CO_2 tension is
   A. 25 to 35 mm Hg.
   B. 30 to 40 mm Hg.
   C. 35 to 45 mm Hg.
   D. 40 to 50 mm Hg.
   E. 45 to 55 mm Hg.

7. Acute alveolar hyperventilation will immediately result in a
   A. low plasma Pco_2.
   B. low arterial pH.
   C. low plasma bicarbonate.
   D. high plasma bicarbonate.
   E. both *A* and *C*.

8. Acute ventilatory failure will result in
   A. changes to pH by buffering.
   B. changes to pH by buffering and renal compensation.
   C. low plasma P_{CO_2}, high arterial pH.
   D. high plasma P_{CO_2}, low arterial pH.
   E. both *A* and *D*.

9. Respiratory compensation of metabolic acidosis occurs over a period of
   A. a few minutes.
   B. a few hours.
   C. 6 to 12 hours.
   D. 24 hours.
   E. several days.

10. Loss of bicarbonate from diarrhea lasting 2 to 3 days may cause
    A. metabolic alkalosis.
    B. metabolic acidosis.
    C. metabolic compensation.
    D. alveolar hypoventilation.
    E. none of the above.

11. If a patient is given sodium bicarbonate during cardiopulmonary resuscitation, which of the following may occur?
    A. respiratory acidosis
    B. respiratory alkalosis
    C. metabolic acidosis
    D. metabolic alkalosis
    E. respiratory and metabolic acidosis

12. Which of the following represents a respiratory compensation for metabolic acidosis?
    A. apnea
    B. eupnea
    C. bradypnea
    D. hypopnea
    E. hyperpnea

13. Complete metabolic compensation for respiratory acidosis may result in a pH of
    A. 7.20.
    B. 7.30.
    C. 7.36.
    D. 7.44.
    E. 7.50.

14. Partial respiratory compensation for metabolic acidosis may result in a pH of
    A. 7.30.
    B. 7.36.
    C. 7.40.
    D. 7.45.
    E. 7.50.

15. The concentration ratio of dissolved CO_2 to carbonic acid is
    A. 1:1.
    B. 20:1.
    C. 100:1.
    D. 800:1.
    E. 1000:1.

16. To maintain the acid-base balance, the concentration ratio of base (bicarbonate) to acid (carbonic acid and dissolved CO_2) is normally
A. 1:1.
B. 20:1.
C. 100:1.
D. 800:1.
E. 1000:1.

17. A compound capable of donating hydrogen ions is called a (an)
A. buffer.
B. base.
C. catalyst.
D. acid.
E. alkali.

18. A compound that can accept hydrogen ions is called a
A. phosphate.
B. base.
C. catalyst.
D. carbonic anhydrase.
E. salt.

19. For every molecule of CO_2 excreted by the lungs, a hydrogen ion is converted to
A. bicarbonate.
B. water.
C. carbonic anhydrase.
D. phosphate.
E. salt.

20. Most carbon dioxide is carried to the lungs as bicarbonate, what type of ion does HCO_3^- react with to revert to CO_2 so that it can be excreted by the lungs?
A. H^+
B. Na^+
C. Cl^-
D. Mg^{++}
E. K^+

ANSWERS TO PRETEST

1. B (F44)
2. B (F53)
3. E (F47)
4. D (F46)
5. C (F45)
6. C (F48)
7. A (F48)
8. E (F49)
9. A (F58)
10. B (F58)
11. D (F58)
12. E (F58)
13. C (F57)
14. A (F58)
15. D (F44)
16. B (F44)
17. D (F45)
18. B (F45)
19. B (F52)
20. A (F52)

FRAME 44. ACID-BASE BALANCE

A subject as complicated as acid-base balance is difficult to describe simply. However, if you can learn the general principles of acid-base balance, you will progress at a more rapid rate later in your studies. In addition to supplying the blood with oxygen, the respiratory system has a major role in maintaining acid-base balance by excreting carbon dioxide. When CO_2 is mixed with body fluids, a small amount is converted into carbonic acid (the ratio of CO_2 to carbonic acid is about 800 : 1). To maintain acid-base balance, the ratio of base (bicarbonate) to acid (carbonic acid and dissolved CO_2) is normally 20 : 1. Changes in this balance of base to acid can produce extreme changes in the rate of cellular chemical reactions, resulting in illness and eventually death.

(Q) The respiratory system maintains acid-base balance by excretion of
- a. bicarbonate (HCO_3^-). 70 a
- b. carbon dioxide. 71 A
- c. bicarbonate and carbon dioxide. 70 A

FRAME 45. NORMAL pH

Many *intrinsic* acids in the body (lactic acid, phosphoric acid, hydrochloric acid) have fairly constant concentrations because of the relationship among acid production, excretion, and the action of certain buffers. However, the never-ending stream of acid end products from metabolism keeps the body working continuously to prevent excess acidity. The acidity of the blood can be measured by its hydrogen ion concentration $[H^+]$.[1] Every acid is a compound capable of donating a specific number of hydrogen ions. The concentration of hydrogen ions present in a solution is defined as pH.[2] The pH of a solution is inversely related to its hydrogen ion concentration—as the hydrogen ions increase, the acidity increases, and the pH decreases. As the hydrogen ions decrease, the alkalinity increases, and the pH increases.

To stabilize the pH, the blood contains a system of buffers that can maintain the concentration of the hydrogen ions only to a limited degree. A compound that can accept a hydrogen ion is called a base. The body must constantly excrete or buffer hydrogen ions to maintain a normal pH. When the processes for eliminating H^+ ions are faulty, the patient develops acidemia from too much acid or alkalemia from too much base or alkali.

(Q) pH refers to the
- a. balance of acids and bases. 70 B
- b. concentration of buffers. 71 B
- c. concentration of hydrogen ions. 71 a

---

[1]The hydrogen ion is a single proton in the nucleus of a hydrogen atom that has lost its single electron.

[2]pH is the negative logarithm of the hydrogen ion concentration per liter of solution, expressed as a positive number.

FRAME 46. ACIDOSIS AND ALKALOSIS

The pH of a solution can be measured in units as symbolized in Figure 2 – 1. Water, which is a neutral solution, has a pH of 7.0. Anything lower than 7.0 indicates acidity. Anything above that indicates the alkalinity of a solution. Although body fluids are mainly water, they contain a mixture of acids and bases, so that the normal arterial blood has a pH range of 7.35 to 7.45. Below 7.35, the patient is considered in acidosis; above 7.45, in alkalosis. Severe abnormalities in the body's pH may cause death.

(Q) Body fluids are normally
- a. neutral. 70 b
- b. slightly acidic. 70 C
- c. slightly alkaline. 71 C

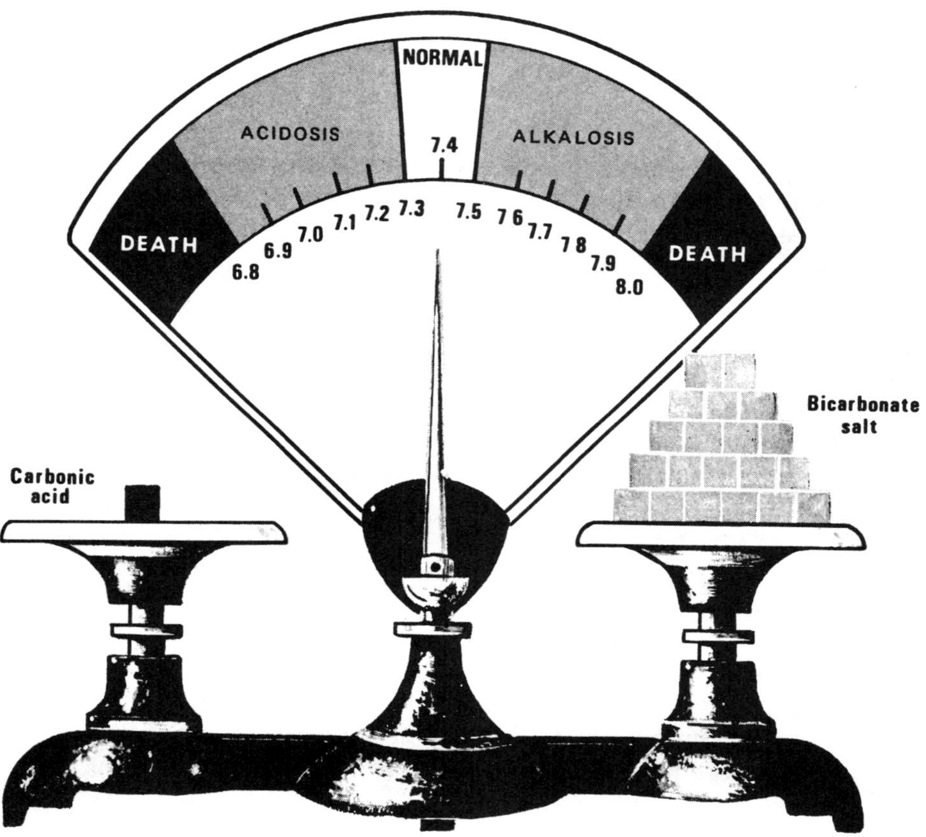

Figure 2 – 1

FRAME 47. BUFFER ACTIVITY

The pH in our bodies is influenced by the food we eat, by liquids we drink, by medications we take, and by many diseases. Maintenance of the acid-base balance consists mainly of prevention of marked alterations in hydrogen ion concentration in our body fluids. There are several ways in which the body maintains this balance: (1) by buffer activity, (2) by respiratory regulation, and (3) by renal regulation.

A buffer is a substance that prevents marked alterations in the hydrogen ion concentration (pH) when a strong acid or alkali is introduced into or removed from a solution (e.g., body fluid). The main buffer systems present in the body are (1) the bicarbonate-carbonic acid system (bicarbonate salt in a ratio of 20:1 with carbonic acid), (2) the phosphate buffer system, (3) the hemoglobin-oxyhemoglobin buffer system, and (4) the protein buffer system. Each of these buffer systems helps to regulate acid-base balance by limiting or buffering large changes in hydrogen ion concentration and thus preventing large shifts in pH.

(Q) Buffer activity tends to

a. neutralize a solution. 71 b

b. prevent marked changes in the acidity or alkalinity of a solution. 77 c

FRAME 48. RESPIRATORY REGULATION OF ACID-BASE BALANCE

The major mechanism for purging the body of excess carbon dioxide and carbonic acid is the respiratory system. With each exhalation, carbon dioxide is excreted, reducing carbonic acid and carbon dioxide in the extracellular fluids. For every molecule of CO_2 excreted by the lungs, a hydrogen ion is converted to water ($H^+ + HCO_3^- \rightarrow H_2CO_3 \rightarrow CO_2 + H_2O$). Overbreathing (hyperventilation) speeds this process. Underbreathing (hypoventilation) slows the process. Normal alveolar ventilation will result in an arterial CO_2 tension that ranges from 35 to 45 mm Hg.

(Q) Hyperventilation will result in

a. a decrease in plasma pH. 70 c

b. an increase in hydrogen ion concentration. 70 D

c. an increase in plasma pH. 76 A

FRAME 49. EFFECT OF METABOLIC RATE

When a person exercises, his or her CO_2 tension and hydrogen ion concentration increase due to the higher metabolic rate. The resultant drop in pH and increase in CO_2 tension cause the patient to breathe deeper and faster, producing a decrease in blood CO_2 tension and an increase in pH. The faster breathing-rate depth may compensate for the higher metabolic rate and return the blood gas values to normal (See Fig. 2–2). Minute volume increases within a few seconds during mild to moderate exercise. Severe exercise causes the minute volume to increase progressively in a linear manner. Increased aerobic metabolism causes an increase in minute volume of 2 to 5 L/mm Hg increase in arterial CO_2 tension. The increased minute volume during mild to moderate exercise is achieved by an increase in tidal volume. Severe exercise results in an increase in both tidal volume (50% of normal vital capacity) and respiratory frequency (40 to 50 breaths per minute).

(Q) The rate and depth of respiration help to determine
- a. the tension of carbon dioxide in the blood. 71 D
- b. the concentration of hydrogen ions in the body fluids. 71 c
- c. both of the above. 77 A

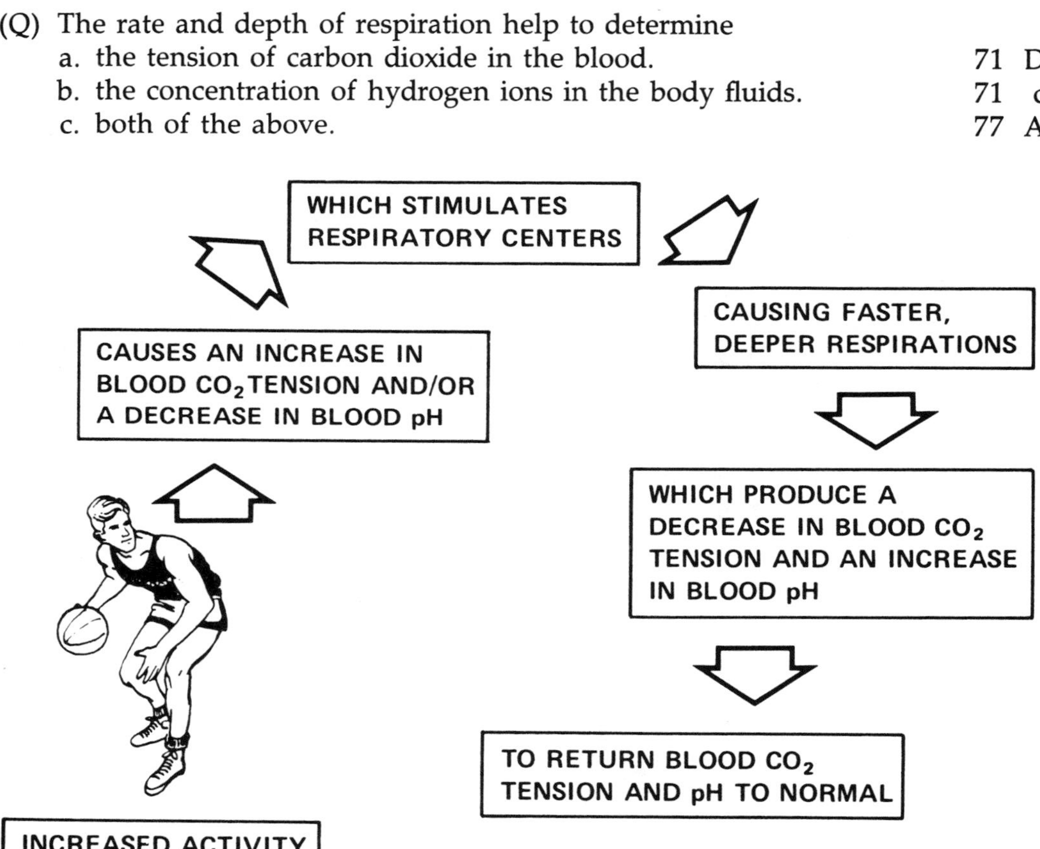

Figure 2–2

FRAME 50. RENAL REGULATION OF ACID-BASE BALANCE

A third mechanism in acid-base balance, in addition to buffer activity and respiratory regulation, is renal (kidney) regulation. The kidneys regulate acid-base balance by eliminating excess hydrogen ions and by reabsorbing bicarbonate.

(Q) Renal regulation of acid-base balance includes the elimination of

a. H^+ ions through urine and reabsorption of all the bicarbonate. 70 d

b. excess hydrogen ions through the urine and reabsorption of bicarbonate from renal tubules as it is needed. 70 E

FRAME 51. RENAL TUBULAR CELLS

The tubular cells of the kidney eliminate the excess hydrogen ions and reabsorb bicarbonate by three distinct mechanisms for pH regulation: (1) acidification of phosphate buffer salts (removing hydrogen ions from the body), (2) reabsorption of bicarbonate (conserving this base for buffer activity), and (3) secretion of ammonium ions (which displace basic ions from salts of various acids, freeing the basic ions for diffusion back into the tubular cells).

Renal mechanisms constitute a device for selectively eliminating hydrogen ions from the body. When blood pH decreases below normal, the kidneys excrete more hydrogen from the blood into the urine via the renal tubules and reabsorb more bicarbonate ions from the renal tubules back into the blood. This decreases urine pH and concurrently returns the blood pH back toward normal.

(Q) When the blood pH rises above normal, less bicarbonate is reabsorbed from the renal tubules into the blood and

a. more hydrogen ions are removed from the blood into the urine. 71 d

b. fewer hydrogen ions are removed from the blood into the urine. 76 B

70A (from page 65, frame 44)
No. Bicarbonate is excreted or reabsorbed by the kidneys. You are partly correct. Return to page 65, frame 44, and select another answer.

70B (from page 65, frame 45)
Generally, yes. But specifically, the pH is an index of the concentration of hydrogen ions in the body fluids or other solutions. Return to page 65, frame 45, and review the material; then select another answer.

70C (from page 66, frame 46)
No. Acidity is below 7.0 on the pH scale. You can see from the illustration that 7.0 would be too low for normal body fluids. Return to page 66, frame 46, and try again.

70D (from page 67, frame 48)
Wrong. Overbreathing causes an excess amount of carbon dioxide to be eliminated from the body, leaving a lower concentration of hydrogen ions in the blood. Return to page 67, frame 48, and select another answer.

70E (from page 69, frame 50)
Correct. An excess of acid is produced during the ordinary course of metabolism. The kidneys compensate for this excess production by secreting acids as components of urine and by reabsorbing bicarbonate, to return it to the blood plasma and extracellular fluid. Consequently, the pH of urine is typically acid. Please continue on page 69, frame 51.

70a (from page 65, frame 44)
No. Bicarbonate is excreted or reabsorbed by the kidneys. Return to page 65, frame 44, and try again.

70b (from page 66, frame 46)
No. Water is a neutral solution that has a pH of 7.0. But body fluids are not neutral. The normal pH of arterial blood is between 7.35 and 7.45. A pH of 7.0 would be far below the pH of body fluids. Return to page 66, frame 46, and try again.

70c (from page 67, frame 48)
Wrong. Overbreathing causes the carbon dioxide to leave the body at an excessive rate, and thus increases the conversion of hydrogen ions to water. The result is a decrease in the hydrogen ion concentration, which affects the pH inversely. Return to page 67, frame 48, and try again.

70d (from page 69, frame 50)
Careful! Remember that the proper acid-base balance must be maintained. If too many hydrogen ions were eliminated or too many bicarbonate ions reabsorbed, the result would be alkalosis. Return to page 69, frame 50, and review the function of the kidneys in maintaining acid-base balance; then select another answer.

71A (from page 65, frame 44)
Correct. By the excretion of carbon dioxide, the respiratory system plays a major role in maintaining the acid-base balance of the body. Please continue on page 65, frame 45.

71B (from page 65, frame 45)
Wrong. The concentration of buffers will partly determine the number of hydrogen ions present, but the pH is a measure of the concentration of hydrogen ions in the body fluids or in other solutions. Please return to page 65, frame 45, and select another answer.

71C (from page 66, frame 46)
Yes. A neutral solution (e.g., water) has a pH of 7.0. But body fluids are not neutral. The normal pH of arterial blood is between 7.35 and 7.45. Since anything above neutral (7.0) is alkaline, the body fluids must remain slightly alkaline to maintain the normal body environment. Please continue on page 67, frame 47.

71D (from page 68, frame 49)
True, but this is not the whole story. Return to page 68, frame 49, and select another answer.

71E (from page 73, frame 55)
No. If the carbon dioxide is increased, the hydrogen ion concentration will increase. Return to page 73, frame 55, and select another answer.

71a (from page 65, frame 45)
Correct. The term *pH* is an index of the concentration of hydrogen ions in a solution. Please continue on page 66, frame 46.

71b (from page 67, frame 47)
Wrong. Remember that the body fluids should normally be slightly alkaline, not neutral. Return to page 67, frame 47, and review the material; then try the question again.

71c (from page 68, frame 49)
True, but this is not the whole story. Return to page 68, frame 49, and select another answer.

71d (from page 69, frame 51)
Careful! Remember, as the blood pH rises it becomes more alkaline, which means that there are not enough hydrogen ions to balance the bicarbonate ions. It is the function of the kidneys to help keep the acid-base ratio at 1:20, 1 part acid to 20 parts base. Return to page 69, frame 51, and select another answer.

71e (from page 75, frame 57)
Wrong. Although buffers in plasma lower the bicarbonate concentration, it will take several days for renal compensation to move blood pH into the normal range of 7.40 to 7.45. Return to page 75, frame 57, and select another answer.

FRAME 52. HYDRATION REACTION

The tubules of the kidneys have the same responsibility as the respiratory system to excrete hydrogen ions, but the respiratory system performs this function faster. The respiratory system indirectly accomplishes this rapid removal of hydrogen ions by excreting carbon dioxide. The removal of CO_2 causes the H^+ ions to combine with HCO_3^- (bicarbonate) to form CO_2 (carbon dioxide) and H_2O (water). As the CO_2 molecules are removed by the respiratory system, the hydrogen ions are changed to water ($H^+ + HCO_3^- \rightarrow H_2CO_3 \rightarrow CO_2 + H_2O$).

The buffer system consists of various chemicals that serve as sponges, absorbing and releasing positive and negative ions to compensate for imbalances and to reduce the "jolt" of excess acids or alkalis introduced into the bloodstream. Thus you can see how the proper functioning of the buffers, kidneys, and lungs is necessary to maintain acid-base balance.

(Q) The acid-base balance in body fluids can be disturbed by

a. an inadequate buffer system. 77 B
b. a respiratory disturbance. 78 A
c. renal (kidney) disturbance. 78 a
d. any one of the above. 76 a

FRAME 53. CARBON DIOXIDE TRANSPORT AS BICARBONATE

Normally, carbon dioxide diffuses from the tissues into the bloodstream and is carried away from the tissues by red cells and plasma. It exists in three forms during transport: (1) as bicarbonate (HCO_3^-), (2) in carbamino forms, and (3) as CO_2 gas physically dissolved in blood.

Bicarbonate, which exists in blood plasma and red cells, accounts for 80% to 90% of carbon dioxide transport. The major portion of carbon dioxide diffuses into the red cells, where it mixes with water and produces carbonic acid (H_2CO_3). This reaction of carbon dioxide and water to produce carbonic acid is called the hydration reaction ($CO_2 + H_2O \rightarrow H_2CO_3$). Normally, it would be a slow process, but an enzyme catalyst (carbonic anhydrase) in red cells speeds the reaction. The carbonic acid undergoes immediate dissociation (separation into smaller molecules) to form bicarbonate and a hydrogen ion in the red cell ($H_2CO_3 \rightarrow H^+ + HCO_3^-$). A major portion of the bicarbonate then diffuses out of the red cells into the plasma. To maintain normal activity and electrical balance, other ions diffuse into the red cells to replace bicarbonate. This process, which occurs in the tissues, is reversed in the lungs. A normal plasma bicarbonate concentration is 24 mEq/L.

(Q) Inadequate excretion of carbon dioxide from the blood results in an excess of carbonic acid (and thus hydrogen ions). This accumulation of CO_2 lowers the pH and produces

a. alkalosis. 76 D
b. acidosis. 76 c

FRAME 54. CARBON DIOXIDE TRANSPORT IN THE CARBAMINO FORMS

About 15% of the carbon dioxide exists in the carbamino forms, as carbon compounds bonded with NH_2 (amino) groups of proteins. The most common carbamino form is carbaminohemoglobin, formed by the bonding of a carbon compound with hemoglobin in the red cells. Reduced hemoglobin has a greater ability to combine with carbon dioxide than oxyhemoglobin.

(Q) Most of the carbon dioxide in blood is in the form of

a. carbamino compounds. 76 C
b. bicarbonate. 77 D
c. dissolved carbon dioxide gas. 76 b

FRAME 55. CARBON DIOXIDE TRANSPORT AS DISSOLVED GAS

A small amount of carbon dioxide exists as CO_2 gas physically in blood or as hydrated carbonic acid. If abnormal ventilation results in inadequate carbon dioxide excretion, then excess amounts of gas will be dissolved in the blood.

(Q) What is the acute effect of this excess CO_2 on the pH of the blood?

a. Hydrogen ions in the blood will *decrease,* thus *increasing* the pH. 71 E
b. Hydrogen ions in the blood will *increase,* thus *increasing* the pH. 78 C
c. Hydrogen ions in the blood will *increase,* thus *decreasing* the pH. 78 c

FRAME 56. CARBON DIOXIDE OUTPUT

Not all of the carbon dioxide that is carried to the lungs by venous blood is removed. Gases in the pulmonary capillaries are in equilibrium with gases in the alveoli. Thus, when the mixed carbon dioxide tension of venous blood is 46 mm Hg and the tension in the alveoli is 40 mm Hg, carbon dioxide diffuses into the alveoli until an equilibrium is reached (Fig. 2–3). A normal systemic arterial carbon dioxide tension of about 40 mm Hg facilitates the normal diffusion of oxygen into the tissues and the elimination of carbon dioxide from the tissues into the bloodstream.

(Q) The normal carbon dioxide pressure in arterial blood is
- a. 46 mm Hg. 77 C
- b. 40 mm Hg. 78 b
- c. 100 mm Hg. 78 B

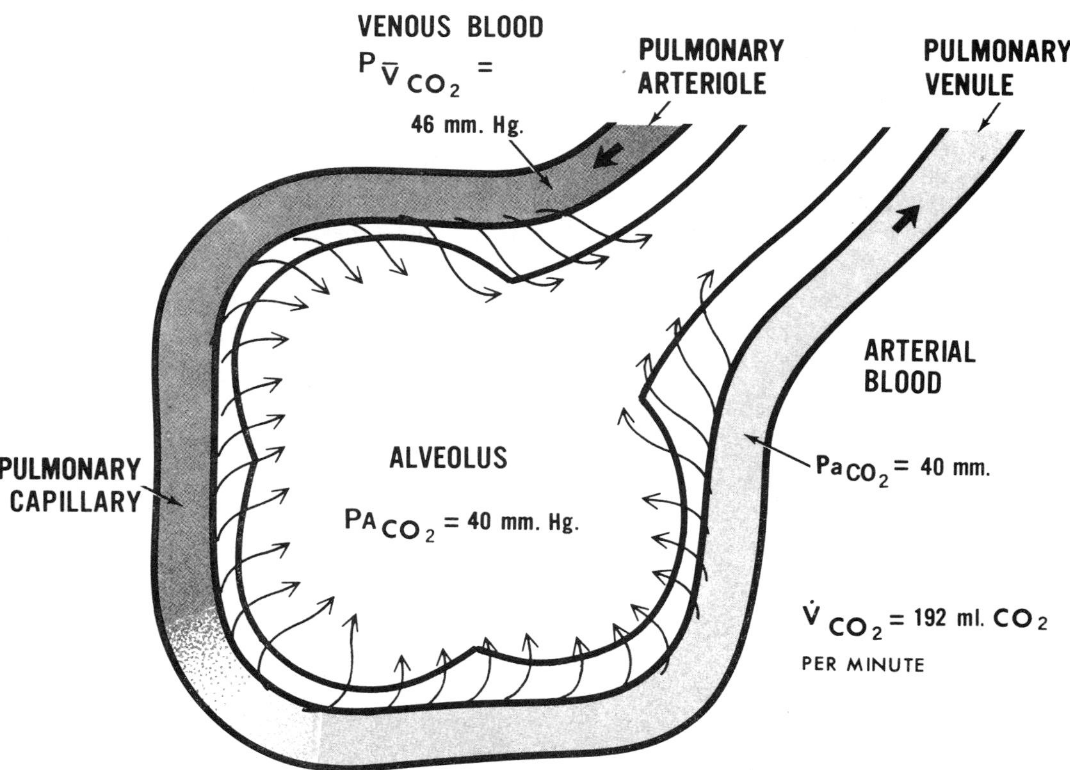

Figure 2–3

FRAME 57. RESPIRATORY DISTURBANCES TO ACID-BASE BALANCE

Respiratory alkalosis and respiratory acidosis will result from disturbances that involve a primary change in alveolar ventilation. When patients hypoventilate, body fluids accumulate CO_2 and the pH drops to an abnormally low level, causing a respiratory acidosis. The initial response to the respiratory acidosis is for the buffer mechanisms to blunt the decrease in pH produced by the increased CO_2. The buffer response is a small increase in plasma bicarbonate occurring in about 10 to 15 minutes. The renal compensatory response becomes apparent in 6 to 18 hours, with a maximal response occuring 5 to 7 days later. Complete metabolic compensation occurs when the pH is restored to the normal range of 7.35 to 7.40.

Respiratory alkalosis occurs when patients hyperventilate, which lowers the CO_2 of body fluids and increases the pH. The buffer response is a small decrease in plasma bicarbonate followed by a larger renal compensatory drop in bicarbonate that does not become apparent until 6 to 18 hours later. This is the opposite of what occurs with respiratory acidosis. *Acute* respiratory alkalosis is defined as a disturbance caused by alveolar ventilation of short duration without any renal compensation.

(Q) Which of the following describes acute respiratory alkalosis?

a. low plasma P_{CO_2}, *high* blood pH, *normal* plasma HCO_3^- 78 d
b. low plasma P_{CO_2}, *high* blood pH, *low* plasma HCO_3^- 77 a
c. low plasma P_{CO_2}, *normal* blood pH, *low* plasma HCO_3^- 71 e

FRAME 58. METABOLIC DISTURBANCES TO ACID-BASE BALANCE

Metabolic acidosis is an abnormal physiological process characterized by a primary gain of strong acid or a primary loss of bicarbonate from the extracellular fluid such as occurs with diarrhea. Metabolic alkalosis is an abnormal physiological process characterized by a primary gain of a strong base or primary loss of a strong acid. Also, the primary gain of bicarbonate by intravenous infusion will cause metabolic alkalosis.

The respiratory system will attempt to compensate for metabolic disturbances by increasing or decreasing alveolar ventilation. A metabolic acidosis would cause the respiratory system to try to compensate by alveolar hyperventilation, which has the effect of lowering CO_2 in body fluids. The opposite respiratory response occurs with metabolic alkalosis and causes the patient to hypoventilate and increase the plasma CO_2 tension. Partial respiratory compensation moves toward a pH of 7.35 to 7.45, but still remains outside the normal range.

(Q) Which of the following would describe acute metabolic acidosis?

a. low blood pH, normal plasma P_{CO_2}, normal alveolar ventilation 77 b
b. low blood pH, high plasma P_{CO_2}, decreased alveolar ventilation 76 d
c. low blood pH, low plasma P_{CO_2}, increased alveolar ventilation 78 D

76A (from page 67, frame 48)
Right. Hyperventilation causes increased excretion of carbon dioxide, resulting in a lower carbon dioxide tension in the blood. This may interfere with gas exchange and other body functions, result in a higher pH, and disturb the acid-base balance. Please continue on page 68, frame 49.

76B (from page 69, frame 51)
Of course! As the blood pH rises it becomes more alkaline, which means there are not enough hydrogen ions to maintain a ratio of 1 part acid to 20 parts base (1 : 20). Thus, fewer hydrogen ions would need to be excreted by the kidneys. Please continue on page 72, frame 52.

76C (from page 73, frame 54)
No. Only about 15% is in the form of carbamino compounds. Return to page 73, frame 54, and select another answer.

76D (from page 72, frame 53)
No. Remember that hydrogen ions concentration is inversely related to the pH. As the hydrogen ion concentration increases, the pH decreases. Acidosis results when the pH decreases below 7.35; alkalosis results when the pH increases above 7.45. Inadequate excretion of carbon dioxide results in an excess of carbonic acid and dissolved CO_2, causing acidosis. Please continue on page 73, frame 54.

76a (from page 72, frame 52)
This is the best answer. Acid-base balance can be maintained only by the proper functioning of all three regulatory mechanisms: (1) the buffers, (2) the lungs, and (3) the kidneys. A disturbance in any one of these could cause an imbalance in the ratio of acid to base in body fluids, which would threaten the life of the patient. Please continue on page 72, frame 53.

76b (from page 73, frame 54)
No. A very small amount of carbon dioxide exists as CO_2 gas physically dissolved in blood. Return to page 73, frame 54, and select another answer.

76c (from page 72, frame 53)
Right. Remember that the hydrogen ion concentration affects the pH inversely. As the hydrogen ion concentration increases, the pH decreases. Inadequate excretion of carbon dioxide (thus increased carbonic acid and dissolved CO_2) results in acidosis. Please continue on page 73, frame 54.

76d (from page 75, frame 58)
Wrong. The respiratory system compensates for metabolic disturbances by changing alveolar ventilation. In this case CO_2 needs to be lowered to compensate for extra hydrogen ions in plasma. Return to page 75, frame 58, and select another answer.

77A (from page 68, frame 49)
Yes. Both of these statements are correct. The rate and depth of respiration help to determine both the tension of carbon dioxide and the concentration of hydrogen ions in the blood and body fluids. Respiratory regulation of arterial CO_2 tension is a very important factor in maintaining the acid-base balance. You should remember from Chapter 1 how gas exchange takes place in the alveoli. Please continue on page 69, frame 50.

77B (from page 72, frame 52)
You're right, but this is not the best answer. Even if the buffer system were adequate, the acid-base balance could still be disturbed. Hypoventilation, for example, would produce an excess of carbonic acid and dissolved CO_2 in the bloodstream. Return to page 72, frame 52, and select another answer.

77C (from page 74, frame 56)
Wrong. You selected the value for the partial pressure of carbon dioxide in mixed venous blood. We're talking about arterial blood. Return to page 74, frame 56, and try again.

77D (from page 73, frame 54)
Yes. Carbon dioxide in amounts of 80% to 90% exists as bicarbonate in the red cells during transport. Please continue on page 73, frame 55.

77a (from page 75, frame 57)
Correct. The plasma buffers lower the plasma bicarbonate concentration within 10 to 15 minutes of the onset of acute respiratory alkalosis. Renal compensation will become apparent 6 to 18 hours later and reach its maximal response 5 to 7 days later. Please continue on page 75, frame 58.

77b (from page 75, frame 58)
Careful! Remember, the respiratory system compensates for metabolic disturbances by changing alveolar ventilation. Return to page 75, frame 58, and select another answer.

77c (from page 67, frame 47)
Yes. Keep in mind that body fluids normally remain slightly alkaline (within a pH range of 7.35 to 7.45). If the hydrogen ion concentration increases suddenly, buffers tend to weaken the effect of this increase. This is accomplished by a chemical reaction that produces a weak acid and a neutral salt from a strong acid. Conversely, if a strong base is added, buffers weaken the effect by a chemical reaction that yields a weakly alkaline salt and water. Thus, buffer activity is one of the ways in which the body prevents a marked change in the pH. However, buffering alone cannot prevent the excretion of large amounts of CO_2 as a result of hyperventilation. Renal compensation is also necessary. Please continue on page 67, frame 48.

78A (from page 72, frame 52)
You're right, but this is not the best answer. Even if the respiratory system were functioning properly, malfunctioning of the kidneys could result in failure to reabsorb enough bicarbonate ions to maintain the balance, or failure to remove excess hydrogen ions from the blood for excretion in the urine. Return to page 72, frame 52, and select another answer.

78B (from page 74, frame 56)
Wrong. You selected the value for partial pressure of oxygen in arterial blood. We're talking about carbon dioxide. Return to page 74, frame 56, and try again.

78C (from page 73, frame 55)
Careful! Remember that the hydrogen ion content affects the pH inversely. Return to page 73, frame 55, and try again.

78D (from page 75, frame 58)
Correct. The respiratory system compensates for acute metabolic acidosis by excreting more CO_2, thereby lowering the CO_2 tension in the blood and body fluids. Please turn to page 79 and complete the chapter exercises.

78a (from page 72, frame 52)
You're right, but this is not the best answer. Even if the kidneys were functioning properly, they could not work fast enough to eliminate the excess carbonic acid and dissolved CO_2 produced by prolonged hypoventilation. Return to page 72, frame 52, and select another answer.

78b (from page 74, frame 56)
Right. The $Paco_2$ is usually around 40 mm Hg. Please continue on page 75, frame 57.

78c (from page 73, frame 55)
Correct. In the hydration reaction, the carbon dioxide mixes with water to produce carbonic acid, which then dissociates into bicarbonate and hydrogen ions. An increase in carbon dioxide results in an increase in hydrogen ion concentration. This affects the pH *inversely*—when the concentration of hydrogen ion increases, the pH decreases; that is, the solution becomes more acidic. If the hydrogen ion concentration is raised, the pH decreases and the solution becomes more acidic. If the hydrogen ion concentration is lowered, the pH is increased and the solution becomes more alkaline. Please continue on page 75, frame 57.

78d (from page 75, frame 57)
Wrong. Remember that the plasma buffer response, while small in comparison to renal compensation, does lower the plasma bicarbonate concentration within 10 to 15 minutes after the onset of acute respiratory alkalosis. Return to page 75, frame 57, and select another answer.

EXERCISES

1. List three examples of common pathologic conditions that can cause a person to hypoventilate.
2. Identify a respiratory disease that may cause a patient to hyperventilate or hypoventilate depending on the stage of the disease.
3. Explain why the kidneys are relatively slow to compensate for a respiratory acid-base disturbance.
4. List two examples of common medical problems that may cause metabolic acidosis.
5. Describe how the respiratory system will try to compensate for metabolic acidosis.
6. Describe how CO_2 is transported from the tissues to the lungs for excretion.
7. Explain the importance of the hydration reaction in facilitating CO_2 transport.
8. Compare and contrast the lungs and the kidneys in terms of their efficiency in maintaining acid-base balance.
9. Describe the role of carbonic anhydrase in maintaining acid-base balance.
10. Explain how the kidneys attempt to adjust acid-base balance.

POSTTEST

This test is designed to evaluate what you learned after completing Chapter 2. Check your answers on page 82 and review the topics where your answer is incorrect.

1. The exrection of CO_2 is the function of the
   A. kidneys.
   B. hemoglobin buffers.
   C. lungs.
   D. erythrocyte bicarbonate.
   E. plasma bicarbonate.
2. The term pH can be defined as the
   A. hydrogen ion concentration.
   B. bicarbonate ion concentration.
   C. positive log of the hydrogen concentration.
   D. negative log of the hydrogen ion concentration.
   E. ratio of bicarbonate to dissolved CO_2 and carbonic acid.
3. A pH of 7.30 in blood plasma is best described as
   A. normal.
   B. alkalemia.
   C. acidemia.
   D. more acidic than H_2O.
   E. alkalosis.
4. How do the kidneys attempt to regulate acid-base balance?
   A. by eliminating *all* hydrogen ions
   B. by eliminating *excess* hydrogen ions
   C. by reabsorbing *all* bicarbonate ions
   D. by *selectively* reabsorbing bicarbonate
   E. both *B* and *D*
5. What effect will a sudden increase in plasma CO_2 have on pH?
   A. The pH will decrease.
   B. The pH will remain at 7.40.
   C. The pH will rise.
   D. The hydrogen ion concentration will decrease.
   E. The ratio of bicarbonate to dissolved CO_2 will increase.
6. Which of the following pH values represent alkalemia?
   A. 7.30
   B. 7.35
   C. 7.40
   D. 7.45
   E. 7.50
7. The normal range for arterial CO_2 tension is
   A. 20 to 30 mm Hg.
   B. 25 to 35 mm Hg.
   C. 30 to 40 mm Hg.
   D. 35 to 45 mm Hg.
   E. 40 to 50 mm Hg.

8. After a sudden metabolic disturbance the respiratory compensation will occur over a period of
   A. minutes to a few hours.
   B. a few hours.
   C. 6 to 12 hours.
   D. 24 hours.
   E. several days.
9. Loss of hydrochloric acid from vomiting may result in
   A. metabolic alkalosis.
   B. metabolic acidosis.
   C. metabolic compensation.
   D. alveolar hyperventilation.
   E. increased acidification of urine.
10. Increased physical exercise without a concurrent increase in alveolar ventilation will cause
    A. respiratory alkalosis.
    B. respiratory acidosis.
    C. metabolic alkalosis.
    D. metabolic acidosis.
    E. both metabolic and respiratory acidosis.
11. The tubular cells of the kidney eliminate excess hydrogen and reabsorb bicarbonate by
    A. acidification of phosphate buffer salts.
    B. increasing pH of urine.
    C. reabsorption of ammonium ions.
    D. reabsorption of hydrogen ions.
    E. all of the above.
12. The hydration reaction that converts CO_2 to bicarbonate occurs primarily in the
    A. blood plasma.
    B. erythrocytes.
    C. proteins.
    D. phosphates.
    E. lungs.
13. Carbonic acid (H_2CO_3) is produced by the reaction of
    A. $H^+ + HCO_3^-$.
    B. $CO_2 + H_2O$.
    C. $H^+ + H_2O$.
    D. $CO_2 + HCO_3^-$.
    E. both *A* and *B*.
14. CO_2 converted to bicarbonate inside red cells will
    A. remain inside red cells.
    B. diffuse out of red cells until HCO_3^- is in equilibrium with plasma.
    C. travel to the lungs as carbonic acid.
    D. attach to hemoglobin molecules.
    E. both *C* and *D*.

15. The plasma bicarbonate concentration will be
    A. higher in venous blood.
    B. higher in arterial blood.
    C. the same in arterial and venous blood.
    D. lower at the tissue level.
    E. negligible in arterial blood.

16. If CO_2 production and alveolar ventilation increase together in a linear manner, the plasma P_{CO_2} will
    A. increase slightly.
    B. increase greatly.
    C. remain at 40 mm Hg.
    D. decrease slightly.
    E. decrease greatly.

17. An abnormal process in which there is a primary decrease in the rate of alveolar ventilation relative to CO_2 production is called
    A. metabolic acidosis.
    B. metabolic alkalosis.
    C. respiratory acidosis.
    D. respiratory alkalosis.
    E. a mixed disturbance.

18. An abnormal process producing a primary gain of strong base or primary loss of acid is called
    A. metabolic acidosis.
    B. metabolic alkalosis.
    C. respiratory acidosis.
    D. respiratory alkalosis.
    E. a mixed disturbance.

19. Which of the following characterizes a compensatory process?
    A. a change in the system *affected* by the primary disturbance
    B. a process that moves pH further *away* from normal
    C. a change in the system *not affected* by the primary disturbance
    D. a primary process that restores the system *affected* to normal
    E. mediation *exclusively* by blood buffers

20. Which of the following primary disturbances is compensated by accelerated excretion of hydrogen ions by the kidneys?
    A. metabolic acidosis
    B. metabolic alkalosis
    C. respiratory acidosis
    D. respiratory alkalosis
    E. a mixed disturbance

ANSWERS TO POSTTEST

1. C (F44)
2. D (F45)
3. C (F46)
4. E (F51)
5. A (F48)
6. E (F46)
7. D (F56)
8. A (F57)
9. A (F58)
10. B (F49)
11. A (F51)
12. B (F53)
13. E (F53)
14. B (F54)
15. C (F53)
16. C (F49)
17. C (F57)
18. B (F58)
19. C (F57)
20. C (F57)

BIBLIOGRAPHY

Barnes, TA: Respiratory Care Practice. Year Book Medical Publishers, Chicago, 1988.

Burton, GG and Hodgkin, JE: Respiratory Care—A Guide to Clinical Practice. JB Lippincott, Philadelphia, 1984.

Collins, RD: Illustrated Manual of Fluid and Electrolyte Disorders. JB Lippincott, Philadelphia, 1976.

Comroe, JH: Physiology of Respiration, ed 2. Year Book Medical Publishers, Chicago, 1974.

Forster, RE, Fisher, AB, DuBois, AB, and Briscoe, WA: The Lung—Physiologic Basis of Pulmonary Function Testing. Year Book Medical Publishers, Chicago, 1986.

Jones, NL: Blood Gases and Acid Base Physiology. Thiemes-Stratton, New York, 1980.

Murray, JF: The Normal Lung, ed 2. WB Saunders, Philadelphia, 1986.

Shapiro, BA, Harrison, RA, Cane, RD, Templin, RK, and Walton, JR: Clinical Application of Blood Gases, ed 4. Year Book Medical Publishers, Chicago, 1988.

Slonim, NB and Hamilton, LH: Respiratory Physiology, ed 5. CV Mosby, St. Louis, 1986.

West, JB: Respiratory Physiology, ed 4. Williams & Wilkins, Baltimore, 1990.

3

Medical Physics

59. Characteristics of a gas
60. Gases in the atmosphere
61. Effect of gravity on gases in the atmosphere
62. Pressure of gases
63. Kinetic energy
64. Effect of temperature on kinetic energy
65. Atmospheric pressure
66. Mercury barometers
67. Partial pressures
68. Measuring small amounts of pressure
69. Boyle's law, Charles's law
70. Gay-Lussac's, Dalton's gas laws
71. The general gas law
72. Recording data on gases
73. Humidity
74. Airway resistance
75. Water-vapor pressure
76. Flow of gases through tubes
77. Compliance
78. Density and viscosity
79. Lateral pressure

PRETEST

This pretest is designed to measure what you already know about medical physics. Check your answers on page 87 and then continue on page 88, frame 59.

1. Which of the following forms of matter can be easily expanded or compressed?
   A. solids
   B. liquids
   C. gases
   D. synthetic solids
   E. none of the above
2. The fractional concentration of oxygen found in the atmosphere is
   A. 1.00.
   B. 0.30.
   C. 0.21.
   D. 0.18.
   E. 0.10.
3. The amount of pressure exerted by a gas may be dependent upon
   A. barometric pressure.
   B. humidity.
   C. temperature.
   D. number of molecules.
   E. all of the above.
4. The kinetic activity of a gas will increase with
   A. decrease in temperature.
   B. decrease in volume.
   C. increase in volume.
   D. increase in temperature.
   E. both *B* and *D*.
5. The normal barometric pressure at sea level is
   A. 300 mm Hg.
   B. 700 mm Hg.
   C. 760 mm Hg.
   D. 800 mm Hg.
   E. 1000 mm Hg.
6. The partial pressure of oxygen in dry air at sea level is normally
   A. 100 mm Hg.
   B. 160 mm Hg.
   C. 300 mm Hg.
   D. 713 mm Hg.
   E. 760 mm Hg.
7. Small pressure changes in the airways are measured in
   A. mm Hg.
   B. mm H_2O.
   C. cm Hg.
   D. cm H_2O.
   E. psig.

8. If temperature and mass of a gas are held constant, what is the final volume (V_2) if $V_1 = 2000$ mL, $P_1 = 760$ mm Hg, and $P_2 = 1520$ mm Hg?
   A. 500 mL
   B. 1000 mL
   C. 2000 mL
   D. 2500 mL
   E. 4000 mL

9. If the pressure and mass of a gas are held constant, what is the final volume (V_2) if $T_1 = 0°C$, $T_2 = 100°C$, and $V_1 = 1000$ mL?
   A. 333 mL
   B. 500 mL
   C. 667 mL
   D. 1000 mL
   E. 1366 mL

10. If volume and mass of a gas are held constant, what is the final pressure (P_2) if $T_1 = 0°C$, $T_2 = 100°C$, and $P_1 = 2200$ psig?
   A. 733 psig
   B. 1100 psig
   C. 1610 psig
   D. 2933 psig
   E. 3006 psig

11. If mass remains constant, what is the final pressure (P_2) if $P_1 = 760$ mm Hg, $T_1 = 0°C$, $T_2 = 100°C$, $V_1 = 1$ L, and $V_2 = 2$ L?
   A. 519 mm Hg
   B. 1038 mm Hg
   C. 1520 mm Hg
   D. 1724 mm Hg
   E. 2077 mm Hg

12. If a gas mixture of oxygen and nitrogen in a 2-liter container has a total pressure of 760 mm Hg and the $Po_2 = 100$ mm Hg, what is the pressure in the container if all the nitrogen is removed?
   A. 20 mm Hg
   B. 100 mm Hg
   C. 380 mm Hg
   D. 760 mm Hg
   E. 1520 mm Hg

13. Pulmonary gas volumes (volume of gases as they exist in the lungs) are recorded as
   A. ATPS.
   B. STPD.
   C. BTPS.
   D. ATPD.
   E. BTPD.

14. The measurement of the actual weight of water in a given volume of gas is called
   A. relative humidity.
   B. body humidity.
   C. humidity deficit.
   D. absolute humidity.
   E. water vapor pressure.

15. If the driving pressure remains constant, decreasing the diameter of a tube will result in
    A. lower gas velocity.
    B. higher gas flow.
    C. lower gas flow.
    D. laminar gas flow.
    E. no change in gas flow.
16. The term used to describe the distensibility of the lungs is called
    A. conductance.
    B. airway resistance.
    C. compliance.
    D. closing volume.
    E. inspiratory capacity.
17. The work done against airway resistance is calculated by dividing flow into a pressure differential determined by subtracting
    A. PEEP from plateau pressure.
    B. CPAP from plateau pressure.
    C. PEEP from peak inspiratory pressure.
    D. plateau pressure from peak inspiratory pressure.
    E. plateau pressure from PEEP.
18. Which of the following gas mixtures would be best to decrease airway resistance caused by turbulent gas flow?
    A. 100% O_2
    B. 21% O_2 and 79% N_2
    C. 70% O_2 and 30% He
    D. 30% O_2 and 70% He
    E. 30% O_2, 60% He, and 10% CO_2
19. A decrease in lateral wall pressure when gas velocity increases is called
    A. Dalton's law.
    B. Bernoulli effect.
    C. Brownian movement.
    D. kinetic energy.
    E. potential energy.
20. A Venturi system that entrains room air will do all of the following *except*
    A. increase total gas flow.
    B. decrease the delivered oxygen concentration.
    C. increase laminar gas flow.
    D. regulate total flow using entrainment port size.
    E. increase turbulent gas flow.

ANSWERS TO PRETEST

1. C (F59)
2. C (F60)
3. E (F62)
4. E (F63)
5. C (F65)
6. B (F67)
7. D (F68)
8. B (F69)
9. E (F69)
10. E (F70)
11. A (F71)
12. B (F70)
13. C (F72)
14. D (F73)
15. C (F76)
16. C (F77)
17. D (F74)
18. D (F78)
19. B (F79)
20. C (F79)

FRAME 59. CHARACTERISTICS OF A GAS

Physics is the science of the laws and phenomena of nature, especially the forces and general properties of matter. Medical physics pertains to the study of diseases and the care of patients. In this chapter we are concerned primarily with gases and how they behave in the respiratory and circulatory systems.

It is necessary for all health personnel working with or around gases to understand their potential, both beneficial and hazardous. This applies not only to the gases used in respiratory care, but to the gases present in the body. Once you learn the principles that goven the behavior of gases, you will be able to predict what will happen to any gas when it undergoes changes in pressure, volume, or temperature.

Because most gases cannot be seen or felt, it is difficult to understand how they can expand or be compressed. As a gas expands, it cools the surrounding atmosphere. When compressed, it produces heat. Under high pressure and low temperature, it can be liquefied or solidified. Technically, however, a gas is considered a gas only in the aeriform (airlike) state, just as water is considered to be water only in the liquid state, not in the form of ice or water vapor.

(Q) A gas is best described as a
- a. a liquid. 92 A
- b. an aeriform fluid. 92 a
- c. a solid. 93 A
- d. any one of the above. 93 a

FRAME 60. GASES IN THE ATMOSPHERE

TABLE 3–1
ATMOSPHERIC GASES

Element	Proportion of the Atmosphere (%)	Trace Amounts
Nitrogen (N_2)	78.08	1. Helium (He)
Oxygen (O_2)	20.95	2. Hydrogen (H_2)
Argon (Ar)	0.93	3. Krypton (Kr)
Carbon dioxide (CO_2)	0.03	4. Neon (Ne)
		5. Ozone (O_3)
		6. Radon (Rn)

The first thing that comes to mind when we talk about "fresh air" is oxygen. You may assume that the atmosphere is composed primarily of oxygen. Accordingly, you should study Table 3–1 (above).

(Q) The gas most prevalent in the atmosphere is
- a. oxygen. 94 A
- b. nitrogen. 95 A
- c. hydrogen. 95 a

FRAME 61. EFFECT OF GRAVITY ON GASES IN THE ATMOSPHERE

Because of the pull of gravity on gas molecules, the density (mass of molecules per liter of volume) of the gases in the atmosphere is greatest close to the earth's surface, decreasing steadily outward toward free space. In spite of this fact, some physicists speculate that the composition of the atmosphere remains relatively the same to a height of some 60 miles. Beyond 60 miles, because of a decrease in turbulence—which keeps the gases well mixed—the elements separate according to their molecular weights. This diffusion separation accounts for the change in the composition of air from what it is at sea level.

(Q) Up to about 60 miles, the composition of the atmosphere remains fairly constant; above that

a. the mass movements of air tend to separate the elements according to their molecular weights. 92 B

b. the decrease in mass movements of air allows the elements to be separated according to their molecular weights. 92 b

FRAME 62. PRESSURE OF GASES

All matter (solids, liquids, and gases) is composed of molecules that are constantly moving at random. A gas is an elastic aeriform fluid in which molecules are separated from one another and so have free paths in which to move. However, they cannot go very far without colliding with one another or with whatever confines them, thus exerting a pressure against the confining container. The container may be as large as the earth's surface or as small as an alveolus in the lung.

The term used to describe the behavior of molecules is *kinetic activity.* The word *kinetic* comes from the Greek *kinetikos,* which refers to motion. Because most gases cannot be seen or felt, it is difficult to imagine all the motion (kinetic activity) going on constantly among the molecules. A demonstration of this motion can be made by substituting Ping-Pong balls for the molecules. If you dropped a bucketful of Ping-Pong balls into a deep box, you can visualize the activity in the first few seconds, with the balls bouncing up and down, from side to side, and against each other. Each collision gives impetus for another collision. With gas molecules, this activity goes on constantly, changing the kinetic energy of the molecules, which affects heat and pressure. The potential energy possessed by a gas is the amount of work the gas can do because of its pressure. The potential energy of the gas will change to kinetic energy as the gas does work (e.g., the gas exerts pressure, causing a piston to move).

(Q) The amount of pressure exerted by a gas depends on

a. the number of molecules. 93 B

b. the frequency of molecular collisions. 94 B

c. both of the above. 95 B

FRAME 63. KINETIC ENERGY

The frequency of molecular collisions within a confined space depends upon the kinetic energy of the molecules. Each collision gives impetus for another collision: the more collisions, the more energy that will be translated into heat and pressure. Since gas molecules are much farther apart than molecules of liquids or solids, it is possible to increase their kinetic energy by compressing them into a smaller space where collisions will be more frequent.

In Figure 3–1, the initial state of the gas is shown in cylinder **A**. At a given temperature, it exerts a given pressure. In cylinder **B**, the gas is being compressed by the piston. Notice the same number of molecules crowded into the smaller space. This causes an increase in molecular collisions, as reflected in a rise in the temperature and pressure of the gas. In cylinder **C**, the piston has been retracted, allowing greater distance between molecules and fewer collisions. The drop in both temperature and pressure signals the decrease in molecular collisions.

(Q) The main purpose of cylinder **B** in the illustration is to demonstrate how

a. heat produces an increase in molecular activity. 93 b

b. increased molecular activity produces heat. 94 C

c. pressure and temperature are increased by compression. 94 a

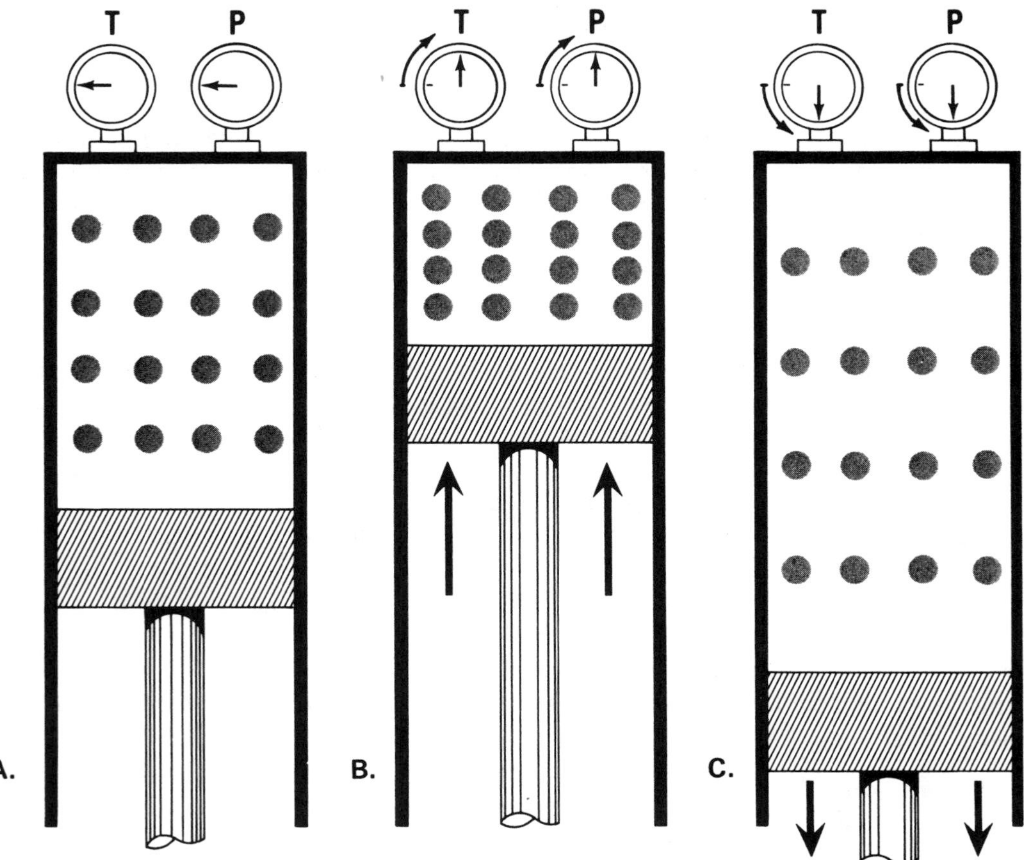

Redrawn from *Fundamentals of Respiratory Therapy* by Donald F. Egan

Figure 3–1

FRAME 64. EFFECT OF TEMPERATURE ON KINETIC ENERGY

As you have learned, the kinetic energy of molecules is dependent upon their collisions in space. The number of collisions and thus the kinetic energy of the molecules varies directly with the number of molecules, and inversely with the volume of space in which they are confined. More molecules increase the chances for collision, since less space for the same number of molecules increases the chances for collision. One additional factor controlling kinetic energy is temperature. A rise in temperature increases molecular activity and thus the chances for molecular collision.

(Q) Which of the following is a correct statement?

a. Kinetic energy increases as the number of molecules per cubic inch increases. 93 c

b. Kinetic energy increases as the number of molecules per cubic inch decreases and the molecules have more room for action. 94 b

c. Kinetic energy decreases as the temperature increases. 95 b

FRAME 65. ATMOSPHERIC PRESSURE

Mercury has a density of 1.36 g/mm^3. At sea level, the average atmospheric pressure will support a column of mercury 760 mm high. Pressure, you will remember, is determined by the height of the mercury in the column multiplied by its density ($P = mm \times g/mm^3$).

(Q) The atmospheric pressure at sea level is

a. $760\ mm \times 1.36\ g/mm^3 = 1034\ g/mm^2$. 94 d

b. $760\ mm \times 1.36\ g/mm^3 = 1034\ g/mm$. 95 C

c. $760\ mm \times 1.36\ g/mm^3 = 1034\ g/mm^3$. 103 A

92A (from page 88, frame 59)
No. Gas can be liquefied (e.g., liquid oxygen), but is considered as *gas* only in its aeriform state. The term *fluid* may have confused you. A fluid is anything that flows, whether liquid or gas. Please continue on page 88, frame 60.

92B (from page 89, frame 61)
No. As long as there is turbulence or mass air movements, the various gases in the atmosphere will remain well mixed. However, when these movements decrease about 60 miles above the earth, the molecules of the different gases separate according to their molecular weights. Please continue on page 89, frame 62.

92C (from page 97, frame 67)
No. While it's true that pressure of a gas varies inversely with the volume, volume is not the *primary* variable. What happens to molecular activity when the volume changes? Return to page 98, frame 67, and try again.

92a (from page 88, frame 59)
Correct. Although a gas can be liquefied (e.g., liquid oxygen) or solidified (e.g., dry ice, which is solid carbon dioxide), it is technically considered a gas only in its aeriform state. Please continue on page 88, frame 60.

92b (from page 89, frame 61)
Yes. Mass air movements will keep the gases well mixed. When the movement decreases in the ionosphere, about 60 miles above the earth, the gases have a tendency to separate according to their molecular weights. Please continue on page 89, frame 62.

92c (from page 97, frame 67)
Right. Kinetic activity is increased when the number of molecules per unit of volume is increased, the volume is decreased, or the temperature is raised. Thus the total atmospheric pressure affects the kinetic activity and the tension or partial pressure exerted by a gas. Please continue on page 98, frame 68.

93A (from page 88, frame 59)
No. Gases can be solidified, as carbon dioxide is solidified into dry ice, but they are technically considered gases only in their aeriform state. Please continue on page 88, frame 60.

93B (from page 89, frame 62)
Yes, the number of molecules within a given space affects the pressure, but there are other factors to consider. Return to page 89, frame 62, and select another answer.

93C (from page 97, frame 67)
No. While it's true that pressure varies directly with the temperature, it is not the primary variable. What happens to molecular activity when the temperature changes? Return to page 97, frame 67, and try again.

93a (from page 88, frame 59)
No. Although a gas can be liquefied (e.g., dry ice, which is solid carbon dioxide), it is technically considered a gas only in its aeriform state. Please continue on page 88, frame 60.

93b (from page 90, frame 63)
No. In this example, the molecular activity is producing the heat, that is, increasing the temperature. Return to page 90, frame 63, and try again.

93c (from page 91, frame 64)
Correct. Kinetic energy increases as the number of molecules per cubic inch increases. Kinetic energy depends upon the frequency of molecular collisions. Molecular collisions increase in direct proportion to increases in temperature and molecular density (number of molecules per unit of volume). Please continue on page 91, frame 65.

93d (from page 96, frame 66)
Wrong. This would be correct if the scale were calibrated in inches, but the example uses millimeters. Return to page 96, frame 66, and try again.

94A (from page 88, frame 60)
Wrong. If you look at the table on page 88, frame 60, you will see that oxygen comprises only about 20.95% of the atmosphere. Return to page 88, frame 60, and try again.

94B (from page 89, frame 62)
Wrong. The frequency with which molecules collide affects the pressure, but there are other variables to consider. Return to page 89, frame 62, and select another answer.

94C (from page 90, frame 63)
True, but what is another result of increased molecular activity when the piston compresses the gas? Return to page 90, frame 63, and try again.

94D (from page 96, frame 66)
Right. If the scale is calibrated in inches, the pressure is determined in pounds per square inch. If the scale is calibrated in millimeters, the pressure must be indicated in grams per square millimeter. Please continue on page 97, frame 67.

94a (from page 90, frame 63)
This is the best answer. It illustrates how compression can increase the kinetic activity, which in turn increases the pressure and temperature of the gas. Please continue on page 91, frame 64.

94b (from page 91, frame 64)
Wrong. Kinetic energy depends upon the frequency of molecular collisions. Remember the Ping-Pong balls? Would the chances of collision be greater if there were only three balls bouncing around in the box or if there were 20 balls bouncing around? Return to page 91, frame 64, and try again.

94c (from page 96, frame 66)
Wrong. In the first place, density is determined by the number of grams per cubic measure (g/mm^3). The formula you have selected represents density as grams per square millimeter (g/mm^2). Secondly, pressure is usually expressed as grams per square centimeter. This formula expresses it as grams per centimeter. Return to page 96, frame 66, and try again.

94d (from page 91, frame 65)
Right. Pressure is determined in pounds per square inch or in grams per square millimeter. Please continue on page 96, frame 66.

95A (from page 88, frame 60)
Right. Many gases as well as water are in the atmosphere, but the four most abundant elements are nitrogen, 78.08%; oxygen, 20.95%; argon, 0.93%; and carbon dioxide, 0.03%. Please continue on page 89, frame 61.

95B (from page 89, frame 62)
Correct. The amount of pressure exerted on the container walls is affected by the number of molecules present, the velocity of the molecules, and the frequency of their collisions. Please continue on page 90, frame 63.

95C (from page 91, frame 65)
Your answer, 1034 g/mm, is not correct. $P = \text{mm} \times \text{g/mm}^3 = \text{g/mm}^2$. Pressure is determined in grams per square millimeter. Return to page 91, frame 65, and try again.

95D (from page 107, frame 74)
Careful, remember airway resistance is reported in liters per second. You must first convert 30 L/min to 0.5 L/s by dividing 30 L by 60 seconds. Return to page 107, frame 74, and select another answer.

95a (from page 88, frame 60)
Wrong. If you look at the table on page 88, frame 60, you will see that there is only a trace of hydrogen in the atmosphere. In fact, hydrogen, neon, helium, krypton, xenon, ozone, and radon altogether comprise only 0.01% of the atmosphere. Return to page 88, frame 60, and try again.

95b (from page 91, frame 64)
Wrong. Heat increases kinetic energy. Cooling slows it down. Return to page 91, frame 64, and select another answer.

95c (from page 107, frame 74)
Correct. The pressure needed to overcome airway resistance is 5 cm H_2O, and when divided by a flow of 0.5 L/s, the correct answer—10 cm H_2O/L per second is determined. Please continue on page 108, frame 75.

95d (from page 107, frame 74)
Not quite, check your math; the pressure needed to overcome airway resistance is 5 cm H_2O and when divided by a flow of 0.5 L/s, the correct answer is determined. Return to page 107, frame 74, and try again.

95e (from page 100, frame 70)
Answers

Boyle's law: With temperature (T) and mass (n) held constant, there is an inverse relationship between volume (V) and pressure (P).

Charles's law: At a constant pressure, the volume of a given mass varies directly with absolute temperature.

Gay-Lussac's law: If volume and mass remain constant, the pressure exerted by a gas varies directly with the absolute temperature of the gas.

Dalton's law: Each gas in a mixture of gases exerts the same pressure it would exert if it occupied the container alone. Please continue on page 101, frame 71.

FRAME 66. MERCURY BAROMETERS

The atmospheric pressure can be measured with a barometer (Fig. 3–2). The principle on which the barometer works is that pressure of the atmosphere on the surface of a reservoir balances the pressure exerted by a column of fluid. The pressure exerted by a column of the fluid is equal to the height of the column times the density of the fluid.

With large volumes of gas such as the atmosphere, pressure is usually expressed as so many grams per square millimeter (g/mm^2) or pounds per square inch (lb/in^2). Remember that pressure is equal to the height of the column multiplied by the density of the fluid in the column. In the metric system, pressure (g/mm^2) equals the height (mm) multiplied by density (g/mm^3). In the English system, pressure (lb/in^2) equals the height (inches) multiplied by density (lb/in^3).

(Q) If the mercury in the barometer reads 40 cm, the formula to use to calculate atmospheric pressure is

a. $P = \text{inches} \times lb/in^3 = lb/in^2$. 93 d
b. $P = \text{cm} \times g/mm^3 = g/mm^2$. 94 D
c. $P = \text{cm} \times g/mm^2 = g/mm$. 94 c

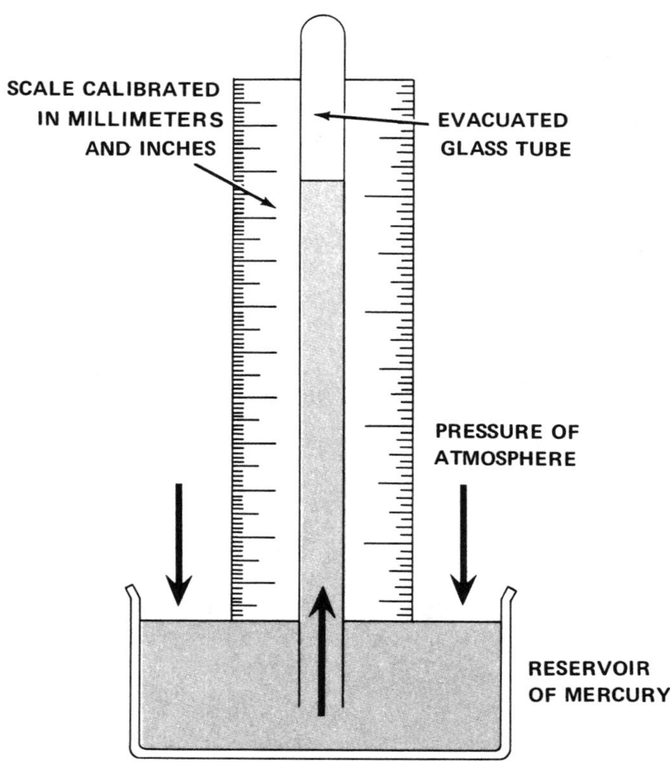

Figure 3–2

FRAME 67. PARTIAL PRESSURES

Examples of pressure exerted by different forces are shown in Figure 3–3. Usually in medical physiology, the pressure of a respiratory gas is referred to as tension or partial pressure (e.g., the tension or partial pressure of oxygen in the blood). Gas tension can exist inside a blood vessel or inside tiny spaces such as alveoli. The partial pressure of a gas is dependent upon the total atmospheric pressure. At very high altitudes such as Denver, Colorado, the total atmospheric pressure is significantly less than pressure found at sea level. The amount of water vapor in the mixture will also directly affect the partial pressure of the gases in the mixture. The equation below expresses the relationship between total atmospheric pressure (P_B), water vapor (P_{H_2O}), fractional concentration of gas (F_X), and the partial pressure of the gas (P_X).

$$P_X = (P_B - P_{H_2O})\, F_X$$

Example: At *sea level*, given P_B 760 mm Hg, P_{H_2O} 20 mm Hg, F_{O_2} 0.21
$P_{O_2} = (760 - 20)0.21$
$P_{O_2} = 155$ mm Hg

Example: *Denver*, given P_B 630 mm Hg, P_{H_2O} 20 mm Hg, F_{O_2} 0.21
$P_{O_2} = (630 - 20)0.21$
$P_{O_2} = 128$ mm Hg

(Q) The primary variable that controls the amount of pressure or tension of a gas is

a. volume. 92 C
b. kinetic activity. 92 c
c. temperature. 93 C

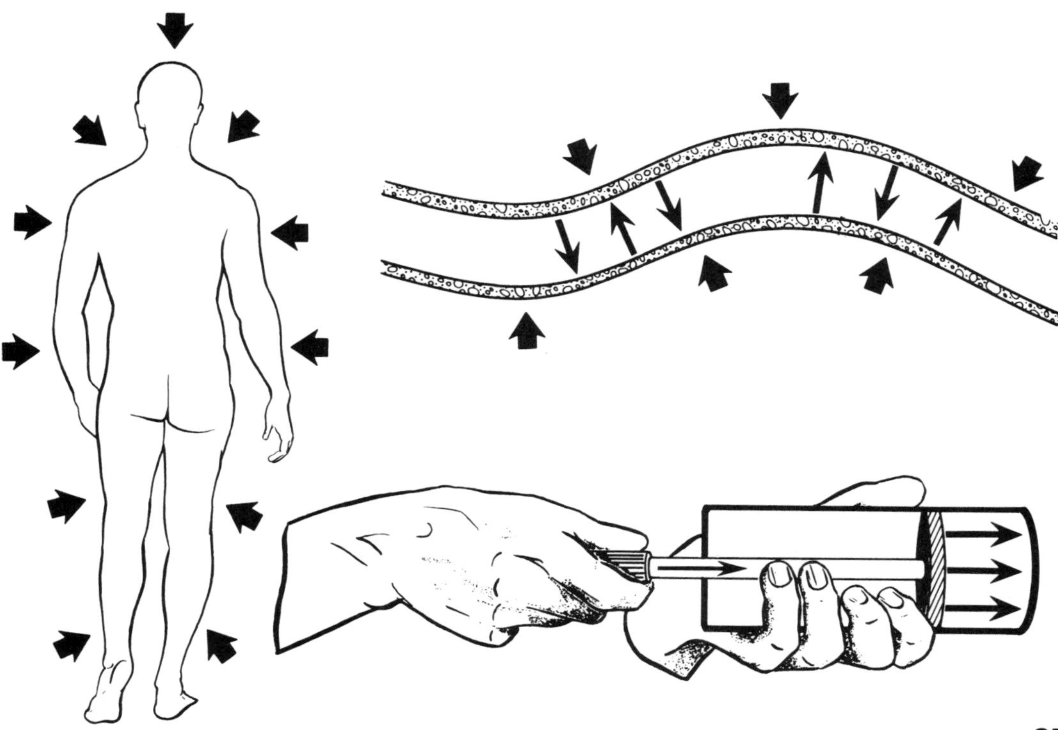

Figure 3–3

FRAME 68. MEASURING SMALL AMOUNTS OF PRESSURE

Until now we have discussed atmospheric pressure. In dealing with small amounts of pressure you will learn to think and talk in terms of millimeters (mm) of mercury (Hg) for blood gases or centimeters (cm) of water (H_2O) for airway pressure. Some physiologists may also refer to 1 mm Hg as 1 *torr*, in memory of the Italian scientist E. Torricelli (1608–1647), who invented the mercury manometer.

If you measure intrapleural pressure using a mercury manometer, it will vary within the thoracic cavity. Gas flows from areas of higher pressure into areas of lower pressure. During inspiration the intrapleural pressure is usually about 6 to 8 mm Hg below atmospheric pressure (760 mm Hg at sea level). Thus, when the pressure in the alveoli is lower than the 760 mm Hg of the atmosphere, air will flow into the lungs until mouth and alveolar pressure are equal.[1]

By the same principle, the partial pressure of carbon dioxide is higher in venous blood than in the alveoli. Thus, the carbon dioxide diffuses across the alveolar capillary membranes into the alveoli. Conversely, the partial pressure of oxygen is higher in the alveoli than it is in the surrounding capillaries. Thus, oxygen diffuses through these membranes into the capillaries. This is how gas exchange takes place with each breath adding oxygen and removing CO_2 from the alveolar space and keeping the arterial blood continually supplied with oxygen and removing excess carbon dioxide.

(Q) Air flows into the lungs during inspiration as a result of the
  a. inflation and contraction of the lungs. 102 A
  b. differences in pressure between the lungs and the atmosphere. 102 a

[1]Atmospheric pressure normally is 760 mm Hg at sea level, less at higher altitudes.

FRAME 69. BOYLE'S LAW, CHARLES'S LAW

Four major principles apply to a given mass of gas.[1] These principles are based on Boyle's, Charles's, Gay-Lussac's, and Dalton's laws and each will be discussed in turn. Three of these laws can be combined to determine what happens when two or three variables change simultaneously (volume, pressure, temperature, and mass).

Boyle's law was named after the English chemist and physicist Robert Boyle (1672–1691). He found there is an inverse relationship between the pressure and volume of a gas, provided the temperature and mass are held constant. In other words, with a given mass of gas, if the temperature remains constant, the pressure increases as the volume is decreased; and the pressure falls as the volume that the gas occupies is increased. This relationship can be expressed by the formula shown below.

$P_1V_1 = P_2V_2$ *when temperature and mass are held constant*

P_1 = initial pressure
P_2 = final pressure
V_1 = initial volume
V_2 = final volume

Jacques Alexandre Cesar Charles (1746–1823) was a French mathematician and physicist who was the first to use hydrogen for inflating balloons. When air was used, a fire had to be built under a balloon to make it rise. Charles noticed that as the heat was increased, the air in the balloon expanded. This increased the volume and decreased the density of the air in the balloon. Since the air in the balloon was less dense than the surrounding atmosphere, the balloon would then rise. By using hydrogen, a lighter-than-air gas, Charles eliminated the need for fire.

Charles theorized that, at a constant pressure, the volume of a given mass varies directly with the absolute temperature—as one increases, the other increases. In calculating the change of volume resulting from the change of temperature, the absolute scale of temperature is used.[2]

$$\frac{V_1}{T_1} = \frac{V_2}{T_2}$$ *when mass and pressure are constant*

where V_1 = initial volume
V_2 = final volume
T_1 = initial temperature
T_2 = final temperature

(Q) Which of the following examples would represent Boyle's law?

a. Building a fire under a balloon will increase the volume. 103 B
b. Compressing a gas decreases its volume and increases the pressure. 103 a
c. Heating a cylinder of gas increases molecular activity, thus increasing the pressure even though the volume remains the same. 104 A

---

[1]Mass can be defined as the quantity of matter contained in a body, that is, the number and size of its molecules.

[2]On the absolute temperature scale, 0° absolute is equivalent to minus 273°C and 273° absolute is equivalent to 0°C, the freezing point of water at sea level (barometric pressure, 760 mm Hg), 373° absolute is equivalent to 100°C, the boiling point of water at 760 mm Hg.

FRAME 70. GAY-LUSSAC'S, DALTON'S GAS LAWS

Joseph Louis Gay-Lussac (1778–1850) was a French chemist and physicist who did research in the expansion of gases. He found that the pressure of a gas varies directly with the absolute temperature, if the volume remains the same—as one increases, the other increases.

$$\frac{P_1}{T_1} = \frac{P_2}{T_2}$$ *when mass and volume are held constant*

The fourth major gas law, Dalton's law, is used to determine partial pressures of gases in a mixture. According to John Dalton (1766–1844), each gas in a mixture of gases exerts the same pressure it would exert if it occupied the container alone. The total pressure of a gas mixture is the sum of the partial pressures of the individual gases. In describing a mixture of gases, you can of course refer to its percentage composition by volume. But if you know the total pressure of the mixture and the percentage that each gas contributes to the mixture, you can refer to the partial pressures exerted by its constituent gases. A gas that comprises 20% of a gas mixture, thus, will exert a partial pressure of 20% of the total pressure.

(Q) Without looking at the book, see if you can write in your own words the four basic gas laws: (1) Boyle's law, (2) Charles's law, (3) Gay-Lussac's law, and (4) Dalton's law. When you have finished, check your responses in answer 95e on page 95.

FRAME 71. THE GENERAL GAS LAW

The four gas laws just discussed will help you understand the behavior of gases as they apply to a given mass (n). In pulmonary physiology, we are concerned not so much with changes in mass but with gas volume when it is subjected to changes in temperature, pressure, or both. To calculate gas volumes that are subjected to different temperatures and/or pressures, it will be necessary to use a combination of the above three gas laws called the *general gas law.*

When gas is subjected to changes in pressure, volume, and/or temperature, the mass remains the same, but changes do occur in one or more of the variables. Once you know the original volume (V_1), the original pressure (P_1), and the original absolute temperature (T_1), you can use the general gas law to calculate the new pressure (P_2), the new volume (V_2), or the new temperature (T_2), provided two of the three variables are known. The formula that combines Boyle's law, Charles's law, and Gay-Lussac's law is as follows:

$$\frac{V_1 \times P_1}{T_1} = \frac{V_2 \times P_2}{T_2}$$

If you want to correct a gas volume for changes in temperature and pressure, for example, you would use the following expression of the general gas law.

$$V_2 = \frac{V_1 \times P_1 \times T_2}{P_2 \times T_1}$$

(Q) The two gas laws dealing with changes in volume are

a. Boyle's law and Gay-Lussac's law. 102 B

b. Charles's law and Boyle's law. 102 b

c. Charles's law and Gay-Lussac's law. 104 a

102A (from page 98, frame 68)
Wrong. The lungs themselves play a passive role in the breathing process. When the lungs are full of air, they are expanded. They contract as the air is exhaled. But why does the air enter the lungs from the atmosphere? Please return to page 98, frame 68, and select another answer.

102B (from page 101, frame 71)
Wrong. Gay-Lussac's law is dependent on a constant volume. If the volume and mass of a gas remain constant, the pressure varies directly with the absolute temperature. We're talking about changes in volume causing changes in temperature or pressure. Return to page 101, frame 71, and try again.

102C (from page 107, frame 73)
This is a true statement, but does your choice indicate that the other option is not true? Return to page 107, frame 73, and select another answer.

102D (from page 108, frame 75)
Correct. When the covered container of water is heated, more water vapor is held above the liquid, increasing the relative humidity and the water vapor pressure. Please continue on page 109, frame 76.

102a (from page 98, frame 68)
Yes. The lungs themselves play a passive role in quiet breathing. Please continue on page 99, frame 69.

102b (from page 101, frame 71)
Correct. Charles's law and Boyle's law both deal with changes in volume. Please continue on page 106, frame 72.

102c (from page 107, frame 73)
This is a true statement, but does your choice indicate the other statement is not true? Return to page 107, frame 73, and select another answer.

102d (from page 110, frame 77)
Of course, gases with different characteristics flow at different rates, just as water flows at a different rate than molasses. But there are other factors involved in the amount of pressure needed to ventilate the lungs. Return to page 110, frame 77, and select another answer.

103A (from page 91, frame 65)
No. Your answer, 1034 g/mm^3, is incorrect. Pressure = cm × g/mm^3 = g/mm^2. The pressure is determined in grams per square centimeter. Return to page 91, frame 65, and try again.

103B (from page 99, frame 69)
Wrong. Remember, Boyle's law requires that temperature and mass be held constant and expresses an inverse, not a direct, relationship between volume and pressure. Return to page 99, frame 69, and review Boyle's law; then make another selection.

103C (from page 110, frame 77)
Yes, but if a gas is flowing in a smooth stream, the flow is greater than if the gas is whirling around eddies at some point. However, other factors are involved in the amount of pressure required to ventilate the lungs. Return to page 110, frame 77, and select another answer.

103D (from page 111, frame 78)
Right. Imagine water flowing freely through the same length of tubing. If the tubing were suddenly constricted at one point, a smaller volume of water per unit of time would flow from the end of the tube. Thus, the rate of flow would be decreased. Please continue on page 112, frame 79.

103a (from page 99, frame 69)
Correct. In Boyle's law, there is an inverse relationship between volume and pressure—as one increases, the other decreases. Please continue on page 100, frame 70.

103b (from page 106, frame 72)
You have it reversed. Lung volumes are reported as BTPS (saturated). Blood gas volumes are reported as STPD (dry). Return to page 106, frame 72, and review the general rules for reporting data on gases; then try again.

103c (from page 110, frame 77)
Naturally, if the airway is clear, the gas will flow more easily than if there is an obstruction in its path. Lungs with a normal compliance will be easier to inflate. However, there are other factors involved in the amount of pressure needed to ventilate the lungs. Return to page 110, frame 77, and select another answer.

103d (from page 111, frame 78)
Not true. Imagine water flowing freely through the same length of tubing. If the tubing were suddenly constricted at one point, would the same volume of water per minute flow from the end of the tube? What would happen to the flow? Return to page 111, frame 78, and try again.

104A (from page 99, frame 69)
Wrong. Remember, Boyle's law requires constant temperature and expresses an inverse (not direct) relationship between volume and pressure. Return to page 99, frame 69, and review Boyle's law; then make another selection.

104B (from page 106, frame 72)
Correct. Lung volumes and capacities are reported as BTPS, and for calculations they must be converted to STPD. Blood gas volumes, on the other hand, are reported as dry gas (STPD). Please continue on page 107, frame 73.

104C (from page 108, frame 75)
Not so. In this case, the relative humidity would be the ratio between the actual water content and the capacity of the entire atmosphere outside the beaker. Would the air trapped beneath the cover of the container have a higher or lower relative humidity and vapor pressure? Return to page 108, frame 75, and select another answer.

104D (from page 109, frame 76)
This would be true only if the respiratory tract were a single straight tube, with no curves or branches. But remember that the airways have approximately 1 million terminal bronchioles and bifuracte 26 times. Return to page 109, frame 76, and select another answer.

104a (from page 101, frame 71)
No. Gay-Lussac's law is dependent on constant volume. If the volume and mass remain constant, the pressure varies directly with the absolute temperature. We're talking about changes in volume causing changes in temperature or pressure. Return to page 101, frame 71, and try again.

104b (from page 107, frame 73)
Correct. Water molecules behave as gases, except water vapor pressure depends entirely upon the temperature and the amount of water available. The pressure of gases is dependent upon the number of molecules present and the frequency of their collisions. Please continue on page 107, frame 74.

104c (from page 109, frame 76)
Right. There are many variables to consider, including flow rate, molecular density and velocity, diameter of the airways, and viscosity of the gas flowing through the airways. Laminar flow will be found in parts of the respiratory tract that are straight with no bifurcations or obstructions. But the tracheobronchial tree has hundreds of branchings, and eddies are created each time the direction of flow is changed. Even in straight passageways, if there is a narrowing or partial obstruction, turbulence and resistance are increased. Please continue on page 110, frame 77.

104d (from page 112, frame 79)
Wrong. Lateral pressure decreases as velocity increases. This is not a direct relationship. Return to page 112, frame 79, and select another answer.

105A (from page 106, frame 72)
No. Blood gas volumes are already recorded as dry gas, so they do not have to be corrected to STPD. Return to page 106, frame 72, and review the general rules for reporting data on gases; then try again.

105B (from page 108, frame 75)
Not really. If you study Figure 3-4, you will see that in the unheated container, vaporization takes place at a much slower rate than in the heated container (there is less molecular activity). Also in the unheated covered container, the molecules leave and return to the reservoir in equal numbers. Return to page 108, frame 75, and select another answer.

105C (from page 109, frame 76)
No. Air flow through the respiratory tract is not entirely turbulent. In parts of the respiratory tract where the airway is straight with no impediments, the flow may be laminar. You must also consider the flow rate, density, velocity, diameter, and viscosity of the gas, which all help to determine if the flow through the airways is laminar or turbulent. Please return to page 109, frame 76, and select another answer.

105D (from page 112, frame 79)
Right. The Bernoulli effect is shown in Figure 3-8A on page 112. The lateral pressure exerted by a steady flow of gas or liquid in a conducting tube varies inversely with the velocity of the fluid. The greater the distance traveled in a given time, the lower the lateral pressure. Please continue on page 113 and complete the chapter exercises.

105a (from page 106, frame 72)
No. Blood gas volumes are reported as STPD. Return to page 106, frame 72, and review the general rules that apply to reporting data on gas volumes; then select another answer.

105b (from page 110, frame 77)
Right. The flow of gas through the airways produces resistance that varies with the characteristics of the gas, the nature of the flow (streamlined or turbulent), and the condition of airways (clear or obstructed, large or small, short or long), and compliance of the lungs and chest wall. Please continue on page 111, frame 78.

105c (from page 111, frame 78)
Not true. Imagine water flowing freely through the same length of tubing. If the tubing were suddenly constricted at one point, would the same volume of water per minute flow from the end of the tube? What would happen to the flow if the original driving pressure remains unchanged? Return to page 111, frame 78, and study Figure 3-7; then select another answer.

FRAME 72. RECORDING DATA ON GASES

Gases are recorded as dry (with no water vapor) or saturated (with a relative humidity of 100% at a given temperature). Since water vapor increases the volume of gas, you can see the importance of distinguishing between a dry gas and a saturated gas when you are considering volumes and pressures. The following general rules apply when data on gases are reported:

1. Volume of gases as they exist in the lungs are reported as BTPS—body, temperature, pressure, saturated. These gas volumes are saturated with water vapor at body temperature and measured at the ambient (surrounding atmospheric) pressure.
2. Gases that undergo a chemical reaction in the body, (such as those measured in blood samples) have their volumes recorded as STPD—standard, temperature, pressure, dry. These are volumes of dry gas at standard temperature (0°C) and standard atmospheric pressure (760 mm Hg).
3. If saturated gas volumes are to be used in calculations, they must first be corrected to dry gas volume measurements. After the calculations are made, the volumes are corrected to their saturated (BTPS) values.

(Q) Which of the following statements is correct?

a. Lung volumes and capacities are reported as STPD and blood gas volumes are reported as BTPS. 103 b

b. Lung volumes and capacities must first be corrected to STPD for calculations, then reported as BTPS. 104 B

c. Lung volumes and capacities and blood gas volumes are first corrected to STPD for calculations, then reported as BTPS. 105 A

d. Lung volumes and capacities and blood gas volumes are reported as BTPS. 105 a

FRAME 73. HUMIDITY

To understand how water vapor affects the measurement of volumes of gases, you must first be able to distinguish among absolute humidity, relative humidity, and water vapor pressure. Humidity is simply a term used to describe moisture in air or gas. Since water vapor occupies space in a mixture of gases, its removal will lower the total pressure exerted by the mixture and its addition will increase the pressure.

Absolute humidity is the measurement of the actual weight of water present in a given volume of air, expressed in grams per cubic meter or mg/L.

Relative humidity is calculated by comparing the absolute humidity with the maximum amount of water the gas could hold if saturated at a given temperature. This ratio of content to capacity is reported as a percentage.

Water-vapor pressure occurs because molecules of water are small enough to behave as a gas, except that the partial pressure of water vapor depends entirely upon temperature and the amount of water available.

(Q) Which of the following statements is true?

a. Gas pressure is dependent upon the number of gas particles present and the frequency of their collisions. 102 C
b. Water-vapor pressure is dependent upon the temperature. 102 c
c. Both *a* and *b* are true. 104 b

FRAME 74. AIRWAY RESISTANCE

Breathing is a dynamic process that requires work to generate a pressure difference not only to distend the lungs but also to overcome resistance to the movement of gas through the airways. Airway resistance can be measured from the concurrent measurement of the *inspiratory flow* ($\dot{V}$) and the pressure required to overcome resistance to gas flow through the airways. The *plateau pressure*[1] must first be determined and subtracted from the *peak inspiratory pressure* to determine the amount of pressure (ΔP) needed to overcome airway resistance, and then the inspiratory flow rate must be determined. The equation shown below is used to calculate *airway resistance* (R_A).

$$R_A = \frac{\Delta P}{\dot{V}}$$

$$\text{Airway resistance} = \frac{\text{peak pressure} - \text{plateau pressure (cm } H_2O)}{\text{inspiratory flow rate (L/s)}}$$

(Q) Calculate airway resistance given a inspiratory flow rate of 30 L/min, peak inspiratory pressure of 40 cm H_2O, and plateau pressure of 35 cm H_2O.

a. 5 cm H_2O/L per second 95 D
b. 10 cm H_2O/L per second 95 c
c. 2.5 cm H_2O/L per second 95 d

[1]For a ventilator patient, this will be the end inspiratory pressure measured after the tidal volume has been delivered but before the patient exhales.

FRAME 75. WATER-VAPOR PRESSURE

The illustration above shows the factors that influence the vaporization of water. In diagram **A** of Figure 3–4, the activity of the water molecules forces molecules into the air, gradually reducing the volume of water in the container. In diagram **B**, the container is covered. Vaporization continues, but when the trapped air becomes saturated, a state of equilibrium is reached. At this point, the trapped air cannot hold any more water molecules and they drop back into the reservoir. In diagram **C**, the open container is heated. Increased molecular activity speeds the rate of vaporization. In diagram **D**, the heated container is covered. Now more vapor crowds into the trapped air, raising the vapor pressure, which is registered on the attached manometer.

(Q) The relative humidity and water vapor pressure are greatest when the container is

a. covered and heated. 102 D
b. uncovered. 104 C
c. covered but unheated. 105 B

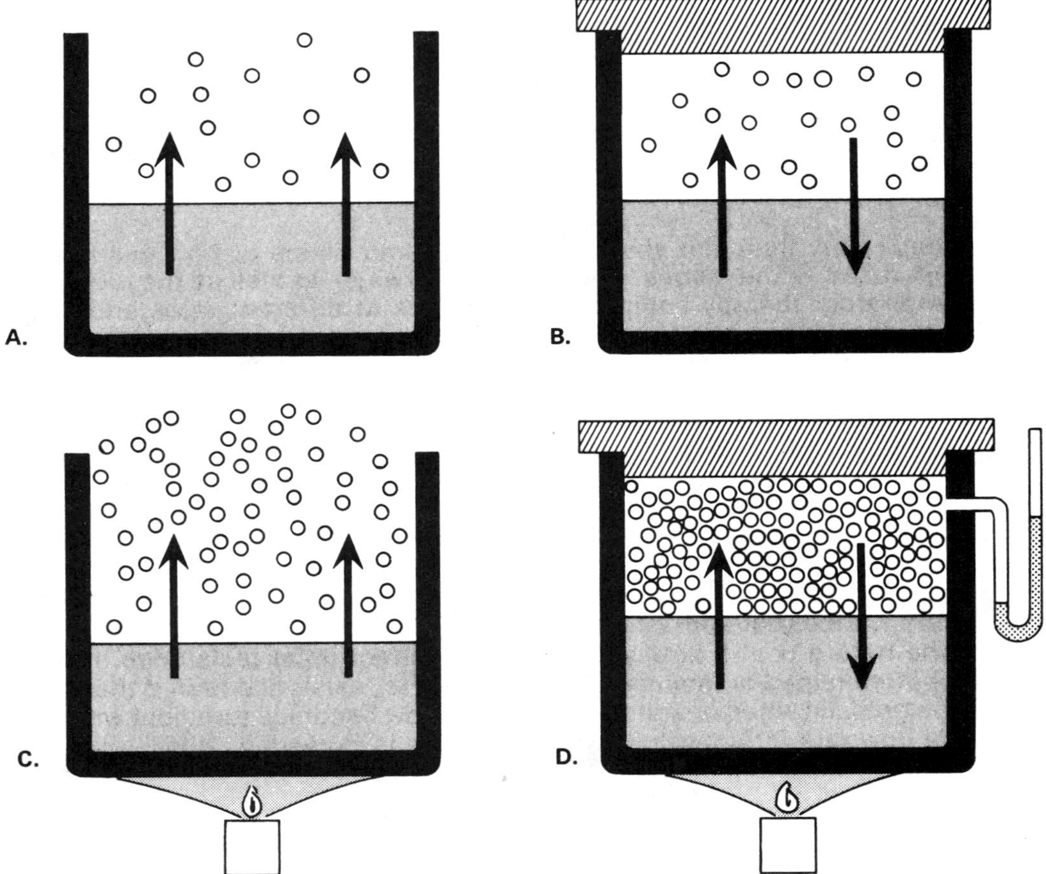

Redrawn from *Fundamentals of Respiratory Therapy* by Donald F. Egan

Figure 3–4

FRAME 76. FLOW OF GASES THROUGH TUBES

The respiratory care practitioner should have some knowledge of how gas flows through tubes such as the airways and circuits of respiratory equipment. Gas flows at different rates and patterns through tubes of different sizes, shapes, and lengths. There are a number of factors that determine the amount of resistance to gas flow through a tube. Just as a driving pressure pumps blood through the arteries, veins, and capillaries (where there is also resistance to flow), a driving pressure must overcome resistance in the airways.

If the airway is a short, wide tube, the resistance will be low. If the flow through this type of tube is small, only minimal driving pressure will be required. By lengthening and narrowing the tube, the resistance will be increased and a greater driving pressure will be needed to produce the same flow in the restricted tube. If a higher flow is needed, a still greater driving pressure will be required.

The nature of the flow also has some effect upon resistance (Fig. 3–5). If the flow is streamlined or laminar, there will be less resistance than if the flow is turbulent (disturbed or agitated). Laminar flow becomes turbulent when a critical flow rate for a particular airway or gas is exceeded. This is usually caused by a change in the direction of the flow or an obstruction in its path.

During inhalation, the alveolar pressure drops below atmospheric pressure, causing air to flow into the lungs. During exhalation, the pressure in the alveoli becomes higher than that of the atmosphere, causing air to flow out of the lungs. As we noted before, some tissues of the lungs and thorax are elastic and can be stretched during inspiration. Exhalation is usually passive during quiet breathing as the distended lung returns to its original shape.

(Q) Gas flow through the airways is usually

a. laminar. 104 D
b. turbulent. 105 C
c. both laminar and turbulent. 104 c

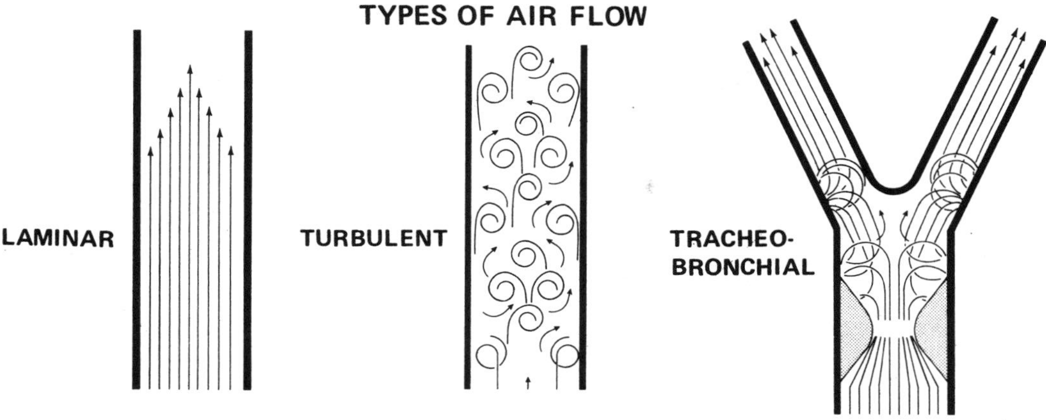

Figure 3–5

FRAME 77. COMPLIANCE

The ability of the lungs to distend with an increase in airway pressure is called lung *compliance.* It may be defined as the volume change per unit of pressure change and is expressed as L/cm H_2O. When the lungs and chest wall are acting together, they require more force (pressure) for expansion than does either component alone. Figure 3-6 below shows that the compliance of the lungs alone is 0.2 L/cm H_2O and the compliance of the lungs and thorax together is 0.1 L/cm H_2O.

$$C = \frac{\Delta V}{\Delta P}$$

$$\text{Compliance} = \frac{\text{exhaled tidal volume}}{\text{plateau pressure} - \text{PEEP}}$$

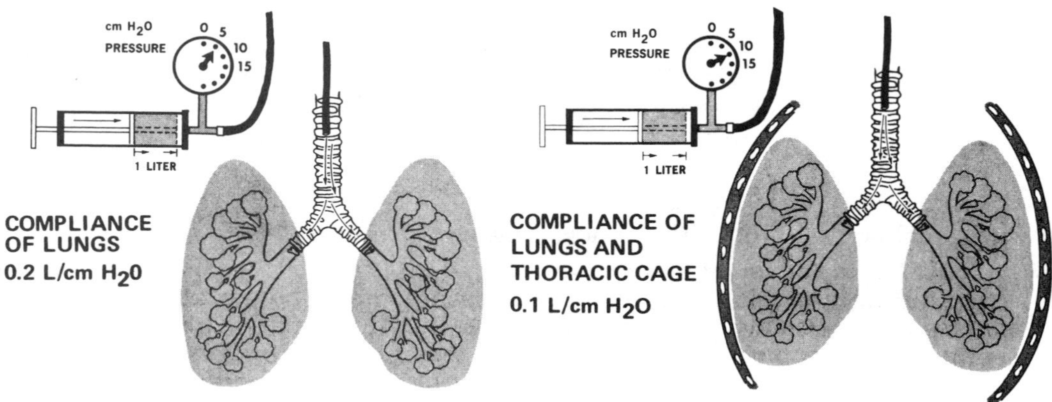

Figure 3-6

The work of breathing equals pressure times volume. When the pressure needed to expand the lungs increases, the work of breathing also increases if the tidal volume does not decrease. Thus, any drop in compliance will increase the amount of work needed to breath, since more pressure will be needed to move the same size tidal volume into the lungs.

In the obstructive pattern of respiratory disease, airway resistance is increased by partial blocking of the airways. A 50% decrease of airway caliber will increase airway resistance by 1600% because flow through tubes is inversely related to fourth power of the radius ($\dot{V} \propto \frac{1}{r^4}$). In adult respiratory distress syndrome (ARDS) the lung parenchyma fills with water, making the lungs difficult to distend, and large pressures are required to ventilate the lungs. This means that lung compliance is lower than normal with ARDS.

(Q) The pressure required to ventilate the lungs depends upon

a. characteristics of the gas. 102 d
b. nature of the flow. 103 C
c. condition of the airways and compliance of the lungs. 103 c
d. all of the above. 105 b

FRAME 78. DENSITY AND VISCOSITY

Just as water flows more easily than molasses, so some gases flow more easily than others because of differences in density and viscosity.[1] The greater a fluid's density and viscosity (resistance to flow under an applied force), the greater its resistance to flow. Where the flow is mainly turbulent, flow rate is influenced more by density than by viscosity. The rate of laminar flow is influenced more by viscosity. Flow rate is not the same as velocity. Flow is a measure of the movement of fluid volume per unit of time (L/min or L/s). Velocity is a measure of the linear movement (speed) of a fluid in a specific direction per unit of time (cm/s or ft/s).

Some respiratory care practitioners use a less dense gas along with oxygen to increase the flow rate with patients with high airway resistance due to retained secretions, exudate, tumors, and other obstructions that cause turbulent gas flow. Since helium is less dense than oxygen, a combination of these two gases (30% O_2 and 70% He) will produce less density than if oxygen is used alone.

Airway obstructions cause the flow to decrease (if the driving pressure is held constant), although the velocity of the gas increases. The increase in the velocity of the gas at the obstruction results in reduced lateral pressure (Fig. 3–7).

(Q) A length of half-inch tubing through which gas is flowing is suddenly constricted at one point to half its diameter. If the original driving pressure remains unchanged, what happens to the gas flow rate through the constriction?

a. Flow decreases. 103 D
b. Flow increases. 103 d
c. Flow remains the same. 105 c

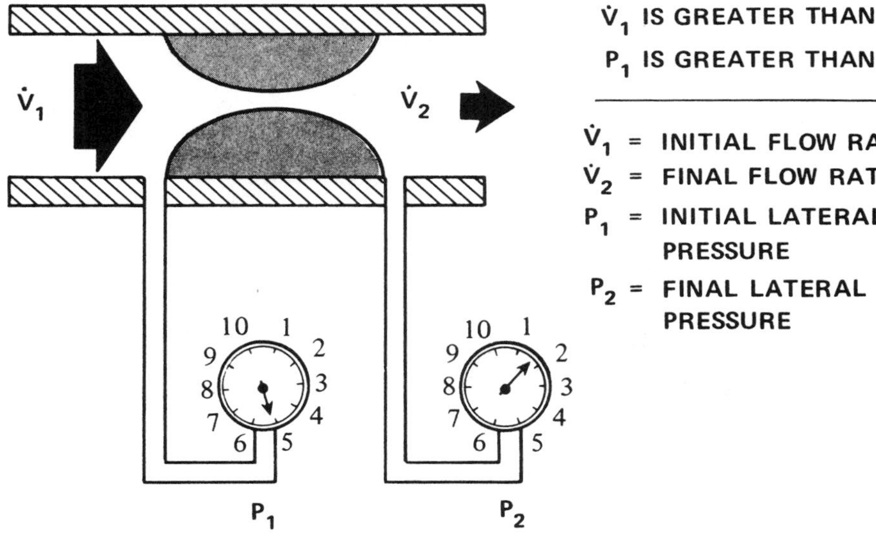

Figure 3–7

[1]When a distorting force is applied to a liquid or gas, the fluid deforms permanently under the force; in other words, it flows. Some gases are more fluid (flow more easily) than others. The viscosity of a gas is its internal resistance to flow.

FRAME 79. LATERAL PRESSURE

If the rate of flow and velocity can be altered by a constriction, what happens to the lateral pressure against the sides of the pipe? Gas flowing through a tube is always moving from a point of higher pressure to a point of lower pressure. As resistance is increased, the applied pressure required to drive the same volume through the tube must be increased. Changes in lateral pressure are dependent on velocity. As the velocity of the gas increases, the pressure it exerts against the sides of a tube (lateral pressure) decreases. With the driving pressure held constant, both liquids and gases flow at a greater velocity through a narrow tube than through a wider tube. Thus, when gas meets a constriction, its velocity is increased even though its flow is decreased. As a result of the increase in velocity, the lateral pressure in the narrower tube is decreased. This is the Bernoulli effect—lateral pressure varies inversely with velocity.

If the flow entering the tube ($\dot{V}_1$) equals the flow leaving the tube ($\dot{V}_2$), the velocity of the fluid must increase as the tube narrows (Fig. 3–8A). The increase in velocity reduces the pressure against the walls of the narrow tube (P_2 is less than P_1).

In respiratory care, a second gas can be mixed with the first where the tube constricts. The lower pressure at the constriction draws in the second gas (Venturi principle). To restore lateral pressure in the tube beyond the constriction and to provide space for the added volume, the tube can be widened after the constriction (Fig. 3–8B). If the angle of the dilation does not exceed 15°, the gas pressure will be restored to its prerestriction level. The second gas will increase the total gas flow and may decrease the delivered oxygen concentration. The mixing of the second gas from the Venturi port with the source gas usually increases the amount of turbulent gas flow. The amount of total gas flow and delivered oxygen concentration can be controlled by regulating the size of the air entrainment port.

(Q) How is the Bernoulli effect demonstrated at a tubing constriction?

a. Lateral pressure varies *inversely* with velocity. 105 D

b. Lateral pressure varies *directly* with velocity. 104 d

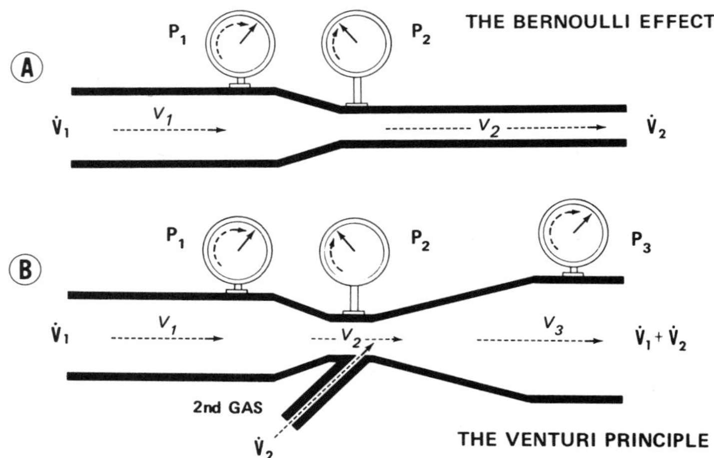

Figure 3–8A and **Figure 3–8B**

EXERCISES

1. Describe the relationship between volume and pressure when temperature and mass are held constant.
2. Describe the relationship between the volume of a given mass and the absolute temperature when pressure is held constant.
3. Describe the relationship between pressure and temperature when volume and mass are held constant.
4. Calculate the change in volume if the pressure is held constant given $V_1 =$ 1000 mL, $T_1 = 0°C$, $T_2 = 100°C$. $V_2 = ?$
5. Calculate the change in pressure if the temperature is held constant given $P_1 = 760$ mm Hg, $V_1 = 1000$ mL, $V_2 = 500$ mL. $P_2 = ?$
6. Calculate the change in temperature if volume is held constant given $T_1 =$ 37°C, $P_1 = 2200$ psig, $P_2 = 15$ psig. $T_2 = ?$
7. Calculate static compliance given peak inspiratory pressure = 40 cm H_2O, plateau pressure (no airflow) = 30 cm H_2O, and V_T = 900 mL, and PEEP = 5 cm H_2O.
8. Calculate airway resistance given peak inspiratory pressure = 40 cm H_2O, plateau pressure (no airflow) = 30 cm H_2O, and flow = 30 L/min.
9. Explain how the Bernoulli effect and the Venturi principle can be used to increase the flow leaving a tube.
10. Describe the difference in the kinetic energy of a gas when its temperature is lowered from 100° to 0°C.

POSTTEST

This test is designed to evaluate what you have learned after completing Chapter 3. Check your answers on page 116 and review the topics where your answer is incorrect.

1. Under what circumstances can a gas be liquified?
   A. low pressure, high temperature
   B. low pressure, low temperature
   C. high pressure, high temperature
   D. high pressure, low temperature
   E. none of the above
2. What proportion of the atmosphere contains carbon dioxide?
   A. 0%
   B. 0.03%
   C. 0.93%
   D. 20.95%
   E. 78.08%
3. The potential energy of a gas is best described as the amount of work that can be done as a result of
   A. heat.
   B. pressure.
   C. moving a piston.
   D. total mass.
   E. total volume.
4. Which of the following is the best example of potential energy of a gas being changed to kinetic energy?
   A. pressure moving a piston
   B. a piston compressing a gas
   C. filling an empty cylinder with gas
   D. cooling a gas
   E. heating a gas
5. At sea level the average atmospheric pressure will support a column of mercury with a height of
   A. 30 cm.
   B. 76 in.
   C. 400 mm.
   D. 760 mm.
   E. 1000 mm.
6. The partial pressure of gases in the blood are measured in units of
   A. cm H_2O.
   B. cm Hg.
   C. mm Hg.
   D. mEq/L.
   E. psig.

7. If a gas mixture has a pressure of 760 mm Hg and P_{H_2O} of 30 mm Hg, what is the P_{O_2} if the oxygen concentration of the mixture is 0.40?
   A. 100 mm Hg
   B. 196 mm Hg
   C. 292 mm Hg
   D. 304 mm Hg
   E. 316 mm Hg

8. If temperture and mass are held constant, what will the final pressure be given $P_1 = 760$ mm Hg, $V_1 = 6$ L, $V_2 = 12$ L. $P_2 = ?$
   A. 180 mm Hg
   B. 380 mm Hg
   C. 600 mm Hg
   D. 760 mm Hg
   E. 1520 mm Hg

9. If the pressure and mass are held constant, what will the final temperature be if $T_1 = 373°K$, $V_1 = 3000$ mL, $V_2 = 6000$ mL. $T_2 = ?$
   A. 0°K
   B. 100°K
   C. 187°K
   D. 373°K
   E. 746°K

10. If the volume and mass are held constant, what is the final temperature if $T_1 = 310°K$, $P_1 = 15$ psig, $P_2 = 2200$ psig. $T_2 = ?$
   A. 2°K
   B. 273°K
   C. 310°K
   D. 373°K
   E. 45,467°K

11. If the mass remains constant, what is the final volume if $P_1 = 15$ psig, $P_2 = 2200$ psig, $T_1 = 300$ K, $T_2 = 310$ K, $V_1 = 210$ ft^3. $V_2 = ?$
   A. 0.59 ft^3
   B. 1.64 ft^3
   C. 1.69 ft^3
   D. 240 ft^3
   E. 248 ft^3

12. What is the total pressure of gas mixture if $P_{O_2} = 100$ mm Hg, $P_{CO_2} = 40$ mm Hg, $P_{N_2} = 573$ mm Hg, $P_{H_2O} = 47$ mm Hg?
   A. 100 mm Hg
   B. 573 mm Hg
   C. 713 mm Hg
   D. 760 mm Hg
   E. 807 mm Hg

13. Gas volumes measured in blood samples are recorded as
   A. BTPS.
   B. ATPS.
   C. STPD.
   D. STPS.
   E. ATPD.

14. The comparison of the absolute humidity with the maximum amount of water that a gas could actually hold if saturated at a given temperature is
    A. water-vapor pressure.
    B. temperature deficit.
    C. humidity deficit.
    D. body humidity.
    E. relative humidity.
15. Which of the following circumstances is likely to result in the most turbulent gas flow?
    A. high flow through the trachea
    B. low flow through the trachea
    C. high flow at the bifurcation of main-stem bronchi
    D. low flow at the bifurcation of main-stem bronchi
    E. low flow through the glottis
16. What is the pulmonary compliance given the following data: exhaled tidal volume 800 mL, peak inspiratory pressure 50 cm H_2O, plateau pressure 45 cm H_2O, and PEEP 5 cm H_2O?
    A. 0.200 L/cm H_2O
    B. 0.100 L/cm H_2O
    C. 0.050 L/cm H_2O
    D. 0.020 L/cm H_2O
    E. 0.018 L/cm H_2O
17. Given the following: flow = 60 L/min, peak airway pressure = 40 cm H_2O, plateau pressure = 30 cm H_2O; what is the airway resistance?
    A. 5 cm H_2O/L per second
    B. 10 cm H_2O/L per second
    C. 15 cm H_2O/L per second
    D. 20 cm H_2O/L per second
    E. 25 cm H_2O/L per second
18. When gas flow is mainly turbulent, the flow is influenced more by
    A. viscosity.
    B. density.
    C. velocity.
    D. internal gas resistance to flow.
    E. both *A* and *C*.
19. Which of the following statements is true?
    A. Lateral pressure varies *inversely* with gas velocity.
    B. Lateral pressure varies *directly* with gas velocity.
    C. Velocity of a gas *decreases* when a tube narrows.
    D. Flow rate of a gas *increases* when a tube narrows.
    E. An increase in flow will *increase* lateral pressure.
20. A Venturi system entrains air into a jet stream because of an
    A. increase in lateral pressure.
    B. increase in jet stream flow.
    C. decrease in lateral pressure.
    D. increase in jet stream flow.
    E. decrease in jet stream velocity.

ANSWERS TO POSTTEST

1. D (F59)
2. B (F60)
3. B (F62)
4. A (F62)
5. D (F65)
6. C (F68)
7. C (F67)
8. B (F69)
9. C (F69)
10. E (F70)
11. C (F71)
12. D (F70)
13. C (F72)
14. E (F73)
15. C (F76)
16. D (F77)
17. B (F74)
18. B (F78)
19. A (F79)
20. C (F79)

BIBLIOGRAPHY

Barnes, TA: Respiratory Care Practice. Year Book Medical Publishers, Chicago, 1988.

Comroe, JH: Physiology of Respiration, ed 2. Year Book Medical Publishers, Chicago, 1974.

Forster, RE, Fisher, AB, DuBois, AB, and Briscoe, WA: The Lung—Physiologic Basis of Pulmonary Function Testing Tests, ed 3. Year Book Medical Publishers, Chicago, 1986.

Kacmarek, RM, Dimas, S, and Mack, CW: The Essentials of Respiratory Therapy, ed 2. Year Book Medical Publishers, Chicago, 1985.

Lane, EE and Walker JF: Clinical Arterial Blood Analysis. CV Mosby, St. Louis, 1987.

Murray, JF: The Normal Lung, ed 2. WB Saunders, Philadelphia, 1986.

Scanlon, C, Spearman, CB, Sheldon, RL, and Egan, DF: Egan's Fundamentals of Respiratory Therapy, ed 5. CV Mosby, St. Louis, 1990.

Shapiro, BA, Harrison, RA, Cane, RD, Templin, RK, and Walton, JR: Clinical Application of Blood Gases, ed 4. Year Book Medical Publishers, Chicago, 1988.

Slonim, NB and Hamilton, LH: Respiratory Physiology, ed 5. CV Mosby, St. Louis, 1986.

West, JB: Respiratory Physiology—the Essentials, ed 4. Williams & Wilkins, Baltimore, 1990.

4

Medical Asepsis

80. The growth of bacteria
81. Shapes of bacteria
82. Properties of bacteria
83. Dirty and clean areas
84. Facilities for cleaning
85. Culture logs
86. Cleaning and disinfecting equipment
87. Hand washing
88. Sterilization of equipment
89. Comparison of steam autoclave and gas sterilization
90. Definition of terms
91. Protocol for bacteriological check
92. Isolation, reverse, and universal precautions

PRETEST

This pretest is designed to measure what you already know about medical asepsis. Check your answers on page 121 and then continue on page 122, frame 80.

1. Which of the following ranges of temperature will allow most pathogens to grow rapidly?
   A. 0° to 32°F
   B. 32° to 50°F
   C. 50° to 110°F
   D. 110° to 170°F
   E. 170° to 212°F
2. Which of the following when located in a microorganism's cell wall may act as a barrier to disinfectants?
   A. fat
   B. NaCl
   C. K^+
   D. HCO_3^-
   E. H_2O
3. Which of the following may cause aerobic bacteria to die?
   A. oxygen
   B. strong light
   C. darkness
   D. heat of 60°F
   E. water
4. Bacteria may be carried in air by
   A. oxygen.
   B. water vapor.
   C. air currents.
   D. particles of dust or moisture.
   E. convection currents.
5. When should equipment returned to the dirty area of a respiratory care department be cultured?
   A. before cleaning
   B. immediately before use
   C. after soaking to remove dry material
   D. after removal from disinfectant solution
   E. after ethylene oxide sterilization
6. A substance that will inhibit the growth and development of microorganisms without necessarily destroying them is called a
   A. disinfectant.
   B. antiseptic.
   C. bactericide.
   D. fungicide.
   E. germicide.

7. An agent that destroys the growing forms of germs but not the resistant spore forms is called
   A. an incomplete disinfectant.
   B. an antiseptic.
   C. a bactericide.
   D. a fungicide.
   E. a germicide.

8. Clean and dirty equipment areas of a respiratory care department should be separated by
   A. a wall.
   B. a partition.
   C. a screen.
   D. a 10-ft counter.
   E. no barrier.

9. Equipment should be placed in sealed packages
   A. upon returning to the dirty area.
   B. after being scrubbed and rinsed.
   C. after gas sterilization.
   D. immediately before gas sterilization.
   E. immediately before liquid chemical sterilization.

10. Nebulizers in use should be replaced with a sterile nebulizer every
    A. 8 hours.
    B. 16 hours.
    C. 24 hours.
    D. 48 hours.
    E. 72 hours.

11. Spot check cultures on respiratory care equipment should be taken
    I. before use.
    II. when in use.
    III. immediately following use.
    A. III only
    B. I and II only
    C. II and III only
    D. I and III only
    E. I, II, and III

12. When taking samples from respiratory care equipment in use for a culture log, you should swab
    A. inner surfaces of tubing and nebulizers.
    B. outer surfaces of tubing and nebulizers.
    C. water in nebulizers.
    D. water in delivery tubes.
    E. all of the above.

13. Which of the following precautions should be taken for strict isolation of a patient with a contagious disease?
    A. gown
    B. gloves
    C. mask
    D. antimicrobial hand washing
    E. all of the above

14. The single most important procedure for preventing infections acquired in hospitals is
    A. reverse isolation.
    B. strict isolation.
    C. hand washing.
    D. patient education.
    E. culture logs.
15. Reverse isolation is used to
    A. protect other patients from contagious diseases.
    B. protect hospital personnel from infection.
    C. isolate the patient's equipment in one location.
    D. allow for special infectious-disease records.
    E. none of the above.
16. Equipment removed from a strict isolation room should be
    A. placed in a bag and taken to the decontamination area.
    B. double bagged and taken to the decontamination area.
    C. taken to the decontamination area and bagged.
    D. placed in a bag and then burned.
    E. disinfected in the room and then removed.
17. Which of the following can be used for antimicrobial hand washing?
    A. soap and water
    B. 30% isopropyl alcohol
    C. glutaraldehyde
    D. iodophors
    E. none of the above
18. In hand washing, soap should be rinsed off with fingers held
    A. up.
    B. down.
    C. 90 degrees to the stream of water.
    D. up and spread apart.
    E. horizontal and spread apart.
19. Which of the following types of equipment is most likely to be a source of hospital-acquired infections?
    A. large passover humidifier for a ventilator
    B. bubble humidifier for a nasal cannula
    C. sidestream medication nebulizer
    D. air-entrainment nebulizer
    E. incentive spirometer
20. The patient most likely to require reverse isolation is a
    A. pediatric patient.
    B. COPD patient.
    C. transplant patient receiving immunosuppressive drugs.
    D. orthopedic patient.
    E. neurosurgical patient.

ANSWERS TO PRETEST

1. C (F80)
2. A (F82)
3. B (F80)
4. D (F80)
5. A (F85)
6. B (F90)
7. A (F90)
8. A (F84)
9. D (F86)
10. C (F85)
11. E (F85)
12. E (F85)
13. E (F92)
14. C (F87)
15. E (F92)
16. B (F92)
17. D (F87)
18. B (F87)
19. D (F85)
20. C (F92)

FRAME 80. THE GROWTH OF BACTERIA

Bacteria and viruses are two of the types of microorganisms responsible for many diseases in man. Both disease-producing (pathogenic) and other bacteria flourish in a variety of environments. They are distributed in nature, living within and upon our bodies, in the food we eat, the water we drink, and the air we breathe.

Although air does not provide a medium for the growth of bacteria, it contains particles of dust and moisture in or on which bacteria can survive and be transferred to the patient through respiratory care equipment (Fig. 4–1). Ventilators and nebulizers using entrainment (air mixed with oxygen) are particularly susceptible to contamination. The air flow keeps the particles suspended until they are trapped in the nebulizer, where bacterial growth can take place.

Please continue on page 123, frame 81.

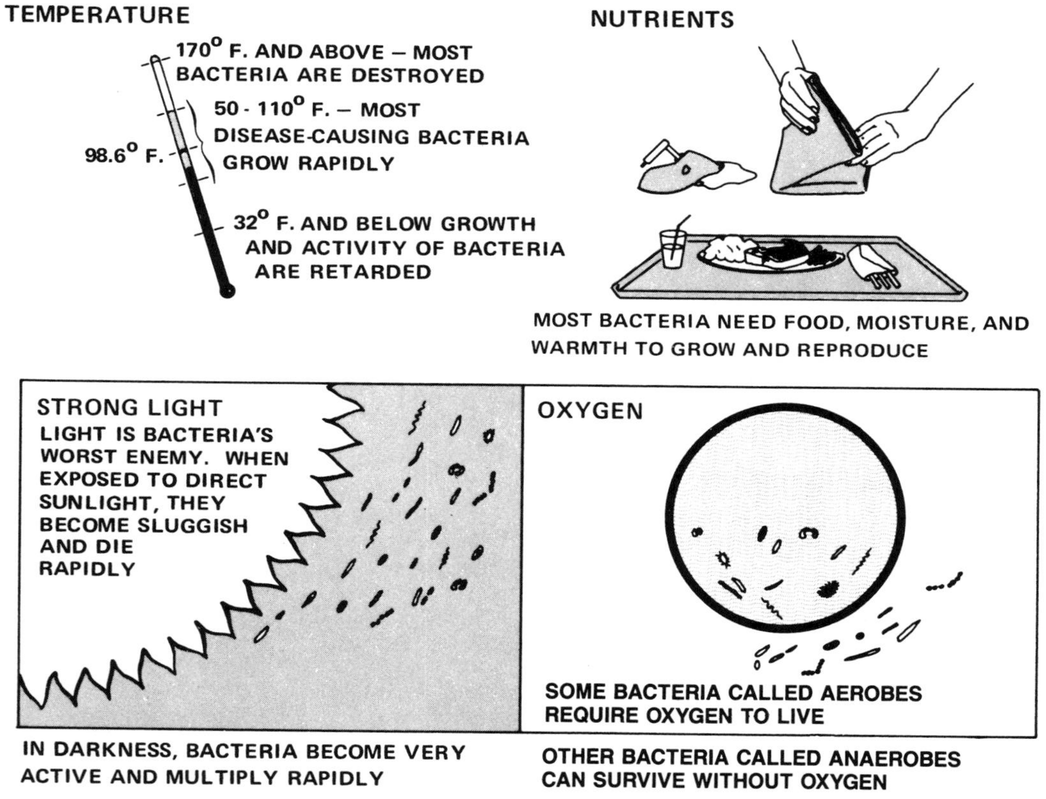

Figure 4–1

FRAME 81. SHAPES OF BACTERIA

The bacteria most commonly found on respiratory care equipment are *Pseudomonas aeruginosa* (su-do-mo-nus air-u-gi-no-sa). This is the same type of bacteria found in pus-producing infections. *P. aeruginosa* can be destroyed by protein coagulation caused by dry or moist heat. It can also be destroyed by certain chemical disinfectants. Gas sterilization, with ethylene oxide, is also effective against *P. aeruginosa.* The shapes and arrangements of various bacteria are shown in Figure 4–2.

(Q) The most effective method for sterilizing a nebulizer that has been contaminated with *P. aeruginosa* is

a. liquid sterilization solutions. 127 a

b. gas sterilization. 136 A

SHAPES AND ARRANGEMENTS OF BACTERIA

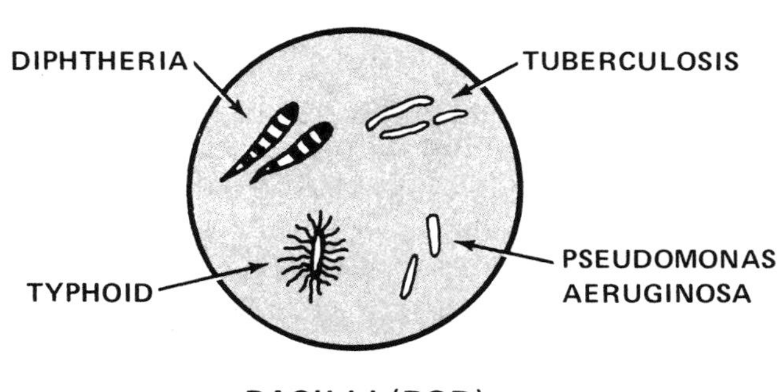

BACILLI (ROD)

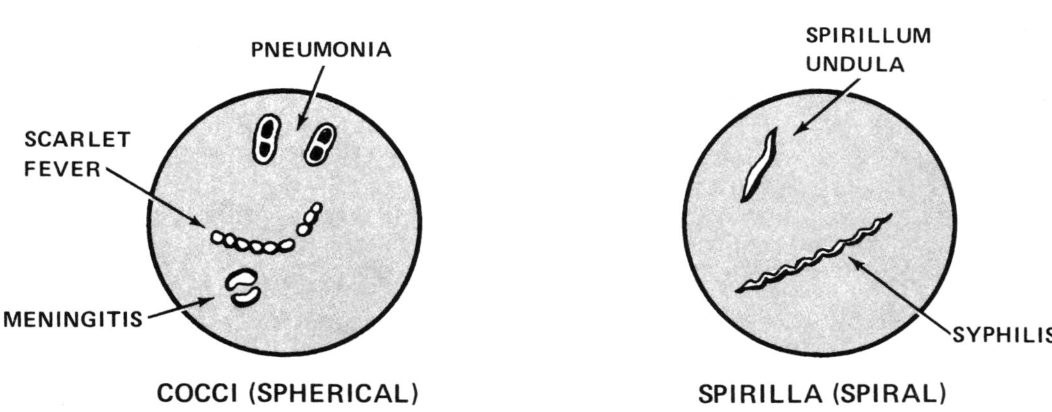

COCCI (SPHERICAL) SPIRILLA (SPIRAL)

Figure 4–2

FRAME 82. PROPERTIES OF BACTERIA

Before a particular bacteria can be destroyed, something must be known about its chemical properties, growth, and reproductive patterns. Several environmental factors enhance or inhibit the growth of microorganisms, including temperature, moisture, osmotic pressure, pH, barometric pressure, gases, radiation chemicals, and the presence of neighboring microbes. Some bacteria have a high fat content in their cell walls, which act as a barrier to disinfectants. However, the vegetative forms of most pathogens are quite easily destroyed by various chemicals or the use of heat to coagulate the proteins in their walls. More viable microorganisms, viruses, and exposed bacterial spores[1] can be killed by high temperature and moisture under pressure.

Disinfection is the act or process of destroying pathogenic microorganisms. *Sterilization* is the process of killing all microorganisms, including spores. A combination of heat, moisture, and pressure, or sometimes heat alone, can effectively sterilize objects of all microorganisms.

(Q) Which of the following statements is true?

a. The temperature needed to kill microbes may vary. 126 A
b. Different disinfectants are used to kill varying types of microbes. 126 a
c. Both *a* and *b* are true. 127 A

FRAME 83. DIRTY AND CLEAN AREAS

The Dirty Area A scrub-and-rinse sink should be covered by an exhaust hood for discharging the toxic fumes given off by some cleaning agents (Fig. 4–3). If this is not possible, adequate ventilation must be provided by some other means. Cleaning equipment, disinfectants, and germicides must be labeled, dated, and provided proper storage space. A pass-through sink should be provided to transfer small pieces of equipment to the clean area without recontamination. All sinks should be operated by foot pedals so that the operator's hands do not touch contaminated faucets.

The Clean Area Equipment that has been scrubbed and disinfected or sterilized in the dirty area is passed into the clean area. These items then are moved to a counter for drying and packaging in preparation for storage or sterilization (autoclave or gas). Separate storage areas should be provided for the many different kinds of equipment, ranging from small mouthpieces to large ventilators. Additional counter space should be set aside for reassembling equipment for use. A hand-scrubbing sink next to the assembly area should be pedal operated.

Please continue on page 125, frame 84.

---

[1]Spores are inactive, resting, or resistant forms of bacteria.

FRAME 84. FACILITIES FOR CLEANING

Preventive measures against harmful bacteria can be successful only if proper equipment and facilities are available. Ideally, the areas where dirty equipment is cleaned and sterilized equipment is stored should be separated from each other by a solid barrier. This is to prevent the use of dirty equipment and to prevent contamination of the clean area. Facilities for cleaning and storing equipment are identified in Figure 4–3.

Facilities for Cleaning

1. Contaminated equipment
2. Scrub brushes
3. Soak, scrub, and rinse
4. Exhaust hood
5. Storage (disinfectants)
6. Disinfectant sink (germicidals)
7. Wall (physical barrier)
8. Rinse sink
9. Work space for drying and packaging for use or sterilization
10. Hand-scrubbing sink
11. Equipment storage area
12. General storage area
13. Assembly area
14. Foot pedals for water and soap dispensers
15. Drying cabinet

(Q) Clean and dirty areas in respiratory care departments should be separated by a

a. wall. 126 b
b. partition. 136 a
c. screen. 136 B

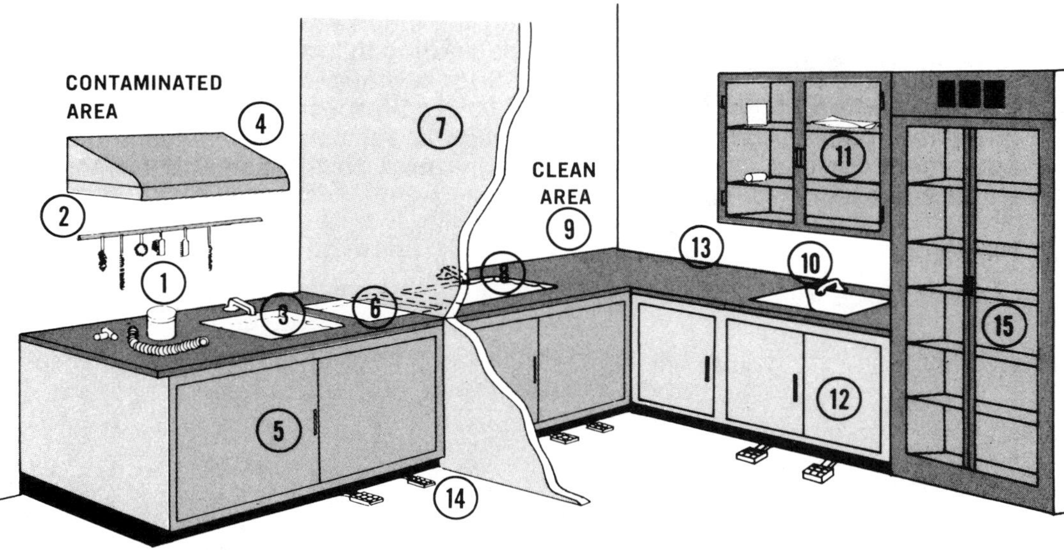

Figure 4–3

126A (from page 124, frame 82)
Right, but does this mean the other statements are false? Return to page 124, frame 82, and select another answer.

126B (from page 128, frame 85)
You are partially correct. The harmful organisms (pathogens) should be traced to their site of origin. The contaminated equipment should be replaced by sterilized equipment. Please continue on page 129, frame 86.

126C (from page 131, frame 88)
Yes. It all depends upon the type of disinfectant used and the organisms present. A *complete* disinfectant, given enough time, will destroy the spores as well as other forms of organisms. Sterilization by heat, chemicals, or gas is the best means of destroying *all microbes* on the object. Please continue on page 132, frame 89.

126D (from page 133, frame 91)
True. However, random cultures must also be taken at predetermined intervals while equipment is in use. If pathogens are found, the equipment should be replaced and the bacteria traced to their site of origin. Return to page 133, frame 91, and select another method.

126a (from page 124, frame 82)
Right, but does this mean the other statements are false? Return to page 124, frame 82, and select another answer.

126b (from page 125, frame 84)
A wall would be the safest. A passageway must be provided for transfer of disinfected equipment from the dirty area to the clean area. Please continue on page 128, frame 85.

126c (from page 130, frame 87)
Careful! Hands should be washed after cleaning dirty equipment. Return to page 130, frame 87, and select another answer.

126d (from page 133, frame 91)
Yes, a culture should be done immediately after use, but it is even more important to determine if the equipment is sterile before use, and if it remains uncontaminated during use. Return to page 133, frame 91, and select another answer.

126e (from page 132, frame 90)

Check Your Definitions Below

Bactericide—An agent that destroys bacteria
Fungicide—An agent that destroys fungus
Germicide—An agent that destroys the growing forms of the microorganism but not the spore forms

Please continue on page 133, frame 91.

127A (from page 124, frame 82)
Correct. Different bacteria react differently to various temperatures and disinfectants. The properties of a bacterium must be known before it can be destroyed or its growth inhibited. Please continue on page 124, frame 83.

127B (from page 128, frame 85)
Correct. Sterilized equipment must be substituted for contaminated equipment and the harmful organisms traced back to their site of origin. Please continue on page 129, frame 86.

127C (from page 129, frame 86)
If you wait until equipment is brought back to the dirty area, it will be difficult to trace the origin of any pathogens that may be found on equipment. They may have been transmitted from another piece of equipment in the dirty area. The best time to take a sample is immediately before equipment is removed from the room for cleaning. Please continue on page 130, frame 87.

127D (from page 131, frame 88)
You can sterilize an object with a *complete* disinfectant (given enough time) and destroy spores as well as other forms of microbes. Return to page 131, frame 88, and select another answer.

127E (from page 133, frame 91)
True, but the equipment must also be checked for contamination that might occur in storage or while being assembled. Return to page 133, frame 91, and select another method.

127a (from page 123, frame 81)
No. Liquid sterilization solutions are not practical because of the many small openings found on nebulizers. Return to page 123, frame 81, and select another answer.

127b (from page 128, frame 85)
Of course, but some effort also should be made to determine where the bacteria came from—the air, the patient, the therapist, or other hospital personnel. Please continue on page 129, frame 86.

127c (from page 129, frame 86)
Correct. If the culture were not taken until the equipment was returned to the respiratory care department, it would be more difficult to trace the origin of any pathogen that might be found on the equipment. Please continue on page 130, frame 87.

127d (from page 131, frame 88)
An incomplete disinfectant will not destroy spores. An object is not sterilized until *all* living microorganisms are destroyed. Some disinfectant solutions will sterilize if equipment is soaked for a predetermined length of time. Return to page 131, frame 88, and find another answer.

127e (from page 134, frame 92)
Careful. Wearing the gown until the equipment decontamination area is reached would expose several areas of the hospital to pathogens from the isolation room. Return to page 134, frame 92, and select another answer.

FRAME 85. CULTURE LOGS

A knowledge of the types of organisms encountered on or in respiratory care equipment is necessary for the equipment to be cleaned properly. Personnel who work with this equipment should realize the importance of keeping a culture log.

The only way you can tell which type of bacteria is present, if any, is to take cultures from the equipment. This is done by swabbing the inner and outer surfaces of the equipment and by taking samples from equipment, such as water from the nebulizer. Samples and swabs should be sent to the laboratory, where a culture can be grown and examined. The laboratory report to the respiratory care department is reviewed and placed in a culture log. Spot-check cultures of respiratory care equipment are taken before use, periodically during use, and immediately after use.

Before Use Equipment in storage should be sterile, but random bacteriological checks should be made during storage, and the results reviewed and recorded in the culture log.

During Use The nebulizers, humidifiers, and their connecting tubing should be spot-checked while in use, and the results reviewed and recorded in the culture log.

Immediately Following Use Spot checks should be made of equipment leaving patient rooms by swabbing equipment and taking a sample of water from the nebulizer.

Even if the equipment is found to be sterile before use, it should be changed every 24 hours or more frequently for patients at special risk to infection. Bacterial contamination of equipment may be caused by the patient or by poor aseptic technique by hospital personnel. Nebulizers are the most likely source of *equipment-related* hospital-acquired infections. They entrain room air, particles of dust, and moisture that may carry bacteria into the nebulizer water and to the patient. Ultrasonic nebulizers produce a high density of stable particles and have the greatest potential for contaminating an area with airborne pathogens. Breathing circuits can be protected from airborne pathogens by placing high-efficiency bacterial filters at air-entrainment ports.

(Q) What should be done if a culture reveals that a piece of respiratory care equipment in use has become contaminated with a pathogen?

a. Replace the item with sterile equipment. 127 b
b. Try to determine the source of contamination. 126 B
c. Both *a* and *b*. 127 B

FRAME 86. CLEANING AND DISINFECTING EQUIPMENT

Contaminated equipment is collected from patient areas, placed in bags, and carried to the dirty area of the respiratory care department as soon as possible to prevent drying of any organic material. The practitioner should wear gloves, gown, and eye protection while cleaning equipment. The equipment should be disassembled, placed in a detergent cleaning solution, and scrubbed until it is free of all foreign material.

The washed pieces are rinsed and then placed immediately into a germicidal (disinfectant) solution for a specified length of time. The disinfectant is any agent (usually chemical) that destroys infective agents or makes them inactive, given enough time. Certain disinfectants will destroy spores as well as vegetative forms of pathogenic microorganisms. After soaking in a disinfectant solution, the equipment is rinsed, dried, and packaged in bags for storage or sterilization. (See Fig. 4–4.) Some hospitals gas-sterilize all or part of their equipment and bypass the disinfectant solution for those items.

Techniques for Cleaning and Disinfection

(Q) A patient's equipment should be cultured

a. in the patient's room before the equipment is bagged and returned to the respiratory care department. 127 c

b. when equipment is brought into the dirty area. 127 C

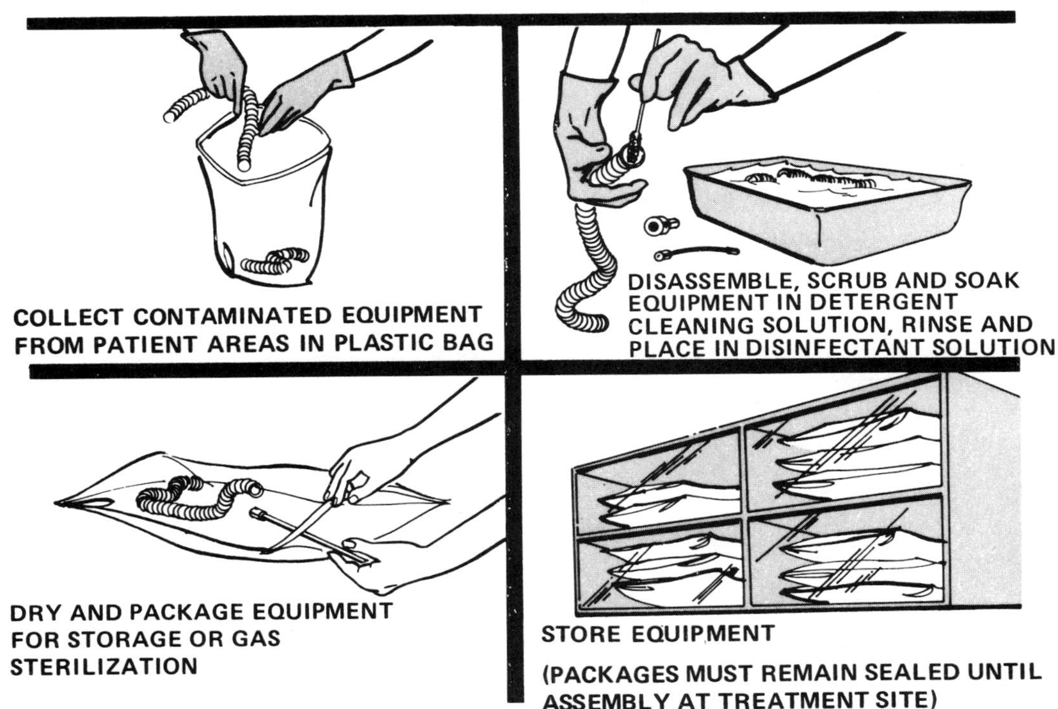

Figure 4–4

FRAME 87. HAND WASHING

When the equipment is ready for use, the package is opened and the pieces are assembled. Once again the equipment is exposed to the air and to the hands of the practitioner. Many hospital personnel are careless about hand washing. Research has revealed that some patients sustain hospital-acquired (nosocomial) infections during their hospital stay. A significant number of hospital personnel also were found to carry resistant strains of infection-producing bacteria. These findings suggest that practitioners must wash their hands properly and use the appropriate techniques when handling clean and dirty equipment.

The single most important procedure for preventing nosocomial infections is hand washing by respiratory practitioners after the care of one patient and before caring for another. Vigorous brief washing with soap under a stream of running water is adequate to remove transient high-virulence pathogens acquired from infected patients. Rings may prevent the removal of pathogens during hand washing and they should not be worn during a tour of duty. Soap should be rinsed off hands with fingers pointed downward to assure that pathogens are not transferred to the wrist and lower arm. After rinsing, remember to dry your hands without touching the faucet handles. Most hospital sinks have foot or knee controls for water faucets. If foot controls are not available, you should turn off the faucet with the paper towel used to dry your hands.

Antimicrobial hand-washing procedures use agents that destroy or prevent the development of microorganisms. This type of hand washing is indicated before all invasive procedures, during the care of patients in isolation, and before entering intensive care units to prevent the spread of pathogens. The most commonly used antimicrobial agents are 70% isopropyl alcohol, iodophors (combination of iodine and a carrier), and chlorhexidene (antibacterial effective against a wide variety of Gram-negative and Gram-positive organisms).

(Q) Which is the correct statement?

a. Hands should be washed before handling dirty equipment and gloves worn for assembling clean equipment. 126 c

b. Hands should be washed after handling dirty equipment and before handling clean equipment. 136 b

c. Gloves should be worn while handling clean equipment. 136 C

FRAME 88. STERILIZATION OF EQUIPMENT

None of the antimicrobial agents can guarantee the complete destruction of *all* living microorganisms, including spore forms. One of the most practical and reliable methods of sterilization is heat in the form of steam under pressure (autoclaving). However, this method cannot be used for all equipment, because some materials used by respiratory care practitioners will be damaged by moisture and high temperature. Gas sterilization (ethylene oxide) can be used with most respiratory care equipment (Fig. 4–5), although it also has certain disadvantages. Boiling for any lengh of time is not a reliable method for killing bacterial spores, especially at high altitudes. At sea level, water boils at 212°F or 100°C; and at an altitude of 5280 ft, it boils at 202°F or 94°C.

(Q) Can an object be sterilized with a disinfectant?

a. yes 127 d
b. no 127 D
c. It depends on the type of agent and how it is used. 126 C

GAS STERILIZATION

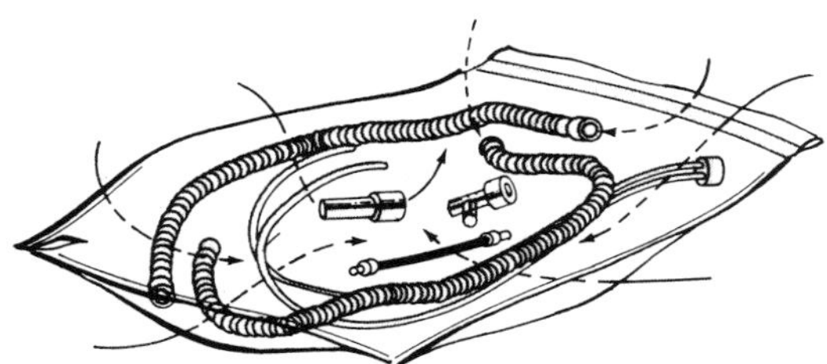

Ethylene Oxide (C_2H_4O) Penetrates Bag and Sterilizes Equipment

- BACTERICIDAL . . NOT MERELY BACTERIOSTATIC
- LETHAL FOR ALL MICROORGANISMS
- PENETRATES MATERIALS OF RELATIVELY LOW PERMEABILITY
- LEAVES LITTLE RESIDUAL GAS . . . EXCEPT IN THICK RUBBER TUBING
- EFFECTIVE AT ROOM TEMPERATURES (70° F)
- ACTIVE AT RELATIVELY LOW HUMIDITY (35%)
- DAMAGES VERY FEW MATERIALS
- COMMERCIALLY AVAILABLE IN QUANTITY

STERILIZATION BY DRY HEAT

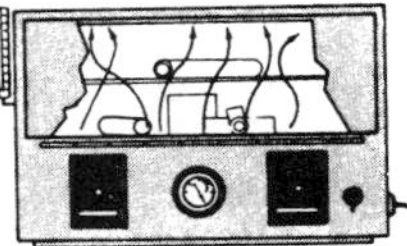

- DESTROYS BACTERIA BY PROTEIN COAGULATION
- KILLS BACTERIA AFTER A MINIMUM OF 160° C. FOR 1 HOUR DURATION

MOIST HEAT

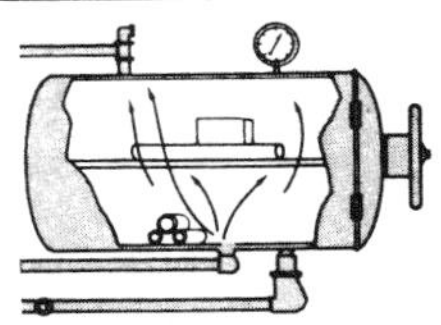

- DESTROYS BACTERIA BY PROTEIN COAGULATION
- A MINIMUM STEAM PRESSURE OF 15 TO 20 POUNDS AND 126.5° C. FOR 15 MINUTES KILLS BACTERIA

STEAM PRESSURE PSI	C°	F°
0	100.0	212.0
20	126.5	259.5
40	141.5	287.0

Figure 4–5

FRAME 89. COMPARISON OF STEAM AUTOCLAVE AND GAS STERILIZATION

The steam autoclave, at a temperature of 260°F (126°C) and under 20 pounds per square inch, can kill all microorganisms in 15 minutes. At autoclave temperature, nearly all plastics except polycarbonate, polyproplyene, nylon, and Teflon have a tendency to melt. Most respiratory care equipment cannot withstand temperatures this high.

The gas sterilizer, using ethylene oxide, can destroy all bacteria within 4 hours at a temperature of 50° to 60°F and a relative humidity of 30% to 50%, but it is expensive, requires special equipment and controlled conditions, and is flammable unless diluted with carbon dioxide or Freon. Prior to sterilization with ethylene oxide, equipment should be dry, disassembled, and sealed in a plastic bag. Ethylene oxide can cause contact irritation and residual gas must be removed after sterilization is complete. The use of heated aeration cabinets reduces the aeration time from more than a week at ambient temperature to 12 hours at 53°C.

(Q) Boiling an object for 3 minutes will

a. partially sterilize it. 136 D
b. not sterilize it. 136 c

FRAME 90. DEFINITION OF TERMS

You should be aware of the differences among several types of cleaning agents. They are often mistakenly substituted for one another. The definition of the terms can be found in their prefixes and suffixes: *anti-* means *"against"* -cide means *"kill"* or *"destroy,"* -stasis and -static mean *"at rest"* or *"in a state of equilibrium."*

1. Disinfectant. Any agent (usually chemical) that destroys pathogenic microorganisms or makes them inactive. A complete disinfectant given enough time, will destroy spores as well as vegetative forms of microorganisms. An incomplete disinfectant destroys vegetative forms but does not destroy spores.
2. Antiseptic. A substance that will inhibit the growth and development of microorganisms without necessarily destroying them. Some common antiseptics are alcohol, boric acid, sodium chloride, and chlorine.
3. Bactericide.
4. Fungicide.
5. Germicide.

(Q) Write a brief definition for items 3 to 5 above. When you finish, turn to page 126e and see how well you have done.

FRAME 91. PROTOCOL FOR BACTERIOLOGICAL CHECK

The danger of contamination of respiratory care equipment cannot be stressed too strongly. If equipment is sterile when taken from storage, it may be contaminated while being assembled for use. While in use an air-entrainment nebulizer may draw in pathogens that mix with the air and aerosol delivered to the patient. Within 24 hours, pathogens from several sources (patient, hands of practitioners, entrained air) may be growing in the reservoir of the nebulizer. Periodic culturing will help identify the pathogens on respiratory care equipment and allow decisions to be made on how often the equipment should be changed. Also, the culture reports can be used to determine the source of the bacteria.

(Q) To determine what kinds of microorganisms are present on respiratory care equipment, when should bacteriological checks (Fig. 4–6) be made?

a. Immediately before respiratory care equipment is used. 126 D
b. At predetermined intervals while equipment is in use. 127 E
c. Immediately after the equipment has been discontinued. 126 d
d. All of the above. 136 d

PROTOCOL OF BACTERIOLOGICAL CHECK

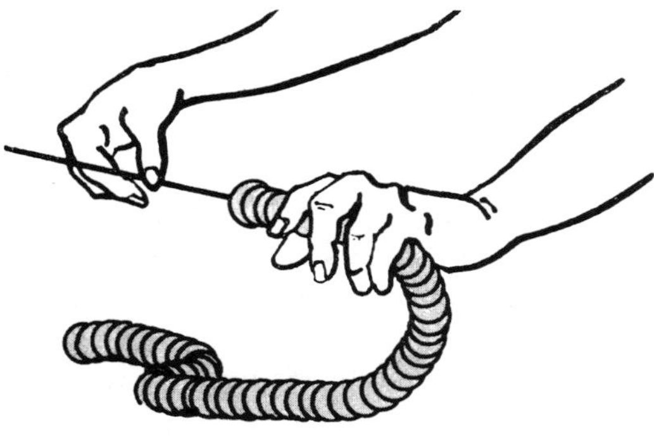

FOR STERILE EQUIPMENT (IMMEDIATELY BEFORE USE)

- USE SWAB DAMPENED WITH SALINE SOLUTION
- SEND SAMPLES TO BACTERIOLOGY LAB FOR CULTURE
- LOG LAB REPORT

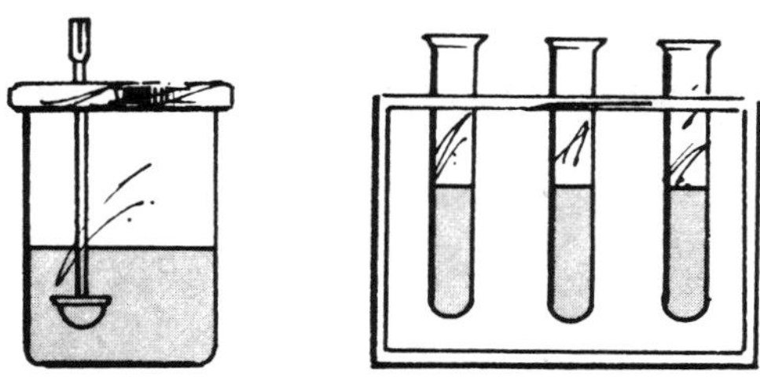

FOR EQUIPMENT IN USE

- OBSERVE TECHNIQUES OF THERAPISTS
- LOG OBSERVATIONS
- CULTURE EQUIPMENT EVERY 24 HOURS
- TAKE SAMPLES OF NEBULIZER WATER
- SEND SAMPLES TO BACTERIOLOGY LAB
- LOG LAB REPORT

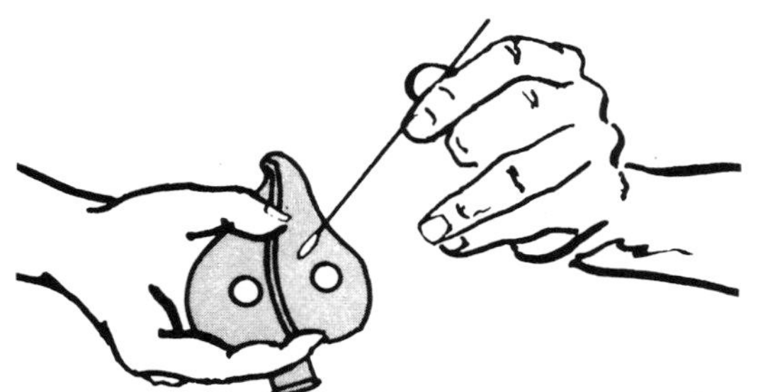

FOR CONTAMINATED EQUIPMENT

- SWAB EQUIPMENT . . . TAKE SAMPLE OF NEBULIZER WATER
- SEND SAMPLE TO BACTERIOLOGY LAB
- LOG LAB REPORT

Figure 4–6

FRAME 92. ISOLATION, REVERSE, AND UNIVERSAL PRECAUTIONS

Strict Isolation Precautions Strict isolation of a patient is designed to break the chain of transmission to and from susceptible patients. If a patient has the potential to spread communicable diseases, a separate room will be required and special precautions must be taken. A mask should be worn by practitioners to block pathogens from entering or leaving the nose or mouth. The mask should remain dry, since pathogens will easily pass through a wet mask. Gloves should be worn to protect personnel from infecting small cuts on their hands. Gowns prevent contamination of the practitioner's clothing, and should be changed before leaving a patient area so that pathogens are prevented from spreading to your clothing. However, gloves should be removed first when leaving the room so that clothing does not become contaminated when removing the gown. Antimicrobial handwashing procedures should be followed upon entering and leaving a patient in strict isolation. Equipment removed from isolation rooms should be double bagged in impervious plastic so that it can be safely carried to the decontamination area.

Reverse Precautions Reverse precautions are designed to protect patients, who have lost their immune response to hospital-acquired infections. Reverse isolation requires all the precautions mentioned for strict isolation except that equipment removed from the room does not need to be double bagged.

Universal Precautions The Centers for Disease Control (CDC) recommends that blood and body-fluid precautions be used for all patients. The CDC has made this recommendation because it is impossible to reliably identify all patients infected with HIV virus or other blood-borne infectious agents. Invasive procedures require the use of gloves and surgical mask to prevent skin and mucous membrane contact with blood and other body fluids. Protective eyewear and gowns are recommended for any procedure that could result in spraying of blood or other body fluids. Health care workers who have exudative lesions or weeping dermatitis should remove themselves from all direct patient care and from handling patient care equipment until the condition is resolved.

(Q) Where should you remove your cap, gown, and gloves when leaving a strict isolation precautions room?

a. inside the room 136 e

b. outside the room 136 E

c. in the equipment decontamination area 127 e

EXERCISES

1. Using a medical dictionary or a microbiology textbook, review Gram's method for identifying Gram-positive, Gram-negative, and acid-fast microorganisms.
2. Compare and contrast factors that tend to inhibit or facilitate the growth of bacteria.
3. Identify the equipment in a respiratory department that should be cultured to check for contamination with pathogens.
4. Visit a respiratory care department's equipment-cleaning area and diagram the flow of equipment from the dirty area through various stages of cleaning, sterilization, and storage.
5. Make three separate lists of equipment that can be safely sterilized by ethylene oxide, steam autoclave, and liquid chemical agents (alkaline glutaraldehyde).
6. Compare and contrast the difference between sterilization and disinfection.
7. Give three reasons for maintaining a culture log with reports on samples taken from respiratory care equipment.
8. Describe when you should wash your hands with soap and water, and identify three situations in which antimicrobial hand-washing procedures should be used.
9. Compare and contrast the differences between the procedures for strict precautions and reverse precautions.
10. Name three agents commonly used for antimicrobial hand washing.

136A (from page 123, frame 81)
Right. Gas sterilization is the best way to kill *P. aeruginosa* or other pathogens in the nebulizer. The many small apertures in a nebulizer make this method of sterilization the most effective. Please continue on page 124, frame 82.

136B (from page 125, frame 84)
A screen would not be best. You must keep in mind that bacteria carried in the air will travel over, under, and around the screen. Return to page 125, frame 84, and select another answer.

136C (from page 130, frame 87)
Gloves may minimize the risk of infection, but they are not always necessary if hands are washed before assembling the equipment. Return to page 130, frame 87, and select another answer.

136D (from page 132, frame 89)
Wrong. There is no such thing as partially sterile. For an object to be sterile, it must be *completely free* of all living microorganisms. Return to page 132, frame 89, and select another answer.

136E (from page 134, frame 92)
Wrong. You risk the chance that disease-spreading agents will be carried to other hospital areas by personnel passing by the isolation room. Return to page 134, frame 92, and select another answer.

136a (from page 125, frame 84)
As long as the air from the contaminated area can rise over the partition, the clean area is at risk of becoming contaminated with airborne pathogens. Return to page 125, frame 84, and find a safer barrier.

136b (from page 130, frame 87)
Yes. This is the best procedure to keep from contaminating the patient and yourself. Keep in mind that even if equipment is sterilized, you may be carrying bacteria on your hands. Please continue on page 131, frame 88.

136c (from page 132, frame 89)
Right. For an object to be sterile, it must be completely free of all living microorganisms. Boiling does not guarantee sterility. Please continue on page 132, frame 90.

136d (from page 133, frame 91)
Correct. Respiratory care equipment should be cultured and the results recorded in a culture log before use, during use, and immediately after use. Please continue on page 134, frame 92.

136e (from page 134, frame 92)
Correct. By keeping the gown inside the room you have reduced the chance that pathogens will be carried to other parts of the hospital. Please continue on page 135, and complete the chapter exercises.

POSTTEST

This test is designed to evaluate what you have learned from completing Chapter 4. Check your answers on page 139 and review the topics where your answer is incorrect.

1. The pathogen most commonly found on respiratory care equipment is
   A. *Staphylococcus aureus.*
   B. *Pseudomonas aeruginosa.*
   C. *Treponema pallidum.*
   D. *Streptococcus pneumonia.*
   E. *Streptococcus pyogenes.*
2. Bacteria that prefer to live without oxygen are called
   A. aerobes.
   B. chemotrophs.
   C. anaerobes.
   D. heterotrophs.
   E. phototrophs.
3. Which of the following will reduce the number of microorganisms on respiratory care equipment?
   A. darkness
   B. oxygen
   C. water
   D. ultraviolet light
   E. warm temperature
4. The temperature range that kills most bacteria is
   A. 0° to 32°F.
   B. 32° to 50°F.
   C. 50° to 110°F.
   D. 150° to 170°F.
   E. 194° to 212°F.
5. If respiratory care practitioners cannot agree on how often to change equipment in use, which of the following can provide data to reach a consensus?
   A. a cost analysis report
   B. a review of cleaning procedures
   C. a report on use of disposable equipment
   D. a culture log
   E. a procedure manual
6. Culture logs contain bacteriological reports regarding
   A. equipment in use.
   B. equipment in supply closets.
   C. ventilators in use.
   D. contaminated equipment.
   E. all of the above.

7. Equipment *dirty areas* should contain
   A. soak, scrub, and rinse sinks.
   B. exhaust hood over disinfectant area.
   C. disinfectant sink or container.
   D. foot- or knee-operated faucets.
   E. all of the above.
8. Personnel disinfecting equipment in a dirty area should wear
   I. Masks.
   II. gowns.
   III. gloves.
   A. I only
   B. II only
   C. III only
   D. II and III only
   E. I, II, and III
9. The first step in disinfecting contaminated respiratory care equipment is to
   A. disassemble it.
   B. soak it in a detergent.
   C. soak it in a disinfectant.
   D. Place it in a drier.
   E. scrub it with brushes.
10. Equipment is moved from the dirty area to the clean area *after* which of the following steps?
   A. sterilization
   B. soaking in a detergent
   C. spraying with an antiseptic
   D. placing in a plastic bag
   E. disassembling
11. Prior to sterilization with ethylene oxide, equipment should be
   A. placed *wet* into muslin packages.
   B. placed *dry* and *disassembled* into a plastic bag.
   C. placed *wet* and *assembled* into a plastic bag.
   D. steam autoclaved.
   E. heated in an oven at 190°F.
12. Wearing gloves while cleaning equipment
   A. removes the need to wash your hands before starting.
   B. removes the need to wash your hands when done.
   C. protects personnel from contaminating each other.
   D. allows you to move in and out of the clean area.
   E. none of the above.
13. Sterilization with ethylene oxide requires the added step of
   A. chemical disinfection.
   B. aeration before use.
   C. dry heat during exposure to gas.
   D. high temperature during exposure to gas.
   E. wrapping equipment in muslin packages.

14. Sterilization by a steam autoclave
    A. takes longer than by dry heat.
    B. takes longer than boiling.
    C. kills microorganisms by desiccation.
    D. kills microorganisms by protein coagulation.
    E. is done at ambient pressure.
15. Which of the following helps to reduce the spread of nosocomial infections related to hand washing?
    A. removing rings from fingers
    B. keeping fingernails short
    C. use of foot pedals on sinks
    D. use of antimicrobial hand lotions
    E. all of the above
16. Hand washing when moving between patients in an intensive care unit requires
    A. soap and water.
    B. 70% isopropyl alcohol.
    C. an iodophor solution.
    D. glutaraldehyde.
    E. 30% isopropyl alcohol.
17. Which of the following pieces of respiratory care equipment carries the greatest risk of contaminating an area with airborne pathogens?
    A. cascade humidifier
    B. small sidestream nebulizer
    C. heated pass-over humidifier
    D. ultrasonic nebulizer
    E. metered dose inhaler
18. Which of the following may help to prevent contamination of breathing circuits by airborne pathogens?
    A. changing circuits every 8 hours
    B. rinsing circuits with sterile water every 8 hours
    C. rinsing circuit with antimicrobial agents every 8 hours
    D. in-line bacterial filters
    E. in-line water traps
19. The chance of contracting an infectious disease from a patient on strict isolation who sneezes and coughs frequently would be reduced by
    A. extra hand washing every 15 minutes.
    B. ultraviolet lamps.
    C. masks.
    D. shoe covers.
    E. none of the above.
20. When preparing to leave a strict isolation room, which of the following should be removed first?
    A. gown
    B. gloves
    C. mask
    D. cap
    E. goggles

ANSWERS TO POSTTEST

1. B (F81)
2. C (F80)
3. D (F80)
4. E (F80)
5. D (F91)
6. E (F85)
7. E (F83)
8. E (F86)
9. A (F86)
10. A (F83)
11. B (F89)
12. E (F86)
13. B (F89)
14. D (F89)
15. E (F87)
16. C (F87)
17. D (F85)
18. D (F86)
19. C (F92)
20. B (F92)

BIBLIOGRAPHY

Anderson, DM: Dorland's Pocket Medical Dictionary, ed 24. WB Saunders, Philadelphia, 1989.

Barnes, TA: Respiratory Care Practice. Year Book Medical Publishers, Chicago, 1988.

Bennington, JL: Saunders Dictionary and Encyclopedia of Laboratory Medicine and Technology. WB Saunders, Philadelphia, 1984.

Burton, GG and Hodgkin, JE: Respiratory Care. A Guide to Clinical Practice, ed 2. JB Lippincott, Philadelphia, 1984.

Burton, GR: Microbiology for the Health Sciences, ed 3. JB Lippincott, Philadelphia, 1988.

Eubanks, DH and Bone, RC: Comprehensive Respiratory Care, ed 2. CV Mosby, St. Louis, 1990.

Riggs, JH: Respiratory Facts. FA Davis, Philadelphia, 1989.

Shapiro, BA, Harrison, RA, Kacmarek, RM, and Cane, RD: Clinical Application of Respiratory Care, ed 3. Year Book Medical Publishers, Chicago, 1985.

Thomas, CL: Taber's Cyclopedic Medical Dictionary, ed 16. FA Davis, Philadelphia, 1989.

5

Initial Assessment and Diagnosis

93. Physician's order
94. Respiratory care plan
95. Spirometry
96. Timed vital capacity
97. Maximum voluntary ventilation
98. Obstructive pulmonary disease
99. Restrictive pulmonary disease
100. Characteristics of obstructive and restrictive disease
101. Applications for the MVV test
102. Bronchodilator evaluation
103. Chest x-rays
104. Breathing patterns
105. Upper airway obstruction
106. Amount and character of sputum
107. Palpation
108. Auscultation
109. Patient interview
110. Maximum inspiratory pressure and peak expiratory flow
111. Calculating minute volume
112. Blood-gas interpretation

PRETEST

This pretest is designed to measure what you already know about initial assessment and diagnosis. Check your answers on page 144 and then continue on page 145, frame 93.

1. Orders for bronchial hygiene therapy should be evaluated
   A. upon discharge from the hospital.
   B. upon transfer from the intensive care unit.
   C. automatically after 48 to 72 hours by standing protocol.
   D. by the medical director of respiratory care.
   E. when the patient reaches 80% of predicted forced vital capacity (FVC).
2. All of the following statements about predicted pulmonary function values are true *except*
   A. the predicted values have a variance of $\pm$ 20%.
   B. the predicted values have a variance of $\pm$ 10%.
   C. a normal FEV_1/FEV (forced expiratory volume) is 83%.
   D. a normal FEV_3/FEV is 97%.
   E. a normal peak expiratory flow is 400 to 600 L/min.
3. While inspecting a recent admission to the emergency room for treatment of multiple injuries from a motor vehicle accident, you observe that the trachea is deviated from midline. What is the most likely explanation?
   A. neck tumor
   B. thyroid enlargement
   C. massive pleural effusion
   D. mediastinal mass
   E. pneumothorax
4. Palpation can be used to assess all of the following *except*
   A. respiratory expansion.
   B. tactile fremitus.
   C. breath sounds.
   D. skin and subcutaneous tissue.
   E. deformities of the chest.
5. Which of the following is associated with vesicular breath sounds heard over the peripheral lung areas?
   I. high pitched and loud
   II. low pitched and soft
   III. I:E ratio of 1:1
   IV. I:E ratio of 1:3
   V. harsh
   A. I and III only
   B. II and V only
   C. II and IV only
   D. I and IV only
   E. I, III, and V only
6. After intubation, which of the following would be most appropriate?
   A. arterial blood-gas study
   B. chest physiotherapy
   C. IPPB with a bronchodilator
   D. bilateral auscultation
   E. bilateral palpation

7. The breathing pattern associated with severe diabetic acidosis and coma that has very deep gasping tidal volumes is called
   A. Biot's respiration.
   B. Kussmaul's respiration.
   C. apneustic respiration.
   D. Cheyne-Stokes respiration.
   E. hypopnea.
8. Which of the following breathing patterns have end-inspiratory pauses followed by periods of apnea?
   A. Biot's respiration
   B. Kussmaul's respiration
   C. apneustic respiration
   D. Cheyne-Stokes respiration
   E. hypopnea
9. Which of the following breathing patterns has shallow tidal volumes that become deeper, then gradually decrease to a period of apnea?
   A. Biot's respiration
   B. Kussmaul's respiration
   C. apneustic respiration
   D. Cheyne-Stokes respiration
   E. hypopnea
10. All of the following are associated with upper airway obstruction *except*
    A. intercostal retractions.
    B. supraclavicular retractions.
    C. "seesaw" movement of the abdomen.
    D. unilateral chest expansion.
    E. extreme agitation.
11. Which clinical entity is associated with sputum that is frothy, thin, and pink?
    A. bronchial asthma
    B. pulmonary edema
    C. bronchiectasis
    D. cystic fibrosis
    E. bronchitis
12. Coarse, discontinuous breath sounds produced during inspiration and expiration by the movement of excessive secretions or fluid in the airways are called
    A. rhonchi.
    B. wheeze.
    C. crackles.
    D. sibilant rales.
    E. none of the above.
13. The term used to refer to vibrations caused by secretions in the airway that can be felt with the fingertips or the ulnar side of the hand when placed against the chest is called
    A. sibilant rhonchi.
    B. sonorous rhonchi.
    C. wheeze.
    D. tactile fremitus.
    E. vocal fremitus.
14. Respiratory care practitioners will be involved most often with which of the following type of patient interview?
    A. complete respiratory history
    B. complete occupational history
    C. interval history
    D. comprehensive health history
    E. comprehensive family history

15. A healthy adult can usually generate a maximum inspiratory pressure within 20 seconds of
   A. 10 cm H_2O.
   B. 20 cm H_2O.
   C. 30 cm H_2O.
   D. 50 cm H_2O.
   E. 80 cm H_2O.
16. The minute volume of a patient with a tidal volume of 400 mL and a respiratory rate of 14/min is
   A. 400 mL.
   B. 560 mL.
   C. 4000 mL.
   D. 5600 mL.
   E. 6000 mL.
17. All of the following must be clearly understood before administering a respiratory care treatment to a patient *except*
   A. indications for therapy.
   B. contraindications of therapy.
   C. hazards of therapy.
   D. comprehensive health history.
   E. therapeutic outcomes expected.
18. Which of the following arterial oxygen tensions would be associated with moderate hypoxemia?
   A. 35 mm Hg
   B. 45 mm Hg
   C. 65 mm Hg
   D. 80 mm Hg
   E. 90 mm Hg
19. What is the acid-base status of a patient if pH = 7.60, $Paco_2$ = 55 mm Hg, HCO_3^- = 51 mEq/L?
   A. uncompensated respiratory alkalosis
   B. partially compensated respiratory alkalosis
   C. partially compensated metabolic alkalosis
   D. compensated metabolic alkalosis
   E. uncompensated respiratory acidosis
20. What is the acid-base status of a patient if pH = 7.38, $Paco_2$ = 76 mm Hg, HCO_3^- = 40 mEq/L?
   A. uncompensated respiratory acidosis
   B. compensated metabolic alkalosis
   C. partially compensated metabolic acidosis
   D. compensated respiratory acidosis
   E. partially compensated respiratory alkalosis

ANSWERS TO PRETEST

1. C (F93)
2. B (F96, 102, 110)
3. E (F107)
4. C (F107)
5. C (F108)
6. D (F108)
7. B (F104)
8. C (F104)
9. D (F104)
10. D (F105)
11. B (F106)
12. C (F108)
13. D (F107)
14. C (F109)
15. E (F110)
16. D (F111)
17. D (F94)
18. B (F112)
19. C (F112)
20. D (F112)

FRAME 93. PHYSICIAN'S ORDER

Before administering respiratory care, the practitioner should review the physician's orders in the patient's chart. Starting at the last entry, the critical elements of the order should be noted with special attention given to the (1) type of treatment, (2) frequency of treatment, (3) type and dose of aerosol medications, (4) amount and type of diluent, and (5) oxygen concentration. Most respiratory care orders need to be reviewed at specific intervals usually within 72 hours and are often automatically discontinued by a standing policy. Once you have reviewed the order sheet, the remaining sections of the patient's medical record (chart) should be quickly reviewed before treating the patient, for example, respiratory treatment notes, physician progress notes, nursing notes, and lab reports.

When reviewing the results of pulmonary function testing it is important to be familiar with normal predicted values. Predicted lung volumes and capacities will vary by gender, height, age, and race. In contrast to other diagnostic studies, such as arterial pH where a slight variance from normal may be meaningful, a variance of 20% from the normal predicted value does not indicate an abnormally low lung volume or capacity.

(Q) Which of the following need to be included in a physician's order for respiratory care?

a. oxygen concentration or flow 150 A
b. type and dose of medication 151 A
c. frequency of treatments 156 D
d. all of the above 156 d

FRAME 94. RESPIRATORY CARE PLAN

Deciding if the respiratory care ordered can be justified based on therapeutic objectives is a major responsibility of respiratory care practitioners. A review of the expected therapeutic outcomes will eliminate some modalities and strongly support the use of others. Also, the hazards and contraindications for some modalities will preclude their use when certain conditions are present. For example, positive end-expiratory pressure (PEEP) may be appropriate for treating refractory moderate hypoxemia resulting from pulmonary edema, but may be hazardous for a patient with chronic obstructive pulmonary disease who already has a greatly increased functional residual capacity. When suggesting changes for a patient being mechanically ventilated, the impact on inspiratory and expiratory times, peak inspiratory flow, and mean intrathoracic pressure must all be taken into account.

A decision to integrate two or more types of therapy may allow a treatment objective to be completed sooner. Indications for respiratory care such as dried retained secretions with weak unproductive cough may suggest a comprehensive approach that includes aerosol therapy, chest physiotherapy, IPPB, and bronchoscopy.

(Q) To determine the appropriateness of an order for PEEP you should

a. review the hazards of PEEP. 156 A
b. review the therapeutic outcomes expected with PEEP. 156 a
c. do both *a* and *b*. 150 E

FRAME 95. SPIROMETRY

It is possible to measure the maximal volume that can be expired (after a maximal inspiration) by the use of simple volume recorders, such as a bellows or a spirometer (spy-*rah*-muh-ter). The spirometer consists of a tube and a mouthpiece connected to a recording device. If a patient inhales maximally and then exhales maximally into a spirometer with a kymograph, the breathing pattern is recorded on a spirogram. The volume that can be exhaled is the vital capacity (VC). The vital capacity is recorded on paper in a tracing called a spirogram. If the patient has a normal pulmonary mechanical ability, the spirogram of his vital capacity will be normal and will look like tracing **A** in Figure 5–1 below. If the patient has a reduced vital capacity, his spirogram will resemble tracing **B** or **C** below.

(Q) From a spirogram, a practitioner can determine the
  a. vital capacity. 156 b
  b. vital capacity as well as the subdivisions expiratory reserve volume (ERV), tidal volume (TV), and inspiratory capacity (IC). 157 A

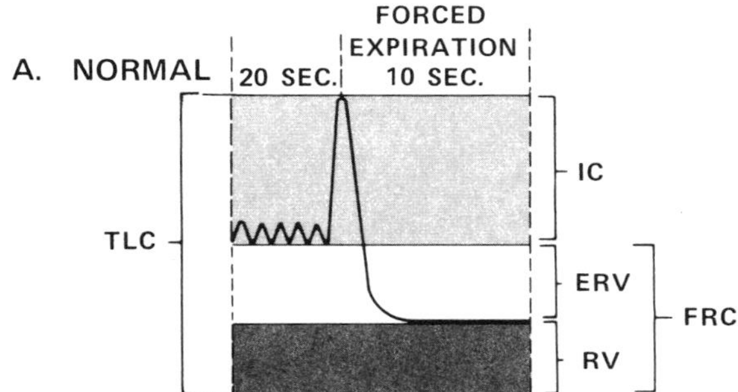

B. RESTRICTIVE

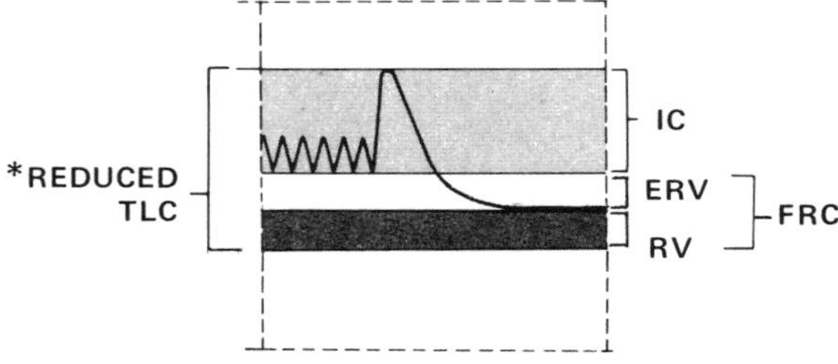

C. OBSTRUCTIVE

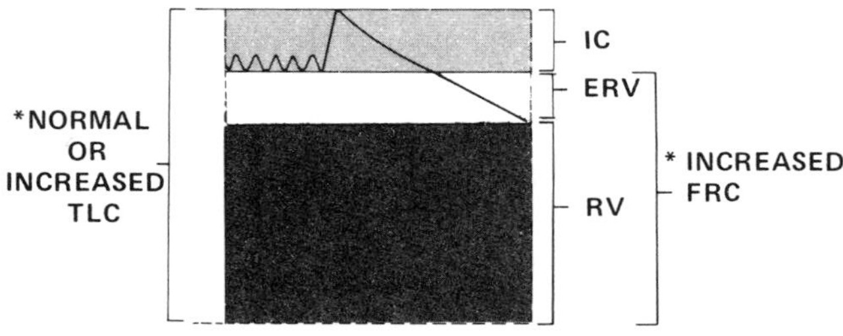

Figure 5–1

FRAME 96. TIMED VITAL CAPACITY

No time limit need be imposed on a vital capacity test as long as exhalation continues until only the residual volume remains. However, in diagnosing respiratory diseases, it is more valuable to use a *timed* vital capacity test to determine how much gas can be exhaled within a specific time period.

Normally, an individual can exhale 70% of his vital capacity in 0.5 second, 83% in 1 second, and 97% in 3 seconds. To determine if the timed vital capacity is normal, a spirometer with a timing mechanism must be used. The timer is set and the spirometer records what volume of the vital capacity is exhaled during 0.5, 1, or 3 seconds. These are symbolized as $FEV_{0.5}$, FEV_1, and FEV_3 respectively. The timed vital capacity is calculated by determining the volume of gas exhaled during the time interval (0.5, 1, or 3 seconds) and dividing the volume by the vital capacity.

(Q) Normally, most of the vital capacity is expired in

a. 0 to 0.5 second. 157 d
b. 0.5 to 1.0 second. 157 B
c. 0.5 to 3.0 seconds. 157 a

FRAME 97. MAXIMUM VOLUNTARY VENTILATION

Pulmonary function testing may include determining the maximum voluntary ventilation (MVV) as well as the vital capacity. The MVV is the maximal volume that can be breathed per minute by voluntary effort. Usually patients with a restrictive pattern of pulmonary disease [low VC and total lung capacity (TLC)] have a normal MVV and the mechanical ability to breathe rapidly. Patients who fall into the obstructive pattern may not have a normal MVV because of airway obstruction.

A patient with a normal MVV may not have adequate ventilation if the tidal volume is too small. Even though the MVV may be normal, a small tidal volume may mean that after the dead space is filled there won't be enough gas left to provide a fresh supply to the alveoli.

Respiratory diseases present one of two general patterns—restrictive or obstructive. It is important for the respiratory care practitioner to be able to recognize the characteristics of each of these patterns.

(Q) Patients who suffer from restrictive pulmonary diseases have

a. abnormal MVV and low VC. 156 c
b. normal MVV and high VC. 157 b
c. normal MVV and low VC. 156 B

FRAME 98. OBSTRUCTIVE PULMONARY DISEASE

The obstructive pattern is defined by an elevated resistance to gas flow and turbulence caused by airway obstructions. Some causes for airway obstruction are constriction of bronchiolar smooth muscle, mucus congestion, edema of bronchiolar tissues, and collapse or kinking of the bronchioles. The obstruction may be caused by a reversible pulmonary abnormality as found early in the course of asthma, or it may be more complex, as with structural diseases of the lung (e.g., emphysema). With chronic airway obstruction, the functional residual capacity and residual volume are increased significantly (due to air trapped behind obstructed airways). If the small airways collapse during exhalation, the vital capacity may be decreased.

A patient with an obstructive pattern of pulmonary disease may not be able to exhale rapidly because of small airway collapse (Fig. 5–2). Patients with emphysema commonly exhale only 50% or less of their vital capacity after 1 second (FEV_1/FVC%). Healthy people can exhale 83% of their vital capacity in 1 second. During normal exhalation, the walls of bronchioles may be slightly narrowed by increased intrathoracic pressure, but the septa of the surrounding alveoli prevent the collapse of small airways. If a disease process destroys the alveolar septa, increased intrathoracic pressure during exhalation may compress the bronchioles and prevent normal airflow from the alveoli.

One way to distinguish between the restrictive pattern and the obstructive pattern of lung disease is to measure total lung capacity. In the restrictive pattern, the TLC is decreased and the functional residual capacity (FRC) and residual volume (RV) are normal or slightly decreased; in the obstructive pattern TLC is normal or increased, and the FRC and RV are increased. Please continue on page 149, frame 99.

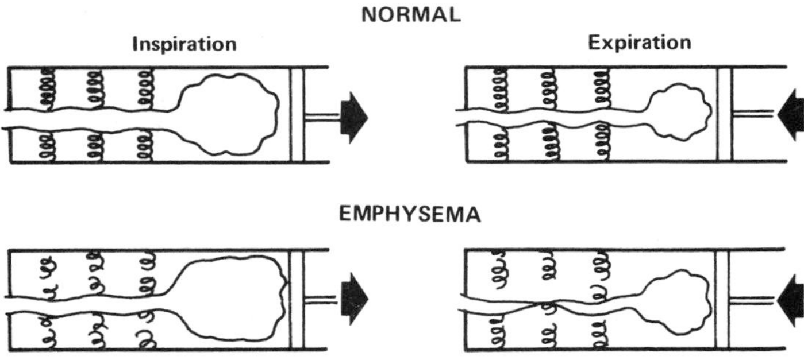

Figure 5–2

FRAME 99. RESTRICTIVE PULMONARY DISEASE

A restrictive pattern results when the lungs cannot expand fully. There are many causes for this pattern, including abnormalities in the thorax, chest, or lung, and immobilization of the diaphragm due to abdominal pathology or late-term pregnancy. Limited lung expansion characterizes the restrictive pattern (Table 5–1).

Since the lungs cannot fully expand in the restrictive pattern, there is obviously a decrease in the vital capacity (Table 5–2). The residual volume may decrease or remain normal. If the patient breathes with quick, small breaths, the MVV may be normal. However, if too much effort is required to overcome restrictive disease, alveolar ventilation may decrease, even though the frequency of breathing increases.

TABLE 5–1
TYPES OF RESTRICTIVE PULMONARY DISEASE

Intrapulmonic
- Interstitial fibrosis
- Pulmonary edema
- Pneumonia
- Vascular congestion
- Adult respiratory distress syndrome
- Pneumoconioses
- Sarcoidosis

Extrapulmonic
- Thoracic
  - Kyphoscoliosis
  - Multiple rib fractures
  - Rheumatoid spondylitis
  - Thoracic surgery
  - Pleural effusion
  - Pneumothorax or hemothorax, or both

Abdominal
- Abdominal surgery
- Ascites
- Peritonitis
- Severe obesity

Neuromuscular defects
- Poliomyelitis
- Guillain-Barré syndrome
- Myasthenia gravis
- Tetanus
- Drugs (e.g., curare, kanamycin)

Respiratory center depression
- Narcotics
- Barbiturates
- Anesthesia

Source: Burton, GG and Hodgkin, JE: Respiratory Care: A Guide to Clinical Practice, ed 2. JB Lippincott, Philadelphia, 1984. Used with permission.

FRAME 100. CHARACTERISTICS OF OBSTRUCTIVE AND RESTRICTIVE DISEASE

TABLE 5–2
PATTERNS OF RESTRICTIVE AND OBSTRUCTIVE DISEASE

NC = No Change ↑ = Increased ↓ = Decreased	Vital Capacity (VC)	Inspiratory Capacity (IC)	Total Lung Capacity (TLC)	Residual Volume (RV)	Functional Residual Capacity (FRC)
RESTRICTIVE PATTERN	↓	↓	↓	NC or ↓	↓
OBSTRUCTIVE PATTERN	NC or ↓	↓	NC or ↑	↑	↑

(Q) An MVV test performed by a patient with the restrictive pattern of pulmonary disease is frequently

a. normal. 157 D
b. abnormal. 157 c

150A (from page 145, frame 93)
Wrong. At a minimum, the frequency of therapy must also be included. Return to page 145, frame 93, and select another answer.

150B (from page 152, frame 102)
Wrong. The 10% increase in forced vital capacity is *not* substantially different from what was seen before the bronchodilator was given. Return to page 152, frame 102, and select another answer.

150C (from page 153, frame 103)
Wrong. You have ignored the need for monitoring during the night when the patient may be at risk from severe hypoxemia resulting from obstructive sleep apnea. Return to page 153, frame 103, and try again.

150D (from page 153, frame 104)
Wrong. Kussmaul's breathing is associated with diabetic acidosis and coma. Return to page 153, frame 104, review the patterns, and try again.

150E (from page 145, frame 94)
Correct. A good understanding of both the expected therapeutic outcomes and the hazards of PEEP is important when recommending its use. Please continue on page 146, frame 95.

150a (from page 152, frame 102)
Almost. FEV_1/FVC has improved substantially following the administration of the bronchodilator. However, there is a better answer choice. Return to page 152, frame 102, and review the improvement seen with FEV_1; then select another answer.

150b (from page 153, frame 103)
Correct. Both ECG and pulse-oximetry monitors should be connected to this patient to alert respiratory care practitioners and nurses to periods of obstructive apnea and desaturation of arterial blood. Monitors with ability to generate hard copy when alarm parameters are crossed will allow a retrospective analysis of the number of apnea-related periods of desaturation at night. A complete study by a sleep laboratory may be indicated for this type of patient. Please continue on page 153, frame 104.

150c (from page 153, frame 104)
No. Although this pattern falls within the broad category of ataxic breathing, a more specific category defines the pattern seen with meningitis. Return to page 153, frame 104, and review the patterns and select another answer.

150d (from page 154, frame 105)
Yes. This is the best choice because the high transpulmonary pressure generated by trying to breathe against an obstructed airway will cause retraction of soft tissue in the intercostal and supraclavicular spaces. Please continue on page 155, frame 106.

151A (from page 145, frame 93)
Wrong. At a minimum, the frequency of therapy must also be included. Return to page 145, frame 93, and select another answer.

151B (from page 153, frame 103)
Wrong. Continuous ECG monitoring should be instituted, but it does not adequately deal with the need to monitor the arterial oxygen saturation at night. Return to page 153, frame 103, and select another answer.

151C (from page 152, frame 102)
Almost. FEV_1 has improved by 43% as a result of administering the aerosolized bronchodilator. However, there is a better answer. Return to page 152, frame 102, and review the improvement seen with FEV_1/FVC; then select another answer.

151D (from page 153, frame 104)
Correct. Biot's breathing is associated with lesions in the medulla, meningitis, basal encephalitis, and increased intracranial pressure. Please continue on page 154, frame 105.

151a (from page 153, frame 103)
Not quite. A patient who has the potential for sudden development of moderate or severe hypoxemia during periods of obstructive apnea should also be monitored for cardiac arrhythmias. Return to 153, frame 103, and select another answer.

151b (from page 152, frame 102)
Correct. Both FEV_1 and FEV_1/FVC have improved substantially and indicate that the patient would benefit from aerosolized bronchodilators. Please continue on page 153, frame 103.

151c (from page 154, frame 105)
Wrong. Abdominal distention is a normal indication of diaphragmatic movement but would be a clinical sign of upper airway obstruction if the lower sternum were retracted inward concurrently, indicating high transpulmonary pressure. Return to page 154, frame 105, and try again.

151d (from page 153, frame 104)
No. Apneustic breathing is associated with a lesion in the lower pontine region of the brainstem. Return to page 153, frame 104; review the patterns and try again.

FRAME 101. APPLICATIONS FOR THE MVV TEST

MVV provides information regarding the mechanics of breathing with many types of cardiopulmonary disease. However, a low value does not determine any particular disease or disorder. The ability of a patient to breathe at sustained high velocity depends upon many factors, some of which include the muscular force available, the compliance of the lungs and thorax, airway resistance, the condition of the lung parenchyma, and patient cooperation.

(Q) A test of maximum voluntary ventilation is important because it can

a. indicate if the lungs and thorax have the mechanical ability to ventilate the lungs adequately. 156 C
b. be used to diagnose certain pulmonary diseases. 157 C

FRAME 102. BRONCHODILATOR EVALUATION

In order to determine if an aerosolized bronchodilator should be ordered, spirometry before and after the administration of the bronchodilator usually is a logical recommendation. The purpose of this type of procedure is to evaluate if there is a meaningful improvement (20% or more) in flow after a bronchodilator is given. In a small number of patients who are overusing bronchodilators a decrement in flow may be observed. The spirometric evaluation compares the pretreatment and posttreatment values of timed vital capacity, peak flow, and forced expiratory volumes. Also, the patient should be monitored for changes in pulse and breath sounds to determine the positive or negative effects of the aerosolized bronchodilator.

(Q) Which of the following pulmonary function results from spirometry before and after an aerosolized bronchodilator indicates that the treatment should be ordered?

a. FVC increases from 3.0 L to 3.3 L. 150 B
b. FEV_1 increases from 2.1 L to 3.0 L. 151 C
c. FEV_1/FVC increases from 60% to 75%. 150 a
d. Both *b* and *c* occur. 151 b

FRAME 103. CHEST X-RAYS

A "stat" chest x-ray is useful for determining endotracheal tube placement and for identifying a pneumothorax or hemothorax when other classical signs such as mediastinal shift, sudden dyspnea, asymmetrical chest excursion, absence of breath sounds, and hyperresonance over affected areas are not definitive. Chest x-rays may help the practitioner determine if air or fluid is present in the pleural space, whether a chest tube should be inserted, oxygen concentration needed, and whether to pull back a tracheal tube positioned in the right main-stem bronchus.

(Q) While charting a patient's arterial oxygen saturation and pulse after a "spot" pulse-oximetry check, you notice that the patient meets the profile for obstructive sleep apnea. Which of the following should be initiated?

a. spot pulse-oximetry checks 150 C
b. continuous ECG monitoring 151 B
c. continuous pulse-oximetry with a hard copy of abnormal events 151 a
d. both *b* and *c* 150 b

FRAME 104. BREATHING PATTERNS

Respiratory care practitioners can gather a large amount of information by simply observing the breathing patterns listed below.

Kussmaul's—Very deep gasping respirations associated with severe diabetic acidosis and coma.

Biot's—Irregular tidal volumes, which may be slow and deep or rapid and shallow, often accompanied by periods of apnea. Biot's respiration is associated with lesions in the medulla, meningitis or basal encephalitis, and increased intracranial pressure. Biot's respiration is a form of ataxic breathing.

Ataxic—Grossly irregular respirations with both deep and shallow tidal volumes caused by a lesion in the dorsomedial part of the medulla.

Cluster—Closely grouped series of gasping respirations followed by irregular periods of apnea. Cluster breathing is associated with a lesion in the lower pontine region of the brainstem.

Cheyne-Stokes—Shallow breathing that becomes deeper, and then gradually tapers off to shallow tidal volumes. The cycle of steplike increase and decrease in tidal volumes regularly alternates with periods of apnea. Cheyne-Stokes respiration has been associated with abnormalities of the central nervous, cardiovascular, and respiratory systems. This type of pattern may also be caused by an overdose of narcotic or hypnotic drugs.

Apneustic—End inspiratory pauses (breath holding) that alternate regularly with periods of apnea. Apneustic breathing is associated with a lesion in the lower pontine region of the brainstem.

(Q) The breathing pattern observed with meningitis is

a. Kussmaul's. 150 D
b. Biot's. 151 D
c. ataxic. 150 c
d. apneustic. 151 d

FRAME 105. UPPER AIRWAY OBSTRUCTION

Respiratory care practitioners must be able to quickly recognize the clinical signs of an upper airway obstruction and take appropriate emergency action to clear the airway. Victims of an upper airway obstruction will not be able to speak, cough, or breathe. They may instinctively raise a hand to the throat and will be extremely agitated. Victims will be using their accessory muscles (sternocleidomastoid and scalene), normally used only during exercise, in an effort to clear the airway. The high transpulmonary pressure caused by vigorous inspiratory efforts with the airway obstructed will cause retraction inward of soft tissue in the intercostal and supraventricular spaces. Also, the lower sternum may retract and the abdomen distend in a "seesaw" fashion as a result of vigorous diaphragmatic contractions.

The Heimlich maneuver is the method of choice when the obstruction is a bolus of food or a foreign body. Other patients may obstruct from flexion of the head, which once hyperextended will open the upper airways. The Heimlich maneuver is performed on a standing adult by standing behind the victim, placing both arms around the waist, and making a fist with one hand. The rescuer positions the thumb side of the fist above the victim's navel, making sure that the fist is well below the xiphoid process. Grabbing this fist with the other hand, the rescuer gives a single, sharp, quick inward and upward compression, which is repeated several times if the obstruction remains after the first thrust.

The Heimlich maneuver is done differently for a victim who collapses to the floor. The victim is turned onto his or her back with the rescuer straddling one or both thighs. The heel of one hand is placed directly above the victim's navel but well below the xiphoid process and the other hand grasps the top of the first hand. The rescuer gives a single, sharp inward and upward thrust, which may need to be repeated 6 to 10 times if the obstruction does not clear after the first thrust.

(Q) Which of the following are signs of increased airway resistance or upper airway obstruction?

a. intercostal and supraclavicular retractions	150	d
b. abdominal distention	151	c
c. severe coughing episodes	162	A
d. use of accessory muscles during exercise	163	B

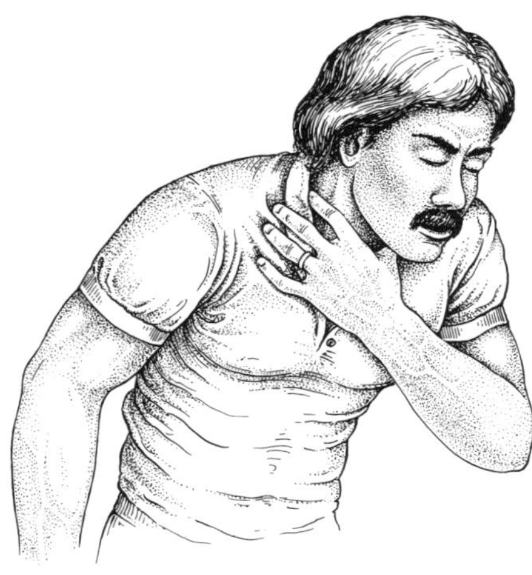

Figure 5–3 Universal sign of choking. (Source: Finucane, BT and Santora, AH: Principles of Airway Management. FA Davis, Philadelphia, 1988. Used with permission.)

FRAME 106. AMOUNT AND CHARACTER OF SPUTUM

The amount and character of sputum provides important information that is helpful in diagnosing respiratory infections and disorders. The volume, color, odor, and consistency of sputum should be charted each time a patient receives a respiratory care treatment. The amount of sputum produced with each respiratory care treatment should be charted. The quantity of sputum produced should be reported in millimeters since descriptors such as "large amount" are open to wide interpretation. Table 5–3 should be studied so that you are familiar with the character of sputum often seen with pulmonary disorders.

TABLE 5–3
DISEASE STATES ASSOCIATED WITH ABNORMAL GROSS APPEARANCE OF THE SPUTUM*

Type of Sputum	Lung Abscess	Acute Bronchitis	Chronic Bronchitis	Pneumonia	Pulmonary Edema	Bronchiectasis	Tuberculosis	Lung Cancer	Pulmonary Infarction	Bronchial Asthma	Cystic Fibrosis	Aspiration Pneumonia
Mucoid (white or clear)			X							X		
Mucopurulent		X	X								X	
Purulent (yellow or green)	X	X		X		X						X
Fetid	X					X					X	X
Bloody		X		X	X	X	X	X	X			
Frothy, sometimes pink					X							

*The most characteristic sputum appearance, consistency, and odor are listed.
Source: Burton, GG and Hodgkin, JE: Respiratory Care—A Guide to Clinical Practice, ed 2. JB Lippincott, Philadelphia, 1984. Used with permission.

(Q) Sputum that is purulent, fetid, and bloody is associated with
a. pulmonary edema. 163 A
b. bronchial asthma. 162 B
c. bronchiectasis. 162 a
d. cystic fibrosis. 163 b

156A (from page 145, frame 94)
Wrong. A review of the hazards and contraindications of PEEP is certainly important, but there is a more complete answer. Return to page 145, frame 94, and select another answer.

156B (from page 147, frame 97)
Correct. The restrictive pattern has a normal MVV because the patient has the mechanical ability to breathe rapidly. The vital capacity and total lung capacity are low because of limited lung expansion, but the percentage of the vital capacity that can be exhaled in a time interval may be normal. Please continue on page 148, frame 98.

156C (from page 152, frame 101)
Yes. Although a low value in the MVV test does not indicate a particular disease or disorder, it can indicate some mechanical malfunction of the lungs and thorax, for example, muscular force available, compliance of the lungs and thorax, airway resistance, or air trapping. Further testing should allow a more specific diagnosis to be made. Please continue on page 152, frame 102.

156D (from page 145, frame 93)
No. You also need to know the type and dose of medication and information on the oxygen concentration. Return to page 145, frame 93, and select another answer.

156a (from page 145, frame 94)
Wrong. A review of the therapeutic outcomes expected with PEEP is certainly critical to its use, but there is a more complete answer. Return to page 145, frame 94, and select another answer.

156b (from page 146, frame 95)
True. But what about the other measurements (ERV, V_T, IC)? Return to page 146, frame 95, and study Figure 5-1. See if you can determine how to calculate the ERV, V_T, and IC from a spirogram.

156c (from page 147, frame 97)
Wrong. In the restrictive pattern (which we will discuss later), the lung expansion is limited, but the patient still has the mechanical ability to breath rapidly and MVV may be normal. Return to page 147, frame 97, and try again.

156d (from page 145, frame 93)
Correct. A physician's order should include the oxygen concentration or flow rate, frequency of treatments, and type and dose of medication. Please continue on page 145, frame 94.

157A (from page 146, frame 95)
Correct. From the spirogram, the practitioner can determine the other volumes and capacities—the ERV, V_T, and IC. Please continue on page 147, frame 96.

157B (from page 147, frame 96)
Wrong. Between 0.5 and 1.0 second, approximately 13% of the vital capacity is exhaled. Return to page 147, frame 96, and review; then try again.

157C (from page 152, frame 101)
Wrong. A test for MVV can reveal decreased pulmonary mechanics, but a low value is not diagnostic of any particular disease. A test for maximum voluntary ventilation is helpful, but other tests will need to be done for a definitive diagnosis. Please continue on page 152, frame 102.

157D (from page 149, frame 100)
Correct. Even if the vital capacity were reduced because of limited lung expansion, the MVV test might be normal if it was performed with quick, small tidal volumes. Please continue on page 152, frame 101.

157a (from page 147, frame 96)
Wrong. Between the 0.5 and 3.0 seconds only 27% is exhaled. Return to page 147, frame 96, and select another answer.

157b (from page 147, frame 97)
Wrong. In the restrictive pattern, the patient has the mechanical ability to breathe rapidly. Thus, the MVV may be normal, but lung expansion is limited. How would this affect the vital capacity? Return to page 147, frame 97, and try again.

157c (from page 149, frame 99)
Not necessarily. If an MVV test is performed with quick, small tidal volumes it may be normal, even if the vital capacity is reduced by limited lung expansion. Please continue on page 152, frame 101.

157d (from page 147, frame 96)
Right. The greatest volume (70%) can be exhaled in the first 0.5 second of exhalation. By the end of 1 second, 83% is exhaled, and by 3 seconds, 97% of the vital capacity is exhaled. Please continue on page 147, frame 97.

FRAME 107. PALPATION

Palpation of the chest can be used to assess chest expansion, tactile fremitus, skin and subcutaneous tissues, and deformities of the thorax. To assess chest expansion place your thumbs along each costal margin toward the xiphoid process and your fingers along the lateral rib cage. On the posterior chest the hands are positioned over the eighth thoracic vertebra. With your thumbs touching after a normal breath, ask the patient to inhale deeply. With normal bilateral expansion, each thumb moves an equal distance from the midline (approximately 3 to 5 cm). Unilateral expansion is seen with lobar consolidation, pneumothorax, atelectasis, and pleural effusion. Diminished expansion on both sides may be the result of neuromuscular disease.

Tactile fremitus refers to vibrations caused by secretions in the airways that can be felt with your fingertips or the ulnar side of your hand when placed against the chest. Vibrations that are created by the vocal cords when the patient is asked to say "99" while the practitioner palpates the chest are called *vocal fremitus*. The flow of air through airways with thick secretions may produce vibrations referred to as *rhonchal fremitus*. A strong cough will often clear the airways of thick secretions and rhonchal fremitus will disappear. Increased tactile fremitus is caused by pneumonia, lung tumor, and atelectasis. Decreased unilateral tactile fremitus is caused by bronchial obstruction, pneumothorax, and pleural effusion. Diminished tactile fremitus is caused by chronic obstructive lung disease and muscular or obese chest wall.

Assessment of skin and subcutaneous tissues is done to check for tenderness, air leaks into subcutaneous tissues, and general condition and temperature of the skin. If air has leaked into the subcutaneous tissue, it will produce a crackling sound when palpated. An air leak into the tissue is called subcutaneous emphysema.

Finally palpation is done to confirm observations, such as suspected deviation of the trachea from the midline position. The trachea can be palpated by pressing the tip of a fully extended index finger into the suprasternal notch. The finger is used to gently probe downward toward the cervical spine touching both sides of trachea when it is midline. If the trachea is pushed over to one side or the other, the finger may not contact the trachea.

(Q) A patient with a pneumothorax is likely to have which of the following clinical signs determined by palpation?

a. increased unilateral tactile fremitus 162 C
b. unilateral reduction in chest expansion 163 D
c. palpation of a midline tracheal position 162 b
d. all of the above 163 a

FRAME 108. AUSCULTATION

In order to better understand abnormal (*adventitious*) breath sounds, you should first review normal (*vesicular*) breath sounds. Vesicular breath sounds, heard over the peripheral lung areas, are low pitched and soft. The inspiratory-to-expiratory (I:E) ratio of vesicular breath sounds heard over the periphery is 1:3. Bronchial breath sounds, heard over the major central airways, are high pitched and loud. The I:E ratio of bronchial breath sounds is 2:3. Breath sounds heard over the trachea are high pitched, very loud, and have an I:E ratio of 5:6. Bronchovesicular breath sounds are heard around the upper part of the sternum and between the scapulae. The pitch and intensity are moderate, and the I:E ratio is 1:1. Wheezes, rhonchi, and crackles are the terms that you should use to describe abnormal breath sounds. Bronchial breath sounds can be classified as abnormal when heard over the peripheral lung areas (Table 5–4).

TABLE 5–4
APPLICATION OF ADVENTITIOUS LUNG SOUNDS

LUNG SOUNDS	MECHANISM	CHARACTERISTICS	CAUSES
Wheezes	Rapid airflow through obstructed airways caused by bonchospasm, mucosal edema	High-pitched; most often occur during exhalation	Asthma, congestive heart failure
Rhonchi	Rapid airflow through obstructed airway caused by excess sputum, bronchospasm	Low-pitched; often occur during exhalation	Bronchitis, asthma
Crackles			
Inspiratory and expiratory	Excess airway secretions moving with airflow	Coarse and often clear with cough	Bronchitis, respiratory infections
Early inspiratory	Sudden opening of proximal bronchi	Scanty, transmitted to mouth; not affected by cough	Bronchitis, emphysema, asthma
Late inspiratory	Sudden opening of peripheral airways	Diffuse, fine; occur initially in the dependent regions	Atelectasis, pneumonia, pulmonary edema, fibrosis

Source: Wilkins, RL, Sheldon RL, and Krider SL: Clinical Assessment in Respiratory Care, ed2. CV Mosby, St. Louis, 1990. Used with permission.

(Q) Diffuse crackles heard over the dependent lung areas of the lung during late inspiration are usually associated with

a. atelectasis, pneumonia, pulmonary edema, fibrosis. 163 C
b. asthma and congestive heart failure. 162 D
c. bronchitis and asthma. 163 c
d. bronchitis and respiratory infections. 162 d

FRAME 109. PATIENT INTERVIEW

Respiratory care practitioners will be actively involved with assessment of patients each time a treatment is administered. The initial comprehensive physical examination and history will usually have been completed by a physician and can be obtained from the patient's chart. The *interval* assessments take the form of an interview with leading questions such as: "Are you feeling better?" "Raising more sputum?" "Has it been easier to cough?" "Do you get short of breath when lying flat?" "Did you sleep sitting up last night?" Attention should be given to changes that occur over these relatively short treatment-to-treatment intervals in order to determine changes in pulmonary function.

One critical finding is how well the patient can follow instructions and cooperate during treatments. Proof that the patient is alert includes the ability to recognize family and acknowledge their presence. However, even alert patients may become confused about their diagnosis and physician's name. Questions that even a confused patient may answer correctly are not very useful. Some things that will interfere with communication are language barrier, medical terminology, mental cognition (understanding), hearing and sight deficits, fear, anxiety, pain, emotional depression, and the influence of medications.

Dyspnea and cough are the chief respiratory complaints for 80% to 90% of patients seen by respiratory care practitioners. Other symptoms include chest pain or discomfort, sputum production, weight loss, hemoptysis, and peripheral edema. Questions related to cough and sputum production should always be asked, since it is important to determine if the cough is productive. The cough should be described in treatment notes in terms of its severity, length, frequency, triggering factors, effect of body position, and type and volume of sputum raised.

Dyspnea is a symptom that only the patient can tell you about; however it should be classified using a scale such as the one described below. To classify the patient's dyspnea (Table 5–5), you will have to ask questions about his or her exercise tolerance and daily living activities.

TABLE 5–5
CLASSIFICATION OF DYSPNEA BY DEGREES OF SEVERITY

Class I	Class II	Class III	Class IV	Class V
Dyspnea only on severe exertion (appropriate)	Can keep pace with person of the same age and body build on the level without breathlessness but not on hills or stairs	Can walk a mile at own pace without dyspnea, but cannot keep pace on the level with a normal person	Dyspnea present after walking about 100 yards on the level or upon climbing one flight of stairs	Dyspnea on even less activity, or even at rest

Source: Burton, GG and Hodgkin, JE: A Guide to Clinical Practice, ed 2. JB Lippincott, Philadelphia, 1984. Used with permission.

(Q) Which of the following will be best to determine a patient's orientation to time, place, and person?

a. Patient recognizes that he or she is in a hospital. 164 A
b. Patient responds to and speaks with relatives. 164 B
c. Patient knows his or her physician's name. 162 c
d. Patient is able to indicate that he or she is in pain. 163 d

FRAME 110. MAXIMUM INSPIRATORY PRESSURE AND PEAK EXPIRATORY FLOW

Maximum Inspiratory Pressure Maximum inspiratory pressure (MIP) along with vital capacity is used to evaluate inspiratory muscle strength. It is used to determine if the patient needs to be mechanically ventilated, especially when it is impossible or difficult to measure the VC. A pressure manometer is placed proximal to the tracheal tube, mask, or mouthpiece, occluding the airway for about 20 seconds. The patient will generate pressure during inspiratory attempts, which should be observed and recorded. Since this procedure may be uncomfortable and frightening, it should be carefully explained to the patient regardless of his or her level of consciousness. The MIP is recorded and used to estimate muscle strength and VC. For example, an MIP of 20 cm H_2O is usually associated with a patient's capability to generate a VC of 15 mL/kg or higher. An MIP within 20 seconds of 20 to 25 cm H_2O indicates that a patient is ready to be weaned from mechanical ventilation. A normal MIP within 20 seconds is 80 cm H_2O. A patient suspected of gradually losing inspiratory muscle strength (as with myasthenia gravis) may have MIP or VC measured serially at specific intervals to evaluate loss of inspiratory reserve volume.

Peak Expiratory Flow The peak expiratory flow (PEF) is the maximum flow that can be achieved by the patient during a forced expiration. It is useful for evaluating the effectiveness of a bronchodilator therapy. An increase in PEF of 20% or more usually indicates a substantial reduction in small airway obstruction. A more sensitive and reliable test is the volume of gas forcibly exhaled in 1 second (FEV_1). However, the PEF can be easily and quickly done and is often used at the bedside, in the emergency room, or in the patient's home for a quick assessment of small airway obstruction. A normal healthy subject can generate a PEF of 400 to 600 L/min; the PEF of a patient with an obstruction may be reduced to 300 L/min or less.

(Q) Which of the following bedside diagnostic procedures indicates that a patient may require mechanical ventilation?

a. an MIP within 20 seconds of 30 cm H_2O 165 A
b. a PEF of 7 L/s 164 C
c. an MIP within 20 seconds of 15 cm H_2O 164 a

FRAME 111. CALCULATING MINUTE VOLUME

To determine the amount of air that a patient breathes per minute you multiply the patient's average V_T by the number of respirations per minute. For example, if V_T is tidal volume, f is respirations per minute, and $\dot{V}_E$ is the minute volume, where V_T = 450 mL, f = 12/min, calculate $\dot{V}_E$.

$$\dot{V}_E = (V_T)\,(f)$$
$$\dot{V}_E = (450\text{ mL})\,(12/\text{min})$$
$$\dot{V}_E = 5400\text{ mL/min}$$

(Q) If a patient has a tidal volume of 300 mL and a minute volume of 10.5 L, what is the respiratory rate per minute?

a. 12/min 165 B
b. 21/min 165 a
c. 35/min 165 b

162A (from page 154, frame 105)
Wrong. If the patient can cough, the upper airway cannot be completely obstructed. Often coughing clears the bolus or foreign body obstructing the airway. Return to page 154, frame 105, and try again.

162B (from page 155, frame 106)
Wrong. The sputum associated with bronchial asthma is described as mucoid (white or clear). Return to page 155, frame 106, and try again.

162C (from page 158, frame 107)
Wrong. A pneumothorax would cause decreased unilateral tactile fremitus. Return to page 158, frame 107, and select another answer.

162D (from page 159, frame 108)
Wrong. Wheezes are associated with asthma and congestive heart failure. Review Table 5–4 on page 159, frame 108, and select another answer.

162a (from page 155, frame 106)
Correct. The sputum associated with bronchiectasis is described as purulent (yellow or green), fetid, and bloody. Please continue on page 158, frame 107.

162b (from page 158, frame 107)
Wrong. A pneumothorax may cause the trachea to be shifted away from the midline. Return to page 158, frame 107, and select another answer.

162c (from page 160, frame 109)
Wrong. While it is true that a patient who knows his or her physician's name may be alert, other patients who are oriented to time, place, and person may simply forget the name of the attending physician—especially if the physician is hospital based and recently assigned to the case. Return to 160, frame 109, and select another answer.

162d (from page 159, frame 108)
Wrong. Crackles during both inspiration and expiration are associated with bronchitis and respiratory infections. Review Table 5–4 on page 159, frame 108, and try again.

163A (from page 155, frame 106)
Wrong. The sputum associated with pulmonary edema is described as bloody, frothy, and sometimes pink. Return to page 155, frame 106, and try again.

163B (from page 154, frame 105)
Wrong. Accessory muscles are normally used during exercise and while they may be used when a victim tries to clear an upper airway obstruction, this is not the best answer. Return to page 154, frame 105, and select another answer.

163C (from page 159, frame 108)
Yes, diffuse crackles heard over dependent areas are associated with atelectasis, pneumonia, pulmonary edema, and fibrosis. Please continue on page 160, frame 109.

163D (from page 158, frame 107)
Correct. A pneumothorax may cause unilateral reduction in chest expansion, decreased tactile fremitus, and a shift of the trachea from midline. Please continue on page 159, frame 108.

163a (from page 158, frame 107)
Wrong. A pneumothorax will not have all three of the clinical signs mentioned. Return to page 158, frame 107, and select another answer.

163b (from page 155, frame 106)
Wrong. The sputum associatd with cystic fibrosis is described as mucopurulent and has a fetid odor. Return to page 155, frame 106, study Table 5-3, and select another answer.

163c (from page 159, frame 108)
Wrong. Rhonchi are associated with bronchitis and asthma. Review Table 5–4 on page 159, frame 108, and select another answer.

163d (from page 160, frame 109)
Wrong. This is not a good indicator of a patient's orientation to time, place, and person. A patient may be able to tell you about his or her pain and still be too confused to follow instructions and cooperate during a treatment. Return to page 160, frame 109, and select another answer.

164A (from page 160, frame 109)
Wrong. Even a disoriented patient may be able to determine that he or she is in a hospital. Return to page 160, frame 109, and select another answer.

164B (from page 160, frame 109)
Correct. A patient who can recognize and respond to questions from family members is usually alert and oriented to time, place, and person. Please continue on page 161, frame 110.

164C (from page 161, frame 110)
Wrong. A peak expiratory flow of 7 L/s is equivalent to 420 L/min and the normal range is 400 to 600 L/min. Return to page 161, frame 110, and select another answer.

164a (from page 161, frame 110)
Correct. A maximum inspiratory pressure of less than 20 cm H_2O is associated with a VC of less than 15 mL/kg ideal body weight. This means that the patient does not have enough respiratory muscle strength to provide adequate spontaneous ventilation and a ventilator is indicated. Please continue on page 161, frame 111.

164b (from page 166, frame 112)
Wrong. The Pao_2 would have to be above 110 torr to be considered overly corrected hypoxemia. The primary acid-base disturbance is to the respiratory system. Return to page 166, frame 112, and try again.

164c (from page 166, frame 112)
Wrong. The Pao_2 would have to be between 40 to 60 torr to be considered moderate hypoxemia. The pH is outside the normal range, indicating that complete compensation has not occurred. Return to page 166, frame 112, and select another answer.

165A (from page 161, frame 110)
Careful. An MIP greater than 25 cm H_2O usually is associated with a vital capacity of 15 mL/kg ideal body weight. This means that the patient has enough respiratory muscle strength to provide adequate ventilation. Return to page 161, frame 110, and select another answer.

165B (from page 161, frame 111)
Wrong. To arrive at the right answer you must isolate the respiratory rate (f) on one side of the equation. Return to page 161, frame 111, check your math, and then select another answer.

165C (from page 166, frame 112)
Yes. The Pa_{O_2} indicates mild hypoxemia and the acid-base status is partially compensated respiratory acidosis. Please continue on page 167 and complete the chapter exercises.

165a (from page 161, frame 111)
Wrong. In order to arrive at the right answer you must isolate the respiratory frequency on one side of the equation. Check your math, then return to page 161, frame 111, and select another answer.

165b (from page 161, frame 111)
Correct. The respiratory rate is determined by dividing the tidal volume into the minute volume; for example, $f = \frac{10{,}500 \text{ mL/min}}{300 \text{ mL}} = 35/\text{min}$. Please continue on page 166, frame 112.

165c (from page 166, frame 112)
Wrong. The Pa_{O_2} would have to be lower than 40 torr to be considered severe hypoxemia, and the pH would have to be higher than 7.45 for this disturbance to be considered an alkalosis. Return to page 166, frame 112, and select another answer.

FRAME 112. BLOOD-GAS INTERPRETATION

A blood-gas study can be used to evaluate a patient's oxygenation and acid-base status. The oxygenation state can be classified as *overly corrected hypoxemia* ($Pa_{O_2} \geq 110$ torr), *normal* ($Pa_{O_2} = 80$ to 110 torr), *mild hypoxemia* ($Pa_{O_2} = 60$ to 80 torr), *moderate hypoxemia* ($Pa_{O_2} = 40$ to 60 torr), and *severe hypoxemia* ($Pa_{O_2} < 40$ torr). The Pa_{O_2} range is lowered 10 torr for each decade over 60 years of age.

A patient's acid-base status can be described as one of four major categories: respiratory acidosis, respiratory alkalosis, metabolic acidosis, or metabolic alkalosis (Table 5–6). The primary disturbance to acid-base balance may be completely or partially compensated by the unaffected process. For example, the respiratory system tries to compensate for a low pH caused by metabolic acidosis by hyperventilation. The renal system compensates for a primary respiratory disturbance to acid-base balance by increasing or decreasing the concentration of bicarbonate (HCO_3^-). Compensation is considered complete if the pH is moved into the normal range of 7.35 to 7.45. Partial compensation occurs when the pH is moved back toward normal but remains outside the normal range.

(Q) What is the oxygenation and acid-base status if $F_{IO_2} = 0.40$, $Pa_{O_2} = 70$ torr, $Pa_{CO_2} = 80$ torr, pH = 7.20, $HCO_3^- = 28$ mEq/L?

a. overly corrected hypoxemia, uncompensated metablic acidosis 164 b
b. moderate hypoxemia, compensated respiratory acidosis 164 c
c. mild hypoxemia, partially compensated respiratory acidosis 165 C
d. severe hypoxemia, partially compensated metabolic alkalosis 165 c

TABLE 5–6
ACID-BASE STATES

	Pa_{CO_2}	HCO_3^-	pH
I. Primary			
Respiratory			
Acidosis	↑	N	↓
Alkalosis	↓	N	↑
Metabolic			
Acidosis	N	↓	↓
Alkalosis	N	↑	↑
II. Compensatory			
Partially compensated			
Respiratory			
Acidosis	↑	↑	↓
Alkalosis	↓	↓	↑
Metabolic			
Acidosis	↓	↓	↓
Alkalosis	↑	↑	↑
Fully compensated			
Respiratory			
Acidosis	↑	↑	N
Alkalosis	↓	↓	N
Metabolic			
Acidosis	↓	↓	N
Alkalosis	↑	↑	N

EXERCISES

1. Draw a sample spirogram for a forced vital capacity and label tidal volume, inspiratory capacity, inspiratory reserve volume, vital capacity, expiratory reserve volume, and the point-of-peak expiratory flow.
2. List five modalities of respiratory care that would be ordered based on chest x-ray reports.
3. List 10 common diagnostic tests ordered for pulmonary patients.
4. Diagram the following breathing patterns: Biot's, cluster, Cheyne-Stokes, apneustic, Kussmaul's, ataxic, eupnea, tachypnea, bradypnea, hypopnea, and hyperpnea.
5. Identify the gas law that helps to explain why the Heimlich maneuver is so successful.
6. List the different colors that may be observed in the sputum of pulmonary patients and describe the pulmonary diseases associated with each color.
7. Compare and contrast the differences between vesicular and adventitious breath sounds that may be heard over peripheral areas of the lung.
8. Describe how subcutaneous emphysema feels when a practitioner palpates an affected area.
9. Practice patient interviewing by checking how quickly you can identify three barriers to communication that a friend simulates. Next, switch roles with your friend using three different barriers to communication.
10. Describe what you will say to a patient to obtain the best effort on a timed vital capacity test.

POSTTEST

This test is designed to evaluate what you have learned from completing Chapter 5. Check your answers on page 170 and review the topics where your answer is incorrect.

1. All of the following should be included in a physician's order for respiratory care *except*
   A. frequency of treatment.
   B. dosage for aerosol medications.
   C. oxygen concentration.
   D. duration of treatment.
   E. type of equipment.
2. A change of ventilation parameters may affect which of the following?
   A. inspiratory time
   B. expiratory time
   C. mean intrathoracic pressure
   D. peak inspiratory flow
   E. all of the above
3. All of the following are associated with the obstructive pattern of pulmonary disease *except*
   A. TLC—50% of predicted.
   B. FRC—150% of predicted.
   C. RV—150% of predicted.
   D. ERV—50% of predicted.
   E. IC—50% of predicted.
4. Which of the following is best to confirm asymmetrical chest expansion?
   A. chest x-ray
   B. palpation
   C. arterial blood-gas study
   D. thoracentesis
   E. timed vital capacity
5. Subcutaneous emphysema can be diagnosed most definitively by
   A. auscultation.
   B. inspection.
   C. palpation.
   D. measurement of $FEV_1/FVC\%$.
   E. none of the above.
6. Which of the following are associated with normal *bronchial* breath sounds?
   I. I:E ratio of 2:3
   II. I:E ratio of 1:3
   III. low pitched and soft
   IV. harsh and loud
   V. high pitched and loud
   A. I and III only
   B. II and III only
   C. I and V only
   D. IV and V only
   E. II and IV only

7. Bronchovesicular breath sounds are heard
   A. over the lung periphery.
   B. over the trachea.
   C. between the scapulae.
   D. over the upper part of the sternum.
   E. over the lower part of the sternum.

8. Which of the following is associated with apneustic breathing?
   A. lesion in the medulla
   B. lesion in the lower pontile area
   C. lesion in central chemoreceptors
   D. lesion in peripheral chemoreceptors
   E. all of the above

9. When performing the Heimlich maneuver the rescuer's fist is placed
   A. above the victim's navel.
   B. below the victim's navel.
   C. over the xiphoid process.
   D. over the middle of the sternum.
   E. to either side of the xiphoid process.

10. Sputum that is mucopurulent and fetid is associated with
    A. streptococcal pneumonia.
    B. staphylococcal pneumonia.
    C. cystic fibrosis.
    D. bronchiectasis.
    E. pneumococcal pneumonia.

11. The best description of sputum from a patient with bronchial asthma is
    A. mucoid, white or clear.
    B. mucopurulent and yellow-green color.
    C. thin and blood streaked.
    D. blood-rust color.
    E. frothy, thin, and pink color.

12. Low-pitched, continuous breath sounds caused by rapid airflow through partially obstructed airways and occurring during exhalation are best described as
    A. rhonchi.
    B. crackles.
    C. sibilant rales.
    D. musical rales.
    E. crepitations.

13. High-pitched, continuous breath sounds caused by rapid airflow through partially obstructed airways caused by bronchospasm and mucosal edema are best described as
    A. rhonchi.
    B. crackles.
    C. sonorous rhonchi.
    D. crepitations.
    E. wheezes.

14. When you assess chest expansion by palpation, each thumb should move an equal distance from midline of
   A. 1 to 2 cm.
   B. 2 to 3 cm.
   C. 3 to 5 cm.
   D. 7 to 10 cm.
   E. 9 to 12 cm.
15. Which of the following is *least* likely to interfere with communication during a patient interview?
   A. hunger
   B. fear
   C. sight deficit
   D. hearing deficit
   E. medical terminology
16. A vital capacity that is greater than 15 mL/kg is associated with the capability to generate a maximum inspiratory pressure of
   A. 10 cm H_2O.
   B. 20 cm H_2O.
   C. 30 cm H_2O.
   D. 50 cm H_2O.
   E. 80 cm H_2O.
17. The normal range of peak expiratory flow is
   A. 50 to 100 L/min.
   B. 100 to 200 L/min.
   C. 200 to 300 L/min.
   D. 300 to 400 L/min.
   E. 400 to 600 L/min.
18. What is the tidal volume if the $\dot{V}_E$ = 12 L/min and f = 30/min?
   A. 250 mL
   B. 300 mL
   C. 400 mL
   D. 500 mL
   E. 750 mL
19. Severe hypoxemia is associated with a Pa_{O_2} of
   A. 35 torr.
   B. 45 torr.
   C. 65 torr.
   D. 80 torr.
   E. 90 torr.
20. What is the acid-base status of the patient if pH = 7.15, Pa_{CO_2} = 50 torr, HCO_3^- = 16 mEq/L?
   A. partially compensated respiratory acidosis
   B. compensated respiratory acidosis
   C. partially compensated metabolic acidosis
   D. compensated metabolic acidosis
   E. respiratory and metabolic acidosis

ANSWERS TO POSTTEST

1. D (F93)	5. C (F107)	9. A (F105)	13. E (F108)	17. E (F110)
2. E (F94)	6. C (F108)	10. C (F106)	14. C (F107)	18. C (F111)
3. A (F100)	7. C (F108)	11. A (F106)	15. A (F109)	19. A (F112)
4. B (F107)	8. B (F104)	12. A (F108)	16. B (F110)	20. E (F112)

BIBILIOGRAPHY

Barnes, TA: Respiratory Care Practice. Year Book Medical Publishers, Chicago, 1988.

Bates, B: A Guide to Physical Examination and History Taking, ed 4. JB Lippincott, Philadelphia, 1987.

Burton, GG and Hodgkin, JE: Respiratory Care: A Guide to Clinical Practice, ed 2. JB Lippincott, Philadelphia, 1984.

Kacmarek, RM, Dimas, S, and Mack, CW: Essentials of Respiratory Therapy, ed 2. Year Book Medical Publishers, Chicago, 1985.

Kacmarek, RM and Stoller, JK: Current Respiratory Care. BC Decker, Philadelphia, 1989.

Ruppel, G: Manual of Pulmonary Function Testing, ed 4. CV Mosby, St. Louis, 1986.

Scanlon, C, Spearman, CB, Sheldon, RL, and Egan, DF: Egan's Fundamentals of Respiratory Therapy, ed 5. CV Mosby, St. Louis, 1990.

Shapiro, BA, Harrison, RA, Kacmarek, RM, and Cane, RD: Clinical Application of Respiratory Care, ed 3. Year Book Medical Publishers, Chicago, 1985.

Shapiro, BA, Harrison, RA, Templin, RK, and Walton, JR: Clinical Application of Blood Gases, ed 4. Year Book Medical Publishers, Chicago, 1988.

Wilkins, RL, Sheldon, RL, and Krider, SJ: Clinical Assessment in Respiratory Care, ed 2. CV Mosby, St. Louis, 1990.

6

Oxygen Therapy

113. Low-flow oxygen therapy
114. High-flow oxygen therapy
115. PEEP and CPAP
116. FIO_2 during mechanical ventilation
117. Practitioner-induced hypoxemia
118. Helium-oxygen therapy
119. Positioning patients to minimize hypoxemia
120. Indications for oxygen therapy
121. Patient response to oxygen therapy
122. Hazards of oxygen therapy

PRETEST

This pretest is designed to measure what you already know about oxygen therapy. Check your answers on page 175 and then continue on page 176, frame 113.

1. All of the following are examples of low-flow oxygen therapy devices *except*
   A. nasal cannula.
   B. simple mask.
   C. rebreathing mask.
   D. Venturi mask.
   E. face tent.
2. Which of the following statements about low-flow oxygen therapy devices is/are true?
   I. Oxygen is delivered at a fixed FIO_2.
   II. Oxygen is delivered at a variable FIO_2.
   III. Gas flow matches the patient's peak inspiratory flow rate.
   A. I only.
   B. II only.
   C. III only.
   D. I and II only.
   E. II and III only.
3. All of the following are examples of high-flow oxygen therapy devices *except*
   A. air-entrainment mainstream nebulizer.
   B. Venturi mask.
   C. rebreathing mask.
   D. continuous-flow intermittent mandatory ventilation (IMV).
   E. oxygen blender.
4. Venturi masks can deliver oxygen concentrations that have a range of
   A. 0.24 to 0.30.
   B. 0.24 to 0.40.
   C. 0.24 to 0.50.
   D. 0.24 to 0.60.
   E. 0.24 to 0.80.
5. Continuous positive-airway pressure (CPAP) or positive end-expiratory pressure (PEEP) improves oxygenation by
   A. increasing vital capacity.
   B. increasing functional residual capacity.
   C. decreasing residual volume.
   D. decreasing FVC.
   E. increasing FEV_1.
6. Which of the following is an indication that *optimal* PEEP may have been exceeded?
   A. PaO_2 does not continue to increase.
   B. Intrapulmonary shunting decreases.
   C. Cardiac output decreases slightly.
   D. Static compliance increases.
   E. Dynamic compliance increases.

7. Until the level of hypoxemia is determined, the initial F_{IO_2} for a ventilator patient should be
   A. 0.21.
   B. 0.30.
   C. 0.40.
   D. 0.50.
   E. 1.00.

8. Which of the following changes should be made for a 60 kg ventilator patient if $F_{IO_2} = 0.60$, PEEP = 5 cm H_2O, V_T = 900 mL, SIMV = 10/min, Pa_{O_2} = 50 torr, Pa_{CO_2} = 38 torr, pH = 7.35?
   A. Increase F_{IO_2} to 0.70.
   B. Increase F_{IO_2} to 0.60.
   C. Increase V_T to 1000 mL.
   D. Increase PEEP to 10 cm H_2O.
   E. Increase PEEP to 15 cm H_2O.

9. Prior to tracheal suctioning, which of the following should be done?
   A. Reinflate the cuff of the tracheal tube.
   B. Manually ventilate the patient with 100% oxygen.
   C. Place patient in a Fowler's position.
   D. Instill 25 mL H_2O into the tracheal tube.
   E. Pull tracheal tube back 0.5 inch.

10. Which of the following is a clinical sign that a patient has become hypoxemic during suctioning of his endotracheal tube?
    A. coughing episode
    B. hypopnea
    C. eupnea
    D. premature ventricular contractions
    E. restlessness

11. An oxygen flowmeter that reads 8 L/min when attached to 70%–30% helium-oxygen will deliver a flow of
    A. 4 L/min.
    B. 6 L/min.
    C. 8 L/min.
    D. 12 L/min.
    E. 14 L/min.

12. Which of the following would be best for administering a 70%–30% helium-oxygen mixture?
    A. nasal cannula
    B. simple face mask
    C. Venturi mask
    D. rebreathing mask
    E. non-rebreathing mask

13. A patient with frank fulminating pulmonary edema will be most comfortable in which of the following positions?
    A. supine
    B. prone
    C. Fowler's
    D. semi-Fowler's
    E. Trendelenburg's

14. Patients with chronic obstructive lung disease will tend to lean forward supporting their scapulae and upper chest with fixed arms in order to
   A. cough more effectively.
   B. use accessory muscles more effectively.
   C. increase diaphragmatic excursion.
   D. stabilize intercostal muscles.
   E. stabilize abdominal muscles.
15. Postoperative patients without chronic obstructive pulmonary disease, should have their arterial oxygen tension held at a level that does not drop below a minimum of
   A. 40 torr.
   B. 50 torr.
   C. 60 torr.
   D. 80 torr.
   E. 100 torr.
16. All of the following are clinical signs that the cardiovascular system is compensating for hypoxemia *except*
   A. tachycardia.
   B. hypotension.
   C. hypertension.
   D. decreased urine output.
   E. decreased skin temperature.
17. All of the following are clinical signs of a positive response to oxygen therapy *except*
   A. normal blood pressure.
   B. warm extremities.
   C. $P\bar{v}O_2$ of 30 torr.
   D. PaO_2 of 90 torr.
   E. improved cognition.
18. A patient who has a PaO_2 of 60 torr and a P_{50} of 27 torr will have a SaO_2 that is
   A. 60%.
   B. 75%.
   C. 80%.
   D. 90%.
   E. 100%.
19. If a chronic obstructive pulmonary disease (COPD) patient (with average weight and height, and a respiratory rate of 20/min) is given 4 L/min of oxygen by nasal cannula, what minute volume should be expected?
   A. 3 L/min
   B. 6 L/min
   C. 8 L/min
   D. 10 L/min
   E. 12 L/min
20. To prevent a toxic response to oxygen, FIO_2 should be below
   A. 0.40.
   B. 0.50.
   C. 0.60.
   D. 0.80.
   E. 1.00.

ANSWERS TO PRETEST

1. D (F113)
2. B (F113)
3. C (F114)
4. C (F114)
5. B (F115)
6. A (F115)
7. E (F116)
8. D (F116)
9. B (F117)
10. D (F117)
11. D (F118)
12. E (F118)
13. C (F119)
14. B (F119)
15. C (F120)
16. B (F120)
17. C (F121)
18. D (F121)
19. A (F122)
20. B (F122)

FRAME 113. LOW-FLOW OXYGEN THERAPY

Oxygen should be delivered in high, moderate, or low concentrations, dependent upon the deficit generated by the disease pathology. The same oxygen concentration used for two different patients may offer one patient complete relief from hypoxemia but produce no beneficial effect in the other.

The decision to administer oxygen must be made by a physician, but she or he may rely upon the respiratory care practitioner for a recommendation on the most effective means of administering oxygen. Oxygen therapy delivery devices are grouped into categories based on their performance characteristics: (1) low flow (variable F_{IO_2}) and (2) high flow (fixed F_{IO_2}). Low-flow devices supply oxygen that is only a portion of all inspired gas. Changes in the size of the tidal and minute volumes and pattern of ventilation will result in variable amounts of room air being mixed with oxygen, and the F_{IO_2} delivered will vary. High-flow devices flood the face with oxygen and prevent air dilution. Thus high-flow devices deliver a preset inspired oxygen concentration that is *not affected* by ventilatory patterns.

One of the most commonly used low-flow oxygen therapy devices is the nasal cannula, a flexible plastic tube with two short extensions that direct oxygen into the nasal pharynx. It is lightweight, easily disposed of, and economical. Maintenance consists of keeping the nasal prongs clean and inserted about 0.5 in into the nares. For patients who need low oxygen concentrations the nasal cannula is a good choice since it is comfortable, easy to place, unconfining, and allows the patient to eat and speak. The major disadvantage is that the inspired oxygen concentration will drop if the patient breathes at a high frequency or gasps for breath. The nasal cannula is used frequently for long-term oxygen therapy with chronic obstructive pulmonary disease (COPD) patients. Some COPD patients retain CO_2 and tend to hypoventilate on high oxygen concentrations but still need supplemental oxygen because of their chronic hypoxemia. The oxygen flow to a nasal cannula for COPD patients who have chronic hypercarbia is usually held to 1 or 2 L/min or less, since their respiratory rate is controlled by a hypoxic drive. Thus giving a COPD patient too much oxygen may result in hypoventilation.

Other low-flow oxygen therapy devices include the simple mask, nasal or tracheal catheters, partial rebreathing mask, and non-rebreathing mask. All of these devices deliver an F_{IO_2} that will vary because of a poor sealing system, variable tidal and minute volumes, low gas flow, or small oxygen reservoir. Oxygen therapy equipment is covered in more detail in Chapter 13.

(Q) Which of the following would be best for a COPD patient for long-term oxygen therapy at home?

a. low-flow oxygen therapy 180 A
b. high-flow oxygen therapy 181 B
c. nasal cannula at 4 L/min 184 A

FRAME 114. HIGH-FLOW OXYGEN THERAPY

The concept behind most high-flow (fixed-performance) oxygen masks is to flood the area around the nose and mouth with gas of a constant F_{IO_2} (Fig. 6–1). The high flow allows the device to meet the inspiratory demand of patients with high respiratory rates and large tidal volumes. The air-entrainment mask is an example of a high-flow device that delivers high total flow by mixing oxygen with entrained air. These masks can deliver oxygen concentrations from 0.24 to 0.50 with a total flow that varies from 33 L/min (F_{IO_2} of 0.50) to 97 L/min (F_{IO_2} of 0.24). An air-driven aerosol can be added to the entrained air to raise the absolute humidity of the inspired gas.

Other high-flow oxygen therapy devices include large-volume nebulizers that provide bland aerosol therapy with some control of the oxygen concentration of the output gas at fixed F_{IO_2} settings (e.g., 0.40, 0.70, 1.00) or are continuously adjustable from 0.30 to 1.00. When higher oxygen concentrations are used, the amount of air dilution is less and total flow drops substantially. For example, when input flow is 15 L/min, the total output flow at 0.40, 0.60, and 0.70 is 63, 30, and 25 L/min, respectively. Thus patients with high inspiratory flow rates may have a much lower F_{IO_2} when nebulizers are set above 0.40 (total flow to the face is decreased). Downstream resistance to output flow such as condensate in lazy loops may cause back pressure, which diminishes the air entrainment and thus raises the F_{IO_2} and lowers total output flow.

(Q) If a severely dyspneic patient has a respiratory rate of 40/min, which of the following oxygen devices is most likely to deliver an F_{IO_2} approaching 0.60 if the input oxygen flow is 15 L/min?

a. mainstream nebulizer set at 100% oxygen 181 A
b. mainstream nebulizer set at 60% oxygen 180 B
c. neither *a* nor *b* 185 A

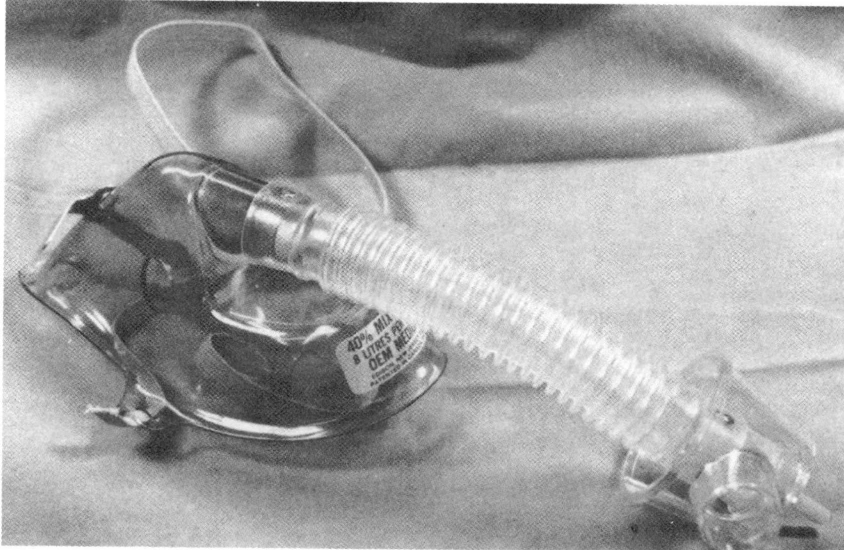

Figure 6–1 Venturi mask with fixed F_{IO_2} with aerosol adapter attached. (Source: Barnes, TA: Respiratory Care Practice. Year Book Medical Publishers, Chicago, 1988. Used with permission.)

FRAME 115. PEEP AND CPAP

Positive end-expiratory pressure (PEEP) and continuous positive-airway pressure (CPAP) are important modalities of respiratory care, which reverse small airway and alveolar collapse. The application of a baseline positive-airway pressure greater than atmospheric pressure to a patient being mechanically ventilated is called PEEP, and when applied to spontaneously breathing patients (without assisted breaths) it is called CPAP. In both applications the principle is the same—oxygenation is improved by increasing the functional residual capacity (FRC).

PEEP or CPAP should be adjusted to a level called *optimal* PEEP. Providing optimal levels of PEEP or CPAP may allow a lower inspired oxygen concentration to be used. In an adult a minimum of 3 to 5 cm H_2O of PEEP will usually be indicated for use when a patient is intubated, since the endotracheal tube holds the larynx constantly open, which leads to some alveolar collapse and reduction in FRC. The safe way to arrive at the optimal level is to start with a baseline of zero and add PEEP or CPAP in 3 to 5 cm H_2O increments while monitoring the criteria used to determine the greatest improvement in oxygen transport. The criteria used to determine the optimal level of end expiratory pressure are (1) substantial improvement in arterial oxygen tension, (2) reduction of intrapulmonary shunt, and (3) minimal reduction in cardiac output (there should be no significant drop in blood pressure). The optimal PEEP or CPAP level will be reached when higher levels of PEEP result in large drops in cardiac output or no substantial change in arterial oxygen tension or shunt is observed.

An alternative method for determining optimal PEEP and CPAP is to measure improvement in static compliance as higher levels are applied. If the compliance does not increase or decreases, the PEEP or CPAP should be lowered to the previous level.

Higher levels of PEEP may be able to be applied with ventilator patients who have pulmonary edema and adult respiratory distress syndrome (ARDS). The extrapulmonary fluid makes the lung wet and heavy and insulates the circulation from increased mean intrathoracic pressure. Other injuries that leave the lungs wet and heavy include left heart failure and chest trauma. Also, for patients receiving high concentrations of oxygen, optimal PEEP or CPAP levels may allow a lower F_{IO_2} to be used. Patients with a flail chest and paradoxical breathing may also benefit from PEEP, which internally splints their chest in a position of function by increasing the FRC.

(Q) Which of the following indicates that PEEP is higher than optimal?

a. Compliance is increased at this level. 184 B
b. Arterial oxygen tension is higher at this level. 185 C
c. Cardiac output decreases substantially at this level. 180 D

FRAME 116. FIO_2 DURING MECHANICAL VENTILATION

Inspired oxygen concentration during mechanical ventilation should be lowered at the first opportunity to minimize the risk of a toxic response to oxygen, which is related to the length of exposure and the partial pressure of oxygen. Patients exposed to a high FIO_2 (>0.50) may develop substernal pain, a nonproductive cough, and a change in breathing pattern. After a long exposure to high concentrations of oxygen (18 to 24 hours and longer), increased lung water may cause a drop in compliance, an increase in right-to-left shunting, and atelectasis. However, until the level of hypoxemia is determined, a patient should receive 100% oxygen.

The FIO_2 should be lowered as soon as possible but dropped in small increments to ensure that the arterial oxygen tension does not drop below 80 torr and arterial saturation is maintained at ≥90%. If the FIO_2 is greater than 0.50, and the disease process has caused generalized intrapulmonary shunting, applying PEEP or increasing its level may allow the FIO_2 to be maintained at a lower level. Once the patient's cardiovascular system is stable, the use of large tidal volumes (15 mL/kg) will help to improve alveolar ventilation.

(Q) Which of the following ventilator changes for a 60 kg patient should be made if $FIO_2 = 0.60$, $PaO_2 = 100$ torr, $PaCO_2 = 36$ torr, $V_T = 900$ mL?

a. $V_T = 1000$ mL, $FIO_2 = 0.70$ 181 C
b. $V_T = 800$ mL, $FIO_2 = 0.40$, PEEP = 10 cm H_2O 184 C
c. $V_T = 900$ mL, $FIO_2 = 0.50$, PEEP = 5 cm H_2O 185 a

FRAME 117. PRACTITIONER-INDUCED HYPOXEMIA

There are respiratory care procedures that may cause hypoxemia if the practitioner does not take preventive action. For example, suctioning secretions from a patient's tracheal tube will also remove oxygen and may cause severe hypoxemia. The hypoxemia may cause premature ventricular contractions, which could lead to ventricular fibrillation (ineffective contractions of the heart). When the heart is fibrillating, blood is *not* pumped from the heart and death may occur (if the patient is not defibrillated). To prevent hypoxemia the patient should always be administered 100% oxygen before and after tracheal suctioning, and monitored for premature ventricular contractions, bradycardia, and hypotension.

Ventilator patients receiving high oxygen concentrations and PEEP are especially at risk of hypoxemia during suctioning. Studies have shown that hypoxemia can develop within 4 minutes if PEEP is removed. Accordingly, when patients are suctioned or when the breathing circuit is changed, they should be manually ventilated with the PEEP valve attached to the exhalation port and with a high oxygen concentration.

(Q) During a ventilator check every 2 hours, the practitioner notes that the ventilator is delivering only 50% of the preset tidal volume. Which of the following actions should be done *first*?

a. Increase tidal volume by 50%. 180 a
b. Remove patient from ventilator and manually ventilate. 181 D
c. Quickly check for large leaks in the breathing circuit. 185 b

180A (from page 176, frame 113)
Correct. Low-flow oxygen therapy devices, such as a nasal cannula, are good choices for long-term oxygen therapy for COPD patients. The need for low-flow oxygen therapy devices is easily met and acceptance is high because they are comfortable. Please continue on page 177, frame 114.

180B (from page 177, frame 114)
Wrong. The total flow will only be 30 L/min and a dyspneic patient's inspiratory flow is often much higher. Thus, air will mix with the output from the nebulizer and lower the FIO_2. Return to page 177, frame 114, and try again.

180C (from page 186, frame 121)
Wrong. A normal $P\bar{v}O_2$ is 40 torr, and it is unlikely that a value of 70 torr would be seen. High inspired oxygen concentrations increase arterial oxygen content by only a very small increment. Return to page 186, frame 121, and select another answer.

180D (from page 178, frame 115)
Correct. A large drop in cardiac output indicates that you have gone higher than the optimal PEEP level and should return to the previous lower level. You would also expect to see little improvement in arterial oxygen tension or a decrease in right-to-left shunt. Also, static compliance will not be increased when compared with the previous PEEP level. Please continue on page 179, frame 116.

180a (from page 179, frame 117)
Wrong. This may not solve the problem if there is a large leak in the circuit. Return to page 179, frame 117, and select another answer.

180b (from page 182, frame 119)
Wrong. This would not help to retard venous return to the heart and may lead to pulmonary edema. Return to page 182, frame 119, and select another answer.

180c (from page 187, frame 122)
Wrong. Symptoms include substernal pain, cough, dyspnea, anxiety, and fatigue, but not necessarily somnolence. Return to page 187, frame 122, and select another answer.

180d (from page 186, frame 121)
Careful. This is the way a patient with chronic pulmonary disease, breathing on a hypoxic drive, would respond if a high concentration of oxygen were administered. Return to page 186, frame 121, and try again.

181A (from page 177, frame 114)
Wrong. Total flow will be only 15 L/min, which means air will mix with oxygen and lower the F_{IO_2} below 0.60. Return to page 177, frame 114, and try again.

181B (from page 176, frame 113)
Wrong. High-flow oxygen devices are relatively uncomfortable, can cause drying if only a bubble humidifier is used, and may increase F_{IO_2} if entrainment ports become occluded. Some low F_{IO_2} air-entrainment masks may be appropriate for inpatient treatment of COPD patients, but they are not commonly used at home for long-term oxygen therapy. Return to page 176, frame 113, and select another answer.

181C (from page 179, frame 116)
Wrong. The tidal volume of 900 mL (15 mL/kg) is at the high end of the recommended range of 10 to 15 mL/kg for this 60 kg patient. The F_{IO_2} should be lowered, since high oxygen concentrations may cause a toxic response. The use of PEEP may improve oxygenation and allow the F_{IO_2} to be lowered. Return to page 179, frame 116, and select a lower F_{IO_2}.

181D (from page 179, frame 117)
Correct. Your first concern should be to maintain adequate ventilation and oxygenation until the problem with the ventilator can be corrected. You must provide an F_{IO_2} equal to or higher than what was set on the ventilator, PEEP must be maintained, and the patient must be ventilated. A manual resuscitator with an oxygen reservoir and PEEP valve will allow you to support the patient while fixing or replacing the ventilator. Please continue on page 182, frame 118.

181a (from page 182, frame 118)
Correct. Patients with upper airway lesions may be ventilated preoperatively with helium-oxygen mixtures in order to reduce the pressure needed. Please continue on page 182, frame 119.

181b (from page 187, frame 122)
Correct. Clinical signs include pulmonary infiltrates, decreased Pa_{O_2}, decreased compliance, pulmonary edema, atelectasis, increased right-to-left shunt, and decreased vital capacity. Symptoms of oxygen toxic response include substernal pain, cough, dyspnea, anxiety, and fatigue. Please continue on page 188 and complete the chapter exercises.

181c (from page 183, frame 120)
Wrong. Restlessness and disorientation are seen in *both* chronic pulmonary disease and acute hypoxemia. Return to page 183, frame 120, and try again.

FRAME 118. HELIUM-OXYGEN THERAPY

The lower density of helium allows lower pressures to be used to ventilate patients with upper airway lesions. The pressure needed to ventilate patients with small-diameter endotracheal tubes can be reduced to approximately one half when an 80%–20% helium-oxygen mixture is used. Air trapping seen with chronic obstructive lung disease leads to an increased FRC. Other uses for helium-oxygen mixtures include treatment of status asthmaticus (intractable bronchospasms) and viral croup that does not respond to other types of treatment.

Several factors need to be kept in mind when administering helium-oxygen mixtures: (1) the mixture must be administered with a tight-fitting closed system (a non-rebreathing mask or via a cuffed endotracheal tube), since helium will escape through small leaks; (2) oxygen flowmeters must be corrected (1.5 × flowmeter for 70%–30% Helox mixtures and 1.8 × flowmeter for 80%–20% Helox mixtures) because of the differences in density of oxygen and helium; and (3) helium-oxygen mixtures are poor carrier gases for aerosol therapy.

(Q) The best indication for use of a 70%–30% helium-oxygen mixture is

a. administration of racemic epinephrine to a child with croup. 185 D
b. oxygen therapy before laser surgery on a laryngeal lesion. 181 a
c. oxygen therapy for treatment of acute asthma. 184 b

FRAME 119. POSITIONING PATIENTS TO MINIMIZE HYPOXEMIA

Placing patients in certain positions will often affect their hypoxemia. For example, patients with pulmonary edema and otherwise normal heart function will often be less hypoxemic in a Fowler's position (sitting at a 45° angle). This position slows the return of blood to the right heart, lowers the blood pressure in the pulmonary circulation, and less fluid may leak from pulmonary capillaries into the lungs.

Extremely obese patients will breathe more easily if their abdomen does not interfere with the movement of their diaphragm. Thus, they will be less hypoxemic and less hypercarbic in a Fowler's position and often sleep in a chair. Patients with chronic lung disease may also sleep in a Fowler's position because they become dyspneic when lying in a supine position. Often patients with chronic obstructive lung disease will tend to lean forward supporting their scapula and upper chest with fixed arms in order to use accessory muscles more effectively.

Turning a patient in bed so that a consolidated area of the lung is placed in a dependent (downward) position may increase intrapulmonary shunting. Turning the patient with the consolidated or atelectatic area down (the good lung is up), gravity will increase blood flow to unventilated alveoli.

(Q) In which of the following positions should a patient with left ventricular failure and acceptable blood pressure be placed?

a. Trendelenburg's 184 a
b. supine 180 b
c. Fowler's 185 c

FRAME 120. INDICATIONS FOR OXYGEN THERAPY

Several factors are analyzed when determining if a patient needs oxygen therapy: (1) Pa_{O_2} (arterial oxygen tension), (2) Sa_{O_2} (saturation of hemoglobin with oxygen in arterial blood), (3) cardiovascular status, (4) work of breathing, and (5) oxygen transport. A Pa_{O_2} below 60 torr is dangerous because it moves you closer to the steep portion of the oxyhemoglobin curve where small changes in oxygen tension result in large drops in hemoglobin saturation.

Checking the cardiovascular status helps to determine if the heart is compensating for hypoxia by trying to pump more blood than normal (e.g., increased heart rate). Hypertension may indicate that the cardiovascular system has directed blood away from nonvital organs such as the skin, kidneys, and gastrointestinal tract. Decreased amounts of oxygen delivered to the brain will affect the patient's ability to think clearly. Thus, disorientation and mental confusion are clinical signs of moderate hypoxemia. The heart may respond to hypoxemia by developing arrhythmias, such as premature ventricular contractions.

Long-term oxygen therapy is indicated when clinical trials demonstrate that low-flow oxygen may provide clinical benefits. The following problems may benefit from long-term supplemental oxygen: (1) cardiac arrhythmias in patients with chronic hypoxemia, (2) chronic congestive heart failure, (3) hypoxemia resulting from exercise, (4) polycythemia, (5) right heart failure (cor pumonale), and (6) pulmonary hypertension.

TABLE 6–1
GENERAL CRITERIA FOR LONG-TERM OXYGEN THERAPY

1. $Pa_{O_2} < 55$ torr or $Sa_{O_2} \leq 85\%$ at rest on room air
2. $Pa_{O_2} < 60$ torr or Sa_{O_2} of 86% to 89% with compensatory polycythemia
3. Evidence of tissue hypoxia:
   - Pulmonary hypertension
   - Compensatory polycythemia
   - Cor pulmonale
4. Evidence of central cyanosis
5. Severe arterial hypoxemia on exercise
6. Improvement of hypoxemic state with low-flow oxygen therapy (1 to 3 L/min; FI_{O_2}, 0.24 to 0.30)

Source: Barnes, TA: Respiratory Care Practice. Year Book Medical Publishers, Chicago, 1988. Used with permission.

TABLE 6–2
SITUATIONS WITH A HIGH INCIDENCE OF HYPOXEMIA

Myocardial infarction
Congestive heart failure
Acute pulmonary disorders
Hypovolemic shock
Sepsis
Blunt chest trauma
Drug overdose (abuse)
Exacerbation of neuromuscular disease
Liver failure
Acute pancreatitis
Head trauma
Extensive general trauma

Source: Barnes, TA: Respiratory Care Practice. Year Book Medical Publishers, Chicago, 1988. Used with permission.

(Q) Evidence of tissue hypoxia observed with patients with chronic lung disease but *not* with acute hypoxemia includes

a. labored breathing, central cyanosis. 185 d
b. restlessness, disorientation. 181 c
c. polycythemia, cor pulmonale. 184 d

184A (from page 176, frame 113)
Careful. Some COPD patients tend to hypoventilate when they breathe higher concentrations of oxygen. The oxygen flow to a nasal cannula for a COPD patient is usually held to 1 or 2 L/min or less. Return to page 176, frame 113, and select another answer.

184B (from page 178, frame 115)
Wrong. The compliance will not change or actually decrease when you have gone higher than the optimal PEEP level. Return to page 178, frame 115, and select another answer.

184C (from page 179, frame 116)
Wrong. You should maintain tidal volume at 900 mL (15 mL/kg) and lower the F_{IO_2} in smaller increments. Also, 10 cm H_2O of PEEP is too large an increase to make in one step. Return to page 179, frame 116, and select another answer.

184a (from page 182, frame 119)
Wrong. This would increase venous return to a heart that is already in failure. Blood pressure in the pulmonary circulation would increase and may cause pulmonary edema. Return to page 182, frame 119, and select another answer.

184b (from page 182, frame 118)
Wrong. The goal of treatment of acute asthma would be to reduce the bronchospasm. If the patient had status asthmaticus, then a helium-oxygen mixture might lower the pressure needed to provide ventilatory support. Return to page 182, frame 118, and select another answer.

184c (from page 186, frame 121)
Correct. Once the arterial oxygen content has increased the systemic blood pressure, the heart rate should return to normal. More oxygen being delivered to the brain may result in the patient becoming less restless and agitated; and respiratory rate, inspiratory flow rate, and minute volume should all decrease toward normal. Please continue on page 187, frame 122.

184d (from page 183, frame 120)
Correct. Polycythemia and cor pulmonale develop as a result of long-term hypoxemia seen with chronic pulmonary disease. Please continue on page 186, frame 121.

185A (from page 177, frame 114)
Correct. The high inspiratory flow rate of a patient breathing 40/min will cause air to mixed with the output of the nebulizer since at settings of 100% and 60% the output flow is 15 and 30 L/min, respectively. Please continue on page 178, frame 115.

185B (from page 187, frame 122)
Wrong. The toxic response to oxygen decreases vital capacity. Return to page 187, frame 122, and select another answer.

185C (from page 178, frame 115)
Wrong. An increase in arterial oxygen tension is a positive sign. The $Pa{O_2}$ will remain unchanged or increase insignificantly when you have gone higher than the optimal PEEP level. Return to page 178, frame 115, and try again.

185D (from page 182, frame 118)
Wrong. Helium-oxygen mixtures are poor choices as a carrier gas for aerosols because helium causes early deposition of the medication in the mask and oropharynx. Return to page 182, frame 118, and select another answer.

185a (from page 179, frame 116)
Correct. The tidal volume should be maintained at 15 mL/kg and the $F{IO_2}$ lowered by 10% to decrease the risk of a toxic response to oxygen. However, 5 cm H_2O is indicated to increase the FRC and improve oxygenation. Please continue on page 179, frame 117.

185b (from page 179, frame 117)
Careful. Finding the leak may take longer than you think and your patient may already be severely hypoxemic. Return to page 179, frame 117 and try again.

185c (from page 182, frame 119)
Correct. The Fowler's position will retard venous return to the heart and may prevent pulmonary edema from developing. Please continue on page 183, frame 120.

185d (from page 183, frame 120)
Wrong. Labored breathing and cyanosis are seen in *both* chronic pulmonary disease and acute hypoxemia. Return to page 183, frame 120, and select another answer.

FRAME 121. PATIENT RESPONSE TO OXYGEN THERAPY

Compensatory mechanisms responding to hypoxemia should change once oxygen therapy has begun provided more oxygen is delivered to and utilized by the tissues. Tissue oxygenation is dependent on adequate amounts of oxygen being carried by arterial blood to the tissues. Assessment of tissue oxygenation includes evaluating the patient's ability to think clearly, blood pressure, extremity (peripheral) temperature, pulses, and mixed venous-oxygen tension ($P\bar{v}O_2$). Unless a patient is critically ill, the $P\bar{v}O_2$ probably will not be available since it requires taking a blood sample from a pulmonary artery (Swan-Ganz) catheter. However, there are several other clinical signs that provide information on the patient's oxygenation status without requiring a pulmonary artery blood sample.

Raising the arterial oxygen tension above 60 torr will move the hemoglobin saturation to the flat portion of the oxyhemoglobin curve and allow arterial oxygen content and saturation to rise to 90% or more of its capacity. Having more oxygen available may reduce or eliminate compensatory hemodynamic changes, which may decrease cardiac work and oxygen consumption. Arrhythmias such as premature ventricular contractions should stop or decrease in number.

Serial arterial blood-gas studies should be done when administering oxygen therapy for acute hypoxemia so that the FIO_2 can be held as low as possible. A PaO_2 over 100 torr should be considered overly corrected hypoxemia and the FIO_2 lowered in small increments until the PaO_2 is between 70 and 100 torr.

Patients with chronic pulmonary disease often breathe on a hypoxic drive. A high-concentration oxygen administered to these patients may result in hypoventilation or apnea. However, low-flow oxygen administration ($FIO_2 < 0.30$) has been shown to decrease hematocrit, lower pulmonary vascular resistance, and decrease the amount of right-heart failure. Low-flow oxygen therapy should allow chronically hypoxemic patients to exercise at a higher level and thus improve their general muscle tone, appetite, and quality of life.

(Q) Which of the following responses would be expected with acute hypoxemia once oxygen therapy is started?

a. decreased heart rate, less agitation 184 c
b. increased heart rate, somnolence 180 d
c. increased $P\bar{v}O_2$ to 70 torr 180 C

FRAME 122. HAZARDS OF OXYGEN THERAPY

Four major complications may arise from the use of oxygen: (1) oxygen-induced hypoventilation, (2) atelectasis, (3) retrolental fibroplasia (retinal detachment syndrome), and (4) oxygen toxic response. Oxygen-induced hypoventilation may occur in patients with an obstructive pattern of respiratory disease because a chronically high arterial CO_2 tension depresses the respiratory centers. Consequently, their stimulus to breathe runs off of peripheral chemoreceptors that respond to arterial oxygen tension of < 60 torr. Administering a high oxygen concentration to these patients may cause oxygen-induced hypoventilation. Atelectasis following surgery may be caused by shallow breathing resulting from lack of ambulation, narcotics for pain, anesthesia, oxygen-induced hypoventilation, and incisional pain.

The hypoxia caused by complete or partial collapse of alveoli (atelectasis) may be improved by the use of oxygen therapy, yet prolonged high concentrations of oxygen can also cause alveoli to collapse. This results from (1) the absence of nitrogen in the lungs and (2) the effect of oxygen on the surfactant in the lungs. High oxygen tensions may promote the inactivation of surfactant that normally lowers the surface tension of alveoli, thus keeping them from collapsing. The chance of oxygen-induced atelectasis is greater in an unconscious or sedated patient who breathes shallowly and does not periodically reinflate collapsed alveoli by sighing.

The formation of fibrous (scar) tissue behind the lens of the eye (retrolental fibroplasia) is another hazard in administering high oxygen concentrations. Premature infants can suffer impaired vision and permanent loss of vision may result from this exposure. To guard against this toxic response, the oxygen concentration of the incubator or oxyhood should be adjusted so that the arterial oxygen concentration of the infant remains in the range of 60 to 80 torr.

Oxygen toxic response occurs in two phases based on pathologic findings: (1) exudative phase (24 to 72 hours) and (2) proliferative phase (after 72 hours). During the early, exudative phase there are changes in the alveolar type-II cells, destruction of endothelial cells in pulmonary capillaries, and necrosis of alveolar type-I cells. All of these changes result in pulmonary edema, hemorrhage, and the formation of hyaline membranes. The later, proliferative phase results in an abnormal increase in the number of alveolar type-II cells found in pulmonary capillaries and fibroblasts. These late changes result in a thickening of the alveolar septa.

The oxygen tension and length of exposure will determine if a toxic response occurs. At one atmosphere of pressure, an $F_{IO_2} < 0.50$ should not result in a meaningful amount of toxic response in adults. Thus, practitioners should administer oxygen at the lowest possible F_{IO_2} and consider using PEEP and CPAP to help maintain adequate oxygenation.

(Q) Which of the following clinical signs may be seen when a toxic response to oxygen occurs?

a. somnolence — 180 c
b. decrease in compliance — 181 b
c. increase in vital capacity — 185 B

EXERCISES

1. List five low-flow and five high-flow oxygen therapy devices.
2. Explain why a non-rebreathing mask is considered to be a low-flow oxygen therapy device.
3. Prepare two graphs that plot PEEP levels against the criteria for optimal PEEP. On the first graph plot Pa_{O_2}, cardiac output, and intrapulmonary shunt against PEEP. On the second graph plot static compliance against PEEP. Identify the optimal PEEP level on each graph.
4. Describe how the use of optimal PEEP may allow lower FI_{O_2} levels to be used during mechanical ventilation.
5. Interview six respiratory care practitioners regarding steps they take to reduce hypoxemia during endotracheal suctioning, postural drainage, and during the change of ventilator breathing circuits.
6. Explain what must be done to effectively administer a 70%–30% helium-oxygen mixture to a patient using a non-rebreathing mask.
7. List three pulmonary diseases where patients assume a unique body position to minimize hypoxemia and dyspnea.
8. List six physiologic benefits of long-term oxygen therapy for patients with chronic hypoxemia.
9. List five physiologic signs of a positive response to oxygen therapy.
10. For each of the four major hazards of oxygen therapy identify the type of patient most often susceptible.

POSTTEST

This test is designed to evaluate what you have learned from Chapter 6. Check your answers on page 191 and review the topics where your answer is incorrect.

1. All of the following are factors that affect the FIO_2 when using low-flow oxygen therapy *except*
   A. tidal volume.
   B. respiratory rate.
   C. inspiratory flow rate.
   D. expiratory flow rate.
   E. oxygen flow rate.

2. Which of the following low-flow oxygen therapy devices allows the patient to eat, talk, and sleep in comfort?
   A. nasal catheter
   B. nasal cannula
   C. simple face mask
   D. partial rebreathing mask
   E. non-rebreathing mask

3. An air-dilution mainstream nebulizer set on an FIO_2 of 0.40 with an oxygen flow of 15 L/min will have a total flow of
   A. 10 L/min.
   B. 14 L/min.
   C. 25 L/min.
   D. 30 L/min.
   E. 60 L/min.

4. A patient with a respiratory rate of 40/min and a tidal volume of 500 mL would receive the highest FIO_2 from
   A. an air-entrainment nebulizer set at 0.40 and O_2 flow of 10 L/min.
   B. a rebreathing mask at O_2 flow of 10 L/min.
   C. a non-rebreathing mask at O_2 flow of 10 L/min.
   D. a nasal cannula at O_2 flow of 5 L/min.
   E. a face tent at O_2 flow of 20 L/min.

5. Which of the following combinations of PEEP and static compliance represent the *optimal* PEEP level?

	Compliance (L/cm H_2O)	PEEP (cm H_2O)
A.	0.010	5
B.	0.020	10
C.	0.030	15
D.	0.050	20
E.	0.050	25

6. Which of the following disorders is likely to require a lower optimal PEEP level?
   A. crushed chest injury
   B. left-heart failure
   C. acute pulmonary edema
   D. Guillain-Barré syndrome
   E. adult respiratory distress syndrome

7. When changing the breathing circuit of an ARDS patient on a ventilator all of the following would help to protect the patient from hypoxemia *except*
   A. preoxygenation with an F_{IO_2} of 1.00.
   B. sigh breaths prior to disconnecting circuit.
   C. manual ventilation at an F_{IO_2} of 1.00.
   D. limiting disconnect time to 20 seconds or less.
   E. manual ventilation with a high F_{IO_2} and PEEP.
8. The effect of high levels of PEEP on the cardiovascular system of critically ill patients can be determined most accurately by monitoring changes in the
   A. cardiac output.
   B. heart rate.
   C. blood pressure.
   D. skin temperature.
   E. urine output.
9. How many minutes does it usually take for the Pa_{O_2} to decrease once PEEP is accidentally dropped to zero?
   A. 4 min
   B. 15 min
   C. 20 min
   D. 30 min
   E. 1 hour
10. A patient who has been mechanically ventilated for one hour on an F_{IO_2} of 1.00 and has a $P(A\text{-}a)O_2$ gradient of 450 torr should have ventilation parameters changed by
    A. decreasing F_{IO_2} to 0.30.
    B. decreasing F_{IO_2} to 0.40.
    C. removing the patient from the ventilator.
    D. decreasing F_{IO_2} to 0.70 and adding PEEP.
    E. maintaining F_{IO_2} at 1.00.
11. All of the following would be indications for 70%–30% helium-oxygen therapy *except*
    A. ventilation before laser surgery on the upper airway.
    B. to reduce the FRC of a COPD patient.
    C. to ventilate a patient in status asthmaticus.
    D. to deliver oxygen during an acute asthma attack.
    E. to deliver oxygen to a patient with epiglottis.
12. To deliver a total flow of 12 L/min of a 70%–30% helium-oxygen mixture, an oxygen flowmeter would be set at
    A. 4 L/min.
    B. 6 L/min.
    C. 8 L/min.
    D. 12 L/min.
    E. 18 L/min.
13. Which position may cause the most hypoxemia with extremely obese patients?
    A. standing
    B. Fowler's
    C. semi-Fowler's
    D. Trendelenburg's
    E. side-lying

14. A patient with a mucus plug blocking ventilation to the right middle lobe may have a drop in Pa_{O_2} if placed in a
    A. right side-lying position.
    B. left side-lying position.
    C. prone position.
    D. supine position.
    E. semi-Fowler's position.
15. All of the following are indications for short-term use of oxygen therapy for a patient breathing room air when examined *except*
    A. $Pa_{O_2} < 60$ torr.
    B. $Sa_{O_2} < 95\%$.
    C. tachycardia.
    D. cardiac arrhythmias.
    E. myocardial infarction.
16. All of the following are signs of tissue hypoxemia *except*
    A. pulmonary hypertension.
    B. polycythemia.
    C. cor pulmonale.
    D. mixed venous-oxygen tension of 40 torr.
    E. evidence of central cyanosis.
17. Overly corrected hypoxemia is best described as a Pa_{O_2} of
    A. 60 torr.
    B. 70 torr.
    C. 80 torr.
    D. 100 torr.
    E. 150 torr.
18. The flat portion (Sa_{O_2} of 90%) of the oxyhemoglobin dissociation curve (assume a P_{50} of 27 mm Hg) will be approached when the Pa_{O_2} is
    A. 40 torr.
    B. 60 torr.
    C. 90 torr.
    D. 100 torr.
    E. 110 torr.
19. Which of the following statements is/are true?
    I. A high Pa_{CO_2} will depress the central (CO_2 sensitive) chemoreceptors in the medulla.
    II. A high Pa_{CO_2} will remove the normal ventilatory response to increased CO_2.
    III. A Pa_{O_2} below 60 torr will stimulate a ventilatory response.
    A. I only.
    B. II only.
    C. III only.
    D. I and II only.
    E. I, II, and III.
20. Atelectasis following surgery may be caused by all the following *except*
    A. ambulation.
    B. narcotics.
    C. anesthesia.
    D. oxygen therapy.
    E. incisional pain.

ANSWERS TO POSTTEST

1. D (F113)
2. B (F113)
3. E (F114)
4. A (F114)
5. D (F115)
6. D (F115)
7. B (F116)
8. A (F116)
9. A (F117)
10. D (F116)
11. D (F118)
12. C (F118)
13. D (F119)
14. A (F119)
15. B (F120)
16. D (F120)
17. E (F121)
18. B (F121)
19. E (F122)
20. A (F122)

BIBLIOGRAPHY

Barnes, TA: Respiratory Care Practice. Year Book Medical Publishers, Chicago, 1988.

Burton, GG and Hodgkin, JE: Respiratory Care: A Guide to Clinical Practice, ed 2. JB Lippincott, Philadelphia, 1984.

Eubanks, DH and Bone, RC: Comprehensive Respiratory Care, ed 2. CV Mosby, St. Louis, 1990.

Kacmarek, RM and Stoller, JK: Current Respiratory Care. BC Decker, Philadelphia, 1989.

Pilbeam, SP and Youtsey, JW: Mechanical Ventilation. CV Mosby, St. Louis, 1986.

Scanlon, C, Spearman, CB, Sheldon, RL, and Egan, DF: Egan's Fundamentals of Respiratory Therapy, ed 5. CV Mosby, St. Louis, 1990.

Shapiro, BA, Harrison, RA, Kacmarek, RM, and Cane, RD: Clinical Appplication of Respiratory Care, ed 3. Year Book Medical Publishers, Chicago, 1985.

Shaprio, BA, Harrison, RA, Templin, RK, and Walton, JR: Clinical Application of Blood Gases, ed 4. Year Book Medical Publishers, Chicago, 1988.

Wilkins, RL, Sheldon, RL, and Krider, SJ: Clinical Assessment in Respiratory Care, ed 2. CV Mosby, St. Louis, 1990.

Witkowski, AS: Pulmonary Assessment: A Clinical Guide. JB Lippincott, Philadelphia, 1985.

7

Humidity and Aerosol Therapy

PRETEST

This pretest is designed to measure what you already know about humidity and aerosol therapy. Check your answers on page 196 and then continue on page 197, frame 123.

1. Which of the following oxygen therapy devices may not require humidification?
   A. nasal cannula at 4 L/min
   B. nasal cannula at 6 L/min
   C. partial rebreathing mask at 10 L/min
   D. non-rebreathing mask at 10 L/min
   E. CPAP system at 30 L/min

2. Most unheated bubbler devices raise humidity to the equivalent of relative humidity at 37°C of
   A. 35% to 45%.
   B. 55% to 65%.
   C. 55% to 85%.
   D. 85% to 95%.
   E. 95% to 100%.

3. All of the following are indications for aerosol therapy *except*
   A. deposition of bronchoactive aerosols.
   B. humidification for ventilator patients.
   C. enhancement of secretion clearance.
   D. sputum induction.
   E. humidification for oxygen therapy.

4. All of the following are categories of bronchoactive drugs *except*
   A. bronchodilators.
   B. mucolytics.
   C. corticosteroids.
   D. diuretics.
   E. decongestants.

5. What size aerosol droplet will be most effective in delivering a drug to the supraglottic mucosa?
   A. 0.5 μm
   B. 3 μm
   C. 5 μm
   D. 10 μm
   E. 15 μm

6. What size aerosol droplet will be most effective in delivering racemic epinephrine to a patient with croup?
   A. 0.1 to 1 μm
   B. 1 to 3 μm
   C. 3 to 5 μm
   D. 5 to 10 μm
   E. 15 to 40 μm

7. To improve deposition to the periphery of the lungs, the breath-hold period should last
   A. 1 second.
   B. 2 seconds.
   C. 3 seconds.
   D. 5 seconds.
   E. 10 seconds.
8. What proportion of aerosol droplets from a metered dose inhaler (without a spacer) will be deposited in the mouth?
   A. 1%
   B. 9%
   C. 50%
   D. 80%
   E. 95%
9. If a patient with an artificial airway breathes room air that has a relative humidity of 50% at 20°C, the absolute humidity deficit will be
   A. 9 mg/L.
   B. 17 mg/L.
   C. 20 mg/L.
   D. 35 mg/L.
   E. 44 mg/L.
10. If a patient breathes dry room air through a tracheal tube, how far into the airways will the gas travel before the humidity deficit is corrected?
    A. carina
    B. main-stem bronchi
    C. lung periphery
    D. second or third bifurcation of the bronchi
    E. fifth or sixth bifurcation of the bronchi
11. The last step in coughing is
    A. glottic closure.
    B. a deep breath.
    C. glottic opening.
    D. increased intrathoracic pressure.
    E. end-inspiratory breath holding.
12. What is the best position to improve aerosol deposition in peripheral airways?
    A. prone
    B. supine
    C. Fowler's
    D. lateral decubitus
    E. Trendelenburg's
13. Which of the following statements about metered dose inhalers is/are true?
    I. A lower dose of drug is ordered per treatment.
    II. Aerosol deposition in the lung periphery is increased when a spacer is used.
    III. Normally five puffs are administered.
    A. I only.
    B. II only.
    C. III only.
    D. I and II only.
    E. II and III only.

14. The normal total dose (two puffs) of Albuterol when delivered by a metered dose inhaler is
    A. 0.13 mg.
    B. 0.18 mg.
    C. 0.40 mg.
    D. 1.30 mg.
    E. 2.50 mg.
15. The mucokinetic action of acetylcysteine is the result of
    A. rupture of disulfide bonds.
    B. reduced viscosity of sputum.
    C. dilution of mucopolysaccharide strands.
    D. alkalinization of mucus.
    E. change in surface tension of gel layer.
16. Alcohol aerosols are used to
    A. dilute mucopolysaccharide strands.
    B. counteract the odor of acetylcysteine.
    C. clear pulmonary edema bubbles.
    D. stabilize aerosol particle size.
    E. reduce bronchospasm.
17. Pulmonary complications of uncompensated humidity deficits occurring with intubated patients may occur when absolute humidity drops below
    A. 12 mg/L.
    B. 17 mg/L.
    C. 30 mg/L.
    D. 37 mg/L.
    E. 44 mg/L.
18. All of the following are advantages of heat and moisture exchangers *except*
    A. low cost.
    B. ease of use.
    C. high absolute humidity.
    D. elimination of water reservoir.
    E. elimination of power or humidity source.
19. All of the following tests may provide evidence that a bronchodilator is effective *except*
    A. FEV_1 (forced expiratory volume).
    B. peak flow.
    C. improved 6-minute walk test.
    D. maximum inspiratory pressure (MIP).
    E. vital capacity (VC).
20. A 50% reduction in airway caliber caused by swelling of dry airway secretions would result in
    A. increased compliance.
    B. 50% reduction in airway conductance.
    C. 16-fold increase in airway resistance.
    D. 50% increase in airway resistance.
    E. eupneic breathing.

ANSWERS TO PRETEST

1. A (F123)
2. A (F123)
3. B (F124)
4. D (F124)
5. E (F125)
6. D (F125)
7. E (F126)
8. D (F126)
9. D (F127)
10. A (F127)
11. C (F129)
12. C (F129)
13. D (F131)
14. B (F131)
15. A (F130)
16. C (F130)
17. C (F128)
18. C (F128)
19. D (F132)
20. C (F132)

FRAME 123. INDICATIONS FOR HUMIDITY THERAPY

Humidification of Dry Medical Gases Oxygen and other medical gases stored in cylinders and central piping systems are dry. A large amount of ambient air is mixed with dry oxygen with low-flow or Venturi-type oxygen therapy devices. Thus, the humidity of inspired gases is similar to that of room air, and there is no need to humidify oxygen at flow rates of 1 to 4 L/min (unless the ambient humidity is unusually dry). Gases delivered to the upper airways at flow rates higher than 4 L/min should be humidified with unheated bubbler devices. If the upper airway is bypassed by a tracheal tube, then dry gases must be raised to a relative humidity of 100% at 37°C. A heated humidifier will be needed when the upper airways are bypassed, since most unheated bubbler devices can deliver only 35% to 45% relative humidity at 37°C.

To deliver gases that have 100% relative humidity at 37°C, the humidifier must actually heat the gas to higher than 37°C to compensate for the cooling that will occur along the length of the delivery tubing. The temperature of inspired gas should be monitored close to a patient's airway and the humidifier adjusted to maintain the temperature between 32°C to 37°C. Special care should be taken not to deliver cool gas mixtures over the face and head of premature infants, since calories are needed for body metabolism rather than for heat production.

Reduction of Airway Resistance Warm, humidified air may reduce airway resistance and may prevent or lessen bronchoconstriction of exercise-induced asthma. Cold air has been reported to increase airway resistance even in normal subjects. A significant decrease in the frequency of cough and sputum has been observed in patients receiving warm, humidified air following upper abdominal surgery. Bronchoconstriction has been observed at night when some asthmatic patients breathe ambient dry air at 23°C and 20% relative humidity. Patients whose asthma is worse at night have benefited by receiving warm, moist air at 37°C and 100% relative humidity.

(Q) Which of the following oxygen therapy devices needs to be connected to a bubbler humidifier?

a. nasal cannula at 4 L/min 202 A
b. a rebreathing mask at 10 L/min 203 B
c. a Venturi mask at 6 L/min 202 C

FRAME 124. INDICATIONS FOR AEROSOL THERAPY

Deposition of Bronchoactive Aerosols The topical administration of bronchoactive agents by aerosol therapy delivers the medication where it is needed and minimizes the systemic exposure. Categories of aerosolized bronchodilator drugs include *bronchodilators, mucolytics, corticosteroids, antiasthmatics, decongestants,* and *antimicrobials.*

Enhancement of Secretion Clearance The nebulization of water and saline results in a productive cough and increased clearance of secretions. It appears that bland aerosols stimulate cough receptors in the trachea and bronchi, and initiate reflex mucus production, cough, and increased airway resistance. Thus, bland aerosols function as expectorants by their general irritant effect on airway mucosa.

Sputum Induction Aerosol therapy can be used to raise sputum by irritating the large airways with an aerosol of water or hypertonic saline. Usually an ultrasonic nebulizer is used to take advantage of its high-density aerosol output and small particle size.

Humidification of Inspired Gases Aerosol therapy is used to provide humidity in some clinical situations because the large surface area of airborne particles promotes evaporation. Aerosol therapy is appropriate for humidifying dry gases used with high-flow air-entrainment nebulizers that deliver a high total flow to an aerosol mask or face tent. The use of a heated nebulizer to deliver a gas at 100% relative humidity at 37°C via an endotracheal tube over a prolonged period may cause pooling of secretions, decreased mucus viscosity, and a medium for growth of organisms. Cold aerosols may cause increased airway resistance, but usually are relatively safe when used to add humidity to high-flow oxygen delivery systems.

Treatment of Upper Airway Inflammation The use of unheated bland aerosols to treat croup has not been proved to have a beneficial effect. The use of topical vasoconstricting agents such as racemic epinephrine is the treatment of choice for croup. Unheated bland aerosols may have a beneficial effect in the case of post extubation edema.

(Q) Which of the following is not an indication for aerosol therapy?

a. bronchoconstriction 202 B
b. humidification of inspired gas of a ventilator patient 203 C
c. clearance of secretions 202 D

FRAME 125. PULMONARY DEPOSITION OF AEROSOLS

Aerosol particles that travel all the way to the lung periphery and deposit in the respiratory bronchioles, alveolar ducts, and alveoli have a range of 1 to 5 μm. In this region of the lung the low flow and large cross-sectional area result in particle deposition due to its weight. Particles that are less than 1 μm are small enough to behave as gases and the mass carried by these particles is too small for therapeutic applications.

If patients breathe through their *mouths*, particles of 5 to 10 μm will reach the first six airway generations; and particles greater than 15 μm do not penetrate beyond the larynx. If patients breathe through their *noses*, particles greater than 10 μm do not penetrate below the larynx. Table 7–1 shows the size of particles that are deposited in different areas of the airways. You should note that large droplets never reach the lung periphery.

(Q) What size aerosol particle will be most effective in delivering a bronchodilator to the small peripheral airways?

a. 0.1 to 1 μm 202 a
b. 1 to 5 μm 203 b
c. 5 to 10 μm 203 A

TABLE 7–1
DEPOSITION OF AEROSOL PARTICLES*

Particle Size μm	MEAN % DEPOSITION			
	Mouth†	N – P‡	T – B‡	P‡
1.0	0	3.6	2.7	25.0
2.0	0	40.6	5.1	34.6
3.0	5	55.2	7.1	30.8
4.0	10	65.4	8.4	23.8
6.0	30	79.9	9.1	10.3
10.0	65	99.2	0.7	0.2
12.0	75			
14.0	85			
> 16.0	100			

Source: Barnes, TA: Respiratory Care Practice. Year Book Medical Publishers, Chicago, 1988. Used with permission.

*N – P = nares to larynx; T – B = trachea to terminal bronchioles; P = respiratory bronchioles to alveoli
†Using mouthpiece, flow = 30 L/min
‡Obtained by calculation, assuming V_T = 750 mL, rate = 15/min

FRAME 126. BREATHING TECHNIQUES FOR AEROSOL THERAPY

Using the proper breathing technique may increase the deposition of aerosols in specific airways. There will be limited deposition between the larger bronchi and the lung periphery because of the decreasing caliber of airways and the high velocity of gas in the upper airways. Varying breathing patterns can direct particle deposition to the nasopharynx, oropharynx, larynx, trachea, first six airway generations, or lung periphery. The variables include inspiratory flow rate, nose versus mouth breathing, lung volume at which inhalation occurs, and length of breath-hold period. Your instructions to the patient will vary according to the targeted site of aerosol deposition. Even with good technique, only 9% of aerosol from a metered dose inhaler (MDI) deposits in the lungs. The remaining particles are accounted for as follows: mouth—80%, MDI actuator—10%, and exhaled—1%.

The lung volume at which a patient should inhale an aerosol may vary from 20% to 80% of vital capacity, and there is little agreement on which end of the range is best. The most important factors are an inspiratory flow of 30 L/min (500 mL/s) and a 10-second breath hold. The following general guidelines have been suggested by research on aerosol deposition:

Periphery

To delivery aerosols to the periphery, a slow inspiratory flow of less than 30 L/min and a 10-second breath hold should be used. The use of an extension tube and reservoir device with MDIs may reduce deposition of particles in the mouth and help the patient to trigger the canister during inspiration.

Nasopharynx

For aerosols that need to be delivered to the nasopharynx a larger particle size of 5 to 15 μm, nose breathing, and normal inspiratory flow of less than 30 L/min will maximize deposition.

Oropharynx, Larynx, Trachea, and First Six Airway Generations

To deliver aerosol droplets to these airways a particle size in the range of 5 to 10 μm should be used and delivered by mouth breathing. Fast inspiratory flow above 30 L/min would increase deposition in the larynx and supraglottic area. Normal flow at 30 L/min would increase deposition in the trachea and the first six generations of airways.

(Q) To deliver a topical anesthetic to the supraglottic tissues prior to intubation, which of the following techniques would be best?

a. Use of an MDI that delivers particles in the range of 1 to 5 μm and slow mouth breathing. 202 b

b. Use a baffled nebulizer that delivers particles in the range of 5 to 10 μm, high inspiratory flow of above 30 L/min, and mouth breathing. 208 A

c. A baffled nebulizer that delivers particles of 10 to 15 μm, high inspiratory flow above 30 L/min, and nose breathing. 209 B

FRAME 127. PREVENTING HUMIDITY DEFICITS

A patient with upper airways intact and normal systemic hydration will be able to humidify inspired air to 100% relative humidity at body temperature (37°C). The amount of water that has to be added is called the humidity deficit. The deficit can be calculated by subtracting the absolute humidity of inspired gas from the absolute humidity of the gas when saturated at body temperature (44 mg/L). For example, if a patient breathes room air with a relative humidity of 25% and a temperature of 20°C, the absolute humidity of the inspired air is approximately 4 mg/L and the humidity deficit is 40 mg/L (44 mg/L − 4 mg/L).

If the upper airway is bypassed by a tracheal tube, the humidity deficit will be corrected by water evaporating from the respiratory mucosa. Inspired gas will be saturated at body temperature by the time it reaches the second or third bifurcation of bronchi. However, the loss of water to correct the deficit may cause decreased ciliary activity and damage to pseudostratified ciliated epithelial cells. A minimum of 12 mg/L should be added to dry gas delivered to the upper airways, and 44 mg/L should be added to gas that is delivered via a tracheal tube. If the gas is delivered at a flow rate below 4 L/min, humidification may not be required. Air-entrainment nebulizers that mix large amounts of air with the dry input gas may not need to be humidified unless the entrained air has a low absolute humidity.

Mechanical ventilators should have humidification systems that deliver 100% relative humidity at body temperature (44 mg/L). In order to ensure that the gas is saturated at body temperature the inspired gas temperature should be monitored.

(Q) If a patient breathes quietly from a non-rebreathing mask that is supplied with oxygen from a flowmeter without a bubbler humidifier, the humidity deficit will be

a. 0 mg/L. 202 c
b. 27 mg/L. 208 B
c. 44 mg/L. 209 A

202A (from page 197, frame 123)
Wrong. There is no need to humidify low-flow oxygen therapy devices when the source gas has a flow rate of 1 to 4 L/min. However, if the room air has low humidity, then a bubbler device should be used. Return to page 197, frame 123, and select another answer.

202B (from page 198, frame 124)
Wrong. Administration of bronchodilators is frequently done by aerosol therapy. Return to page 198, frame 124, and select another answer.

202C (from page 197, frame 123)
Wrong. There is no need to humidify Venturi devices because of the large amount of room air that is entrained and mixed with the oxygen. However, if the room air has low humidity, then a bubbler device should be used. Return to page 197, frame 123, and select another answer.

202D (from page 198, frame 124)
Wrong. Mucolytic and bland aerosol therapy may improve the clearance of secretions. Return to page 198, frame 124, and select another answer.

202a (from page 199, frame 125)
Careful. Remember aerosol droplets below 1 μm behave like a gas and will be exhaled. Return to page 199, frame 125, and try again.

202b (from page 200, frame 126)
Wrong. Metered dose inhalers that produce aerosols with a particle size of 1 to 5 micrometers are designed to deliver medications to the peripheral airways. Slow mouth breathing also enhances deposition in the periphery. Return to page 200, frame 126, and select another answer.

202c (from page 201, frame 127)
Wrong. This is the absolute humidity of dry oxygen. The question asks about the amount of water needed to bring the gas to 100% relative humidity at body temperature. Return to page 201, frame 127, and try again.

202d (from page 205, frame 130)
Wrong. Alcohol is used to clear pulmonary edema bubbles that block small airways, but will not have any important effect on loosening retained airway secretions. Return to page 205, frame 130, and select another answer.

203A (from page 199, frame 125)
Wrong. Particles in this range will deposit in the first six generations of the tracheal-bronchial tree. They are large enough to be affected by the high velocity and turbulence found in larger airways. Return to page 199, frame 125, and select another answer.

203B (from page 197, frame 123)
Correct. Low-flow oxygen therapy devices with flow rates over 4 L/min need to use bubbler humidifiers. Please continue on page 198, frame 124.

203C (from page 198, frame 124)
Correct. Administration of heated water aerosols to humidify dry gas for a ventilator patient over a prolonged period may result in pooling of secretions, decreased mucus viscosity, and a medium for growth of organisms. Please continue on page 199, frame 125.

203a (from page 206, frame 131)
Wrong. Cromolyn sodium is used to prevent asthma attacks by stabilizing cellular membranes of mast cells. Mast cells release histamine and other agents that induce bronchospasm. Cromolyn sodium is of no use during an acute asthma attack. Return to page 206, frame 131, and review Table 7–2; then select another answer.

203b (from page 199, frame 125)
Correct. Particles in this range will deposit in the small peripheral airways. Please continue on page 200, frame 126.

203c (from page 204, frame 129)
Wrong. A larger breath is needed to produce an effective cough. Return to page 204, frame 129, and select another answer.

203d (from page 207, frame 132)
Wrong. The dyspnea is caused by the irritant effect of the high density of particles produced by an ultrasonic nebulizer and swelling of dry secretions. What could be done to allow the treatment to continue? Return to page 207, frame 132, and select another answer.

FRAME 128. ARTIFICIAL AIRWAY HUMIDIFICATION

Bypassing upper airways with a tracheal tube requires the use of heated humidifiers. This is especially important when a patient is mechanically ventilated, since oxygen and air are usually obtained from pipeline systems that have little or no absolute humidity. The Emergency Care Research Institute (ECRI) recommends an absolute humidity of at least 37 mg/L, which can be compared to the absolute humidity for saturated gas at body temperature of 44 mg/L. To deliver an absolute humidity of 37 mg/L, gas must be saturated with water vapor at a temperature of 93°F, when measured proximal to the airway (inspiratory limb next to the Y-connector). Pulmonary complications related to an uncorrected humidity deficit may occur when absolute humidity drops below 30 mg/L (equivalent to saturated gas at 86°F).

Heat and moisture exchangers are the newest technology for airway humidification. They provide absolute humidity that falls below the 30-mgL level of absolute humidity needed to avoid drying airway mucosa. Advantages of heat and moisture exchangers (artificial nose) are their low cost, ease of use, and elimination of the need for water. Precautions in their use include lower humidity, two joints for possible disconnection, and increased dead space.

(Q) Patients who are being transported to special procedures or surgery and require ventilation may benefit from a
- a. heat and moisture exchanger. 208 c
- b. heated humidifier delivering gas at 85°F. 208 b
- c. humidification from an unheated mainstream nebulizer. 209 c

FRAME 129. AEROSOL THERAPY FOR BRONCHIAL HYGIENE

Delivery of aerosols to the periphery of the lung to mobilize secretions that may be obstructing small airways requires the use of a nebulizer that produces particles in the range of 1 to 5 μm. The patient should be placed in a position that encourages deep breathing, such as the Fowler's position, so that the weight of abdominal organs will not restrict movement of the diaphragm. Placing the patient in a postural drainage position, once retained secretions have been hydrated or broken by mucolytics, may help the patient use gravity to raise sputum. The patient should be encouraged to breathe slowly and deeply through the mouth and to pause at the end of inspiration. Abdominal breathing should be encouraged to improve deposition of particles in the lung periphery.

Many patients do not know how to cough effectively and practitioners should routinely review the five steps of producing a strong cough: (1) a deep inspiration, (2) an inspiratory pause, (3) glottic closure, (4) increased intrathoracic pressure, and (5) glottic opening.

Assessment of aerosol therapy involves inspection of respiratory pattern and rate, sputum collection, and chest auscultation. The patient should be asked questions about breathing patterns and sputum production. Chest x-rays and sputum culture reports should be reviewed as they become available.

(Q) How deep a breath does a patient need to take to cough effectively?

a. 7 mL/kg 203 c
b. 10 mL/kg 208 C
c. 15 mL/kg 209 D

FRAME 130. MUCOKINETIC AEROSOL THERAPY

Mucokinetic aerosol medications are used to loosen retained airway secretions. The most commonly used mucolytic, acetylcysteine (Mucomyst), works by rupturing the disulfide bonds of long chains of mucoprotein molecules. Acetylcysteine should be diluted to a 10% solution with isotonic saline because it is irritating to the airway mucosa and a higher concentration is not more effective. A bronchodilator is frequently added to the solution to counteract bronchospasm that may occur when the agent is applied to the airways. Acetylcysteine has a foul sulfurous odor and an unpleasant taste. The odor and irritant effect of acetylcysteine on oropharyngeal mucosa may induce gagging, nausea, or vomiting. Since 80% of the aerosol droplets impact in the oropharynx, patients should rinse their mouths with water or mouthwash after a treatment.

The degree to which water and weak electrolyte solutions (NaCl and $NaHCO_3$) reduce the viscosity of sputum has been questioned since the mucous gel layer is relatively impervious to absorption of water. Bland aerosols may trigger reflex mucus production, cough, and increased airway resistance by stimulating cough receptors in the trachea and bronchi. The result of using bland aerosols is similar to what is seen during sputum induction.

Water and weak electrolyte solutions are used by some practitioners to reduce the viscosity of sputum by diluting mucopolysaccharide strands. When sodium bicarbonate is aerosolized in low concentrations (2%), it makes the mucus alkaline; this tends to break the amino bonds of mucus. Glycerol and propylene glycol have been used in the past to stabilize aerosol particle size, but ultrasonic nebulizers have reduced the need for their use. Alcohol aerosols (diluted to less than 50%) are used to clear small airways blocked by pulmonary edema bubbles. The alcohol lowers the surface tension of the bubbles, causing them to burst and thus opening the airways and improving ventilation.

(Q) Which of the following solutions when nebulized will loosen retained airway secretions?

a. 25% alcohol 202 d
b. 20% acetylcysteine and 2% $NaHCO_3$ (equal parts) 208 a
c. 10% acetylcysteine and 0.5% (1:200) isoproterenol 209 b

FRAME 131. BRONCHOACTIVE AEROSOL MEDICATIONS

Drugs given by aerosol therapy for topical treatment of the pulmonary system are called bronchoactive drugs. Several bronchoactive drugs are listed in Table 7-2 by their categories: bronchodilators, mucolytics, corticosteroids, antiasthmatics, decongestants, and antimicrobials. The dosages listed are per administration, and it should be recalled that only approximately 9% from MDIs will actually be deposited in the lungs with 80% depositing in the mouth. Holding the mouthpiece $1\frac{1}{2}$ in from the mouth reduces impaction in the throat and increases the amount of drug delivered to the lung periphery. Gas-powered nebulizers deliver less aerosol than an MDI, especially when a spacer is used with an MDI to keep the actuator away from the mouth. The dose of bronchodilator given by an MDI is much smaller and reflects a more controlled delivery. The dosage and use for several bronchoactive drugs listed in Table 7-2 should be carefully reviewed.

(Q) Which of the following bronchoactive drugs would be a good choice to treat an acute asthma attack?

a. cromolyn sodium 203 a
b. isoetharine 208 D
c. racemic epinephrine 209 C

TABLE 7-2
BRONCHOACTIVE AEROSOL DRUGS—DOSAGE* AND USE

	Nebulizer	MDI	USE
Bronchodilators			
Isoproterenol	1.25–2.5 mg	0.125–0.250 mg	Short-term bronchodilator
Isoetharine	2.5–5.0 mg	0.34–0.68 mg	Short-term bronchodilator
Metaproterenol	15 mg	1.3–1.95 mg	Maintenance bronchodilator
Terbutaline	- - -	0.40 mg	Maintenance bronchodilator
Albuterol	2.5 mg	0.18 mg	Maintenance bronchodilator
Atropine	0.05 mg/kg	- - -	Anticholinergic
Ipratropium	- - -	0.036 mg	Anticholinergic
Mucolytics			
Acetylcysteine	200–300 mg		Reduce viscosity of mucus
Corticosteriods			
Dexamethasone	- - -	0.3 mg	Anti-inflammatory, asthma
Beclomethasone	- - -	0.1 mg	Anti-inflammatory, rhinitis
Triamcinolone	- - -	0.4 mg	Anti-inflammatory
Flunisolide	- - -	0.5 mg	Anti-inflammatory
Antiasthmatic			
Cromolyn sodium			Asthma prophylaxis
Decongestants			
Racemic epinephrine	5.6–11.3 mg	- - -	Vasoconstriction and reduction of mucosal edema
Phenylephrine	2.5–5.0 mg	- - -	Vasoconstriction and reduction of mucosal edema
Lidocaine	40–60 mg	- - -	Anesthesia, upper airway
Antimicrobials			
Kanamycin	250 mg		Gram-negative pulmonary infections
Gentamicin	80 mg		
Polymixin B	5–10 mg		
Amphotericin B	5 mg/day		Fungal pulmonary infections
Nystatin	100,000 units		Fungal pulmonary infections

*Dosages are per administration. For example, flunisolide is 0.5 mg per 2 puffs.

Source: Barnes, TA: Respiratory Care Practice. Year Book Medical Publishers, Chicago, 1988. Used with permission.

FRAME 132. EVALUATING AEROSOL AND HUMIDITY THERAPY

Evaluating aerosol and humidity therapy will require assessing the patient for the expected pharmacologic response and recognizing and dealing with the potential hazards associated with the agents being delivered to the airways. A pretreatment evaluation of the patient will provide a baseline for determining if the aerosol therapy is effective. For example, measuring forced expiratory volume in 1 second (FEV_1), forced vital capacity (FVC), or peak expiratory flow (PEF) before administering a bronchodilator and after the treatment will indicate if there has been a substantial decrease in bronchospasm. Pre- and posttreatment evaluation will provide information regarding which aerosol agent, dose, or delivery device (gas-powered inhaler or metered dose inhaler) results in the best patient response.

The potential hazards of aerosol therapy include cardiac beta-1 side effects seen with some beta-adrenergic bronchodilators. Tachycardia, palpitation, and flushing of the skin are side effects that will vary according to how much beta-1 effect the agent has and the amount of drug administered. Other side effects of aerosols include precipitation of bronchospasm, since aerosols can be irritants to the lung. The higher the aerosol density of aerosol delivered, the more likely that bronchospasm will develop. Thus, patients should never be left unattended when receiving aerosol therapy from high output devices, such as ultrasonic nebulizers. Often a bronchodilator is added to bland solutions that are delivered by ultrasonic nebulizers to reduce the amount of bronchospasm that occurs. Ultrasonic nebulizers may cause a fluid overload with infants because of the high aerosol output delivered by these devices.

Swelling of dried secretions during ultrasonic treatments will seriously increase airway resistance, since small changes in the caliber of airways results in exponential changes in conductance; for example, a 50% reduction in airway caliber would result in a 16-fold increase in air resistance. Steps should be taken to mobilize hydrated secretions by scheduling ultrasonic nebulizer treatments with chest physiotherapy, such as postural drainage, chest percussion, vibrations, and shaking.

The volume, color, tenacity, and odor of sputum raised during aerosol therapy should be evaluated and charted. Lung sounds should be assessed before, during, and after the aerosol therapy. The work of breathing as exhibited by respiratory rate, breathing pattern, and the use of accessory muscles should be noted. Chest x-rays should be reviewed to check for changes in segmental atelectasis.

(Q) Which of the following recommendations should be made if a patient develops dyspnea while receiving bland aerosol by ultrasonic nebulizer?

a. Discontinue treatment and recommend another type of nebulizer. 203 d

b. Add a bronchodilator to the bland aerosol and continue treatments. 208 d

c. Integrate chest physiotherapy with ultrasonic nebulizer treatments and add a bronchodilator to the bland aerosol and continue treatments. 209 a

208A (from page 200, frame 126)
Correct. A nebulizer that produces particles in the range of 5 to 10 μm will result in deposition in the supraglottic tissue. A fast inspiratory flow rate will result in more deposition in this area due to increased impaction caused by turbulent gas flow. Please continue on page 201, frame 127.

208B (from page 201, frame 127)
Wrong. The oxygen is completely dry and there is very little or no room air mixed with oxygen. Return to page 201, frame 127, and try again.

208C (from page 204, frame 129)
Wrong. A larger inspiration is needed to produce an effective cough. Return to page 204, frame 129, and select another answer.

208D (from page 206, frame 131)
Correct. Isoetharine (Bronkosol, Dilabron) is a clinically effective adrenergic drug that can be used to treat the bronchospasm seen during an acute asthma attack. It has the advantage of only minor beta-1 effects at therapeutic doses. Please continue on page 207, frame 132.

208a (from page 205, frame 130)
Careful. The equal portion of $NaHCO_3$ will lower the acetylcysteine to a safe 10% concentration, but it will not help counteract the bronchospasm that usually develops. Return to page 205, frame 130, and try again.

208b (from page 204, frame 128)
Wrong. Transporting a water-filled humidifier is difficult and it would remain unheated when away from electrical service. Return to page 204, frame 128, and select another answer.

208c (from page 204, frame 128)
Correct. This is good application of a heat and moisture exchanger, since using water-filled humidifiers would be difficult during transport. Although the heat and moisture exchanger does not increase the absolute humidity to more than 20 to 30 mg/L, it would be better than ventilating the patient with dry gas. Please continue on page 204, frame 129.

208d (from page 207, frame 132)
Almost. Adding a bronchodilator to a bland aerosol solution should reduce the bronchospasm induced by airborne particles. However, what is being done to mobilize and remove hydrated secretions? Return to page 207, frame 132, and select another answer.

209A (from page 201, frame 127)
Correct. Since the oxygen is completely dry and very little if any room air is inhaled, the deficit will be 44 mg/L. However, by the time the gas reaches the carina it will reach 100% relative humidity at body temperature by means of warming by convection and humidification by evaporation of water from the upper airways. Please continue on page 204, frame 128.

209B (from page 200, frame 126)
Wrong. Particles this large will impact before reaching the supraglottic tissues. Nose breathing at rapid inspiratory flow rates will result in most particles depositing in the nasopharynx. Return to page 200, frame 126, and select another answer.

209C (from page 206, frame 131)
Wrong. Racemic epinephrine is a vasoconstrictor and has a small bronchodilator effect. The problem during an acute asthma attack is smooth muscle spasm and bronchoconstriction. Return to page 206, frame 131, review Table 7–2, and try again.

209D (from page 204, frame 129)
Correct. A large inspiration of 15 mL/kg or larger is needed to produce an effective cough. Please continue on page 205, frame 130.

209a (from page 207, frame 132)
Correct. Adding a bronchodilator to the aerosolized bland solution should reduce any bronchospasm induced by aerosol particles. Starting chest physiotherapy concurrently should help to mobilize and remove recently hydrated secretions, and the patient's dyspnea should subside. Please continue on page 210 and complete the chapter exercises.

209b (from page 205, frame 130)
Correct. The 10% concentration of acetylcysteine is safe and effective, and the isoproterenol will help to counteract any bronchospasm that develops. Please continue on page 206, frame 131.

209c (from page 204, frame 128)
Wrong. Transporting a patient with a water-filled nebulizer is not practicable and would require a gas source for operating the nebulizer. Also, a nebulizer may deliver more water than necessary and cause pooling of secretions. Return to page 204, frame 128, and select another answer.

EXERCISES

1. List 10 devices that can be used to administer oxygen therapy and identify the type of humidifier that would be used or describe how a humidity deficit would be prevented for devices used without a humidifier.
2. Describe how aerosol therapy can be used for sputum induction.
3. Identify the best size of aerosol particle for deposition in each of the following: peripheral airways, first six generations of bronchi, larynx, oropharynx, and nasopharynx.
4. Describe how you would instruct a patient to breathe to maximize aerosol deposition in each of the following areas: peripheral airways, subglottic mucosa, and nasopharyngeal mucosa.
5. Calculate the absolute humidity in air at room temperature of 20°C and a relative humidity of 25%, 50%, and 75%.
6. Ask a friend to cough, evaluate the strength of the cough, review the five steps for producing a strong cough with him or her, and then re-evaluate your friend's ability to cough effectively.
7. Compare and contrast the advantages and disadvantages of delivering bronchoactive drugs by aerosol therapy compared with other routes of administration.
8. Explain how acetylcysteine, water, weak electrolyte solutions, and alcohol are used to loosen retained airway secretions.
9. Compare and contrast the advantages and disadvantages of heated mainstream humidifiers with heat and moisture exchangers. Identify three applications for heat and moisture exchangers.
10. Outline a plan of action for treating dyspnea that occurs 5 minutes after bland aerosol therapy is administered with an ultrasonic nebulizer.

POSTTEST

This test is designed to evaluate what you have learned from completing Chapter 7. Check your answers on page 213, and review the topics where your answer is incorrect.

1. Patient's with artificial airways should have medical gases delivered with 100% relative humidity at a temperature of
   A. 26° to 31°C.
   B. 28° to 33°C.
   C. 30° to 35°C.
   D. 32° to 37°C.
   E. 34° to 42°C.
2. Cool gas mixtures should *not* be delivered to
   I. premature infants.
   II. patients with asthma.
   III. patients recently extubated.
   A. I only
   B. II only
   C. III only
   D. I and II only
   E. II and III only
3. Aerosol therapy for sputum induction is best administered with
   A. an ultrasonic nebulizer.
   B. a gas-driven sidestream nebulizer.
   C. a gas-driven mainstream nebulizer.
   D. a metered dose inhaler.
   E. a heated jet humidifier.
4. Which of the following is the most appropriate for treating croup?
   A. unheated bland aerosols
   B. racemic epinephrine
   C. beclomethasone
   D. cromolyn sodium
   E. isoetharine
5. The particle size with maximal deposition in peripheral airways is
   A. 0.1 to 1 μm.
   B. 1 to 5 μm.
   C. 5 to 10 μm.
   D. 10 to 15 μm.
   E. 15 to 20 μm.
6. If a patient breathes through his or her nose, what proportion of 10 μm particles will deposit above the larynx?
   A. 1%
   B. 5%
   C. 25%
   D. 50%
   E. 99%

7. Which of the following statements about aerosol deposition are true?
   I. Inspiratory flow rate affects particle deposition in upper airways.
   II. A breath-hold period increases deposition in peripheral airways.
   III. Particle deposition in peripheral airways occurs by settling.
   IV. Particle deposition in upper airways occurs by impaction.
   A. I and III only.
   B. II and IV only.
   C. II and III only.
   D. I, III, and IV only.
   E. I, II, III, and IV.

8. To increase aerosol deposition in the larynx and supraglottic area, inspiratory flow should be
   A. 15 L/min.
   B. 20 L/min.
   C. 25 L/min.
   D. 30 L/min.
   E. 40 L/min.

9. The minimum absolute humidity that a gas delivered to a patient's upper airway should have is
   A. 0 mg/L.
   B. 4 mg/L.
   C. 12 mg/L.
   D. 20 mg/L.
   E. 44 mg/L.

10. Mechanical ventilators should deliver gas with absolute humidity of
   A. 21 mg/L.
   B. 30 mg/L.
   C. 33 mg/L.
   D. 44 mg/L.
   E. 50 mg/L.

11. How should a patient breathe for maximal deposition of aerosol delivered by an MDI?
   A. fast inspiratory flow, small tidal volume, and no breath hold
   B. slow inspiratory flow, large tidal volume, and no breath hold
   C. slow inspiratory flow, large tidal volume, and a 10-second breath hold
   D. fast inspiratory flow, large tidal volume, and a 10-second breath hold
   E. slow inspiratory flow, normal tidal volume, and a 5-second breath hold

12. Which of the following should be evaluated for a patient receiving aerosol therapy for bronchial hygiene?
   I. respiratory pattern and rate
   II. sputum production
   III. chest x-ray
   IV. sputum culture
   V. lung sounds
   A. I, II, and IV only
   B. I, III, and V only
   C. I, II, IV, and V only
   D. II, III, IV, and V only
   E. I, II, III, IV, and V

13. Which of the following bronchodilators is/are used to provide long-term maintenance of bronchodilator therapy?
   I. Isoproterenol
   II. Terbutaline
   III. Albuterol
   A. I only
   B. II only
   C. III only
   D. I and II only
   E. II and III only

14. Which of the following may be used to treat Gram-negative pulmonary infections?
   A. dexamethasone
   B. cromolyn sodium
   C. phenylephrine
   D. kanamycin
   E. amphotericin B

15. What concentration of acetylcysteine has proved to be effective as a mucolytic?
   A. 1%
   B. 5%
   C. 10%
   D. 20%
   E. 50%

16. Which of the following mucokinetic aerosol solutions works by destabilizing amino acid bonds in mucus by raising the pH of mucus?
   A. acetylcysteine
   B. alcohol
   C. propylene glycol
   D. glycerol
   E. sodium bicarbonate

17. The range of absolute humidity created by heat and moisture exchangers is
   A. 20 to 30 mg/L.
   B. 25 to 35 mg/L.
   C. 30 to 40 mg/L.
   D. 35 to 45 mg/L.
   E. 40 to 50 mg/L.

18. To monitor delivery of adequate humidity by a ventilator, inspired temperature should be monitored at the
   A. humidifier outlet.
   B. humidifier inlet.
   C. inspiratory limb proximal to Y-connector.
   D. expiratory limb proximal to exhalation valve.
   E. expiratory limb proximal to Y-connector.

19. When should FEV_1 be measured when evaluating the effectiveness of bronchodilator aerosol therapy?
   I. before the treatment
   II. during the treatment
   III. immediately after the treatment
   A. I only
   B. II only
   C. I and III only
   D. II and III only
   E. I, II, and III

20. The aerosol delivery device most likely to cause bronchospasm is the
   A. MDI.
   B. gas-powered sidestream nebulizer.
   C. gas-powered mainstream nebulizer.
   D. ultrasonic nebulizer.
   E. MDI with spacer.

ANSWERS TO POSTTEST

1. D (F123)	5. B (F125)	9. C (F127)	13. E (F131)	17. A (F128)
2. D (F123)	6. E (F125)	10. D (F127)	14. D (F131)	18. C (F128)
3. A (F124)	7. E (F126)	11. C (F129)	15. C (F130)	19. C (F132)
4. B (F124)	8. E (F126)	12. E (F129)	16. E (F130)	20. D (F132)

BIBLIOGRAPHY

Aloan, CA: Respiratory Care of the Newborn: A Clinical Manual. JB Lippincott, Philadelphia, 1987.

Barnes, TA: Respiratory Care Practice. Year Book Medical Publishers, Chicago, 1988.

Bell, CW, Blodgett, D, Goike, CA, Green, M, Kieffer, J, and Smith, M: Home Care and Rehabilitation in Respiratory Medicine. JB Lippincott, Philadelphia, 1984.

Burton, GG and Hodgkin, JE: Respiratory Care: A Guide to Clinical Practice, ed 2. JB Lippincott, Philadelphia, 1984.

Eubanks, DH and Bone, RC: Comprehensive Respiratory Care, ed 2. CV Mosby, St. Louis, 1990.

Finucane, BT and Santora, AH: Principles of Airway Management. FA Davis, Philadelphia, 1988.

Kacmarek, RM and Stoller, JK: Current Respiratory Care. BC Decker, Philadelphia, 1989.

Koff, PB, Eitzman, DV, and Neu, J: Neonatal and Pediatric Respiratory Care. CV Mosby, St. Louis, 1988.

Scanlon, C, Spearman, CB, Sheldon, RL, and Egan, DF: Egan's Fundamentals of Respiratory Therapy, ed 5. CV Mosby, St. Louis, 1990.

Shapiro, BA, Harrison, RA, Kacmarek, RM, and Cane, RD: Clinical Application of Respiratory Care, ed 3. Year Book Medical Publishers, Chicago, 1985.

8

Airway Care

133. Maintenance of patent airways
134. Oral and nasopharyngeal airways
135. Endotracheal tubes
136. Confirming endotracheal tube position
137. Tracheal tube cuff inflation
138. Tracheal suctioning
139. Cough evaluation and instruction
140. Indications for chest physical therapy
141. Chest percussion and vibration
142. Postural drainage positions
143. Complications and hazards of airway care
144. Indications for IPPB
145. Relative contraindications and hazards of IPPB
146. IPPB—patient instruction
147. Monitoring patient response to IPPB
148. Control interaction during IPPB
149. Etiology and pathophysiology of atelectasis
150. Indications for incentive spirometry
151. Incentive spirometry—patient instruction
152. Breathing exercises

PRETEST

This pretest is designed to measure what you know about airway care. Check your answers on page 218 and continue on page 219, frame 133.

1. Which of the following would be best to prevent atelectasis from developing postoperatively?
   A. intermittent positive-pressure breathing (IPPB)
   B. breathing exercises
   C. incentive spirometry
   D. postural drainage
   E. aerosol therapy

2. Oral airways should be used in which of the following situations?
   A. conscious patient prior to tracheal intubation
   B. conscious patient receiving nasotracheal suctioning
   C. obtunded patient during bag and mask ventilation
   D. conscious patient with a nasotracheal tube in place
   E. obtunded patient following tracheotomy

3. What size suction catheter is appropriate for use with a size 7 endotracheal tube?
   A. 6 Fr (French dimensions)
   B. 8 Fr
   C. 10 Fr
   D. 12 Fr
   E. 14 Fr

4. What is the most accurate method of determining if an endotracheal tube is properly placed?
   A. end-tidal CO_2 monitoring
   B. metabolic cart monitoring
   C. stat chest x-ray
   D. auscultation of the epigastrium
   E. auscultation of the chest bilaterally

5. Tracheal tube cuff pressure will stop lymphatic flow and cause mucosal edema when the pressure exceeds
   A. 5 mm Hg.
   B. 15 mm Hg.
   C. 20 mm Hg.
   D. 25 mm Hg.
   E. 30 mm Hg.

6. The vacuum applied to the suction catheter of an adult patient should be limited to
   A. − 20 to − 50 mm Hg.
   B. − 50 to − 80 mm Hg.
   C. − 80 to − 120 mm Hg.
   D. − 120 to − 160 mm Hg.
   E. − 160 to − 200 mm Hg.

7. A strong cough will generate expiratory flow of
   A. 30 L/min.
   B. 50 L/min.
   C. 60 L/min.
   D. 100 L/min.
   E. 300 L/min.

8. Of the following at least risk for developing a need for chest physical therapy is
   A. ventilator patients.
   B. abdominal surgery.
   C. thoracic surgery.
   D. intracranial surgery.
   E. chronic obstructive pulmonary disease (COPD).
9. Which postural drainage position would be best to drain the anterior segment of the right upper lobe?
   A. prone Trendelenburg's
   B. supine Trendelenburg's
   C. modified sideways with left side down
   D. semi-Fowler's
   E. Fowler's
10. Which of the following chest physiotherapy procedures produce(s) mechanical energy that is delivered to the patient's chest during both inspiration and expiration?
   A. vibration
   B. percussion
   C. segmental breathing exercises
   D. lateral costal breathing exercises
   E. abdominal breathing exercises
11. The minimal leak technique should be used to inflate endotracheal tube cuffs so that the inflation pressure is as low as possible and no higher than
   A. 5 mm Hg.
   B. 15 mm Hg.
   C. 20 mm Hg.
   D. 25 mm Hg.
   E. 35 mm Hg.
12. IPPB is indicated to promote coughing with patients who have a forced vital capacity less than
   A. 7 mL/kg.
   B. 10 mL/kg.
   C. 13 mL/kg.
   D. 15 mL/kg.
   E. 20 mL/kg.
13. All of the following are hazards or contraindications of IPPB *except*
   A. recent myocardial infarction.
   B. recent intracranial surgery.
   C. pneumothorax.
   D. weak cough.
   E. hemoptysis.
14. Which of the following would be the best way for a patient to breathe when receiving IPPB?
   A. fast, deep inhalation followed by slow exhalation
   B. slow, deep inhalation followed by fast exhalation
   C. slow, deep inhalation, pause, followed by fast exhalation
   D. fast, medium-size inhalation, pause, followed by slow exhalation
   E. slow, deep inhalation, pause, followed by slow exhalation
15. All of the following should be monitored before, during, and after IPPB *except*
   A. pulse.
   B. temperature.
   C. breath sounds.
   D. abdominal distention.
   E. ability to cough effectively.

16. Controls on an IPPB machine that affect inspiratory time include
    I. cycling pressure.
    II. flow.
    III. sensitivity.
    IV. apnea timer.
    A. I only
    B. II only
    C. I and II only
    D. I, II, and III only
    E. I, II, III, and IV
17. Increasing transpulmonary pressure leads to
    I. alveolar inflation and expansion.
    II. lung and alveolar collapse.
    III. decreased expiratory reserve volume.
    A. I only
    B. II only
    C. III only
    D. II and III only
    E. I and III only
18. Why is incentive spirometry more appropriate than IPPB to treat or prevent atelectasis?
    A. Patients breathe deeply with incentive spirometry.
    B. Recently inflated alveoli may collapse within 60 minutes.
    C. IPPB machines cost more.
    D. Incentive spirometers are disposable.
    E. IBBP machines spread nosocomial infections.
19. How many sustained maximal inspirations should a patient using incentive spirometry perform each waking hour?
    A. 1
    B. 2
    C. 5
    D. 12
    E. 20
20. Which of the following breathing exercises will increase lower lobe expansion and diaphragmatic excursion without restricting the movement of the abdomen?
    A. pursed-lip breathing
    B. diaphragmatic breathing
    C. relaxation exercises
    D. lateral costal breathing
    E. segmental breathing

ANSWERS TO PRETEST

1. C (F133)
2. C (F134)
3. C (F135)
4. E (F136)
5. A (F137)
6. C (F138)
7. E (F139)
8. D (F140)
9. C (F142)
10. B (F141)
11. D (F143)
12. D (F144)
13. D (F145)
14. E (F146)
15. B (F147)
16. C (F148)
17. A (F149)
18. B (F150)
19. C (F151)
20. D (F152)

FRAME 133. MAINTENANCE OF PATENT AIRWAYS

Several important principles are involved in maintaining patent airways such as: (1) humidification of inspired gases, (2) inflammatory response of pulmonary mucosa to secretions, (3) effect of partial or complete plugging of airways, and (4) effect of stasis of secretions. Chapter 7 covers the humidification of inspired gases when artificial airways bypass upper airways. A humidity deficit will result in increased water loss from the pulmonary tree, which leads to disruption of the continuous layer of mucus covering the airways. The cilia in the airway epithelium move this mucus layer constantly upward toward the pharynx, which keeps the lungs free of airborne particles. A humidity deficit or dehydration will dry this mucus belt and disrupt this protective mechanism. When drying of the mucus belt occurs, cilia are less effective in moving secretions upward and the more tenacious secretions partially or completely block bronchioles, which leads to atelectasis. Secretions trapped behind plugged airways are an ideal culture medium, which may cause bacterial infiltration of mucosa and pneumonia.

Prophylactic and therapeutic respiratory care procedures used to keep the airways patent are called bronchial hygiene therapy. Incentive spirometry is the prophylactic treatment of choice and is considered more effective than intermittent positive-pressure breathing (IPPB) or chest physical therapy for the *prevention* of atelectasis. To mobilize retained secretions, reinflate areas of absorption atelectasis, and reduce the chance of bacterial infection or pneumonia; a combination of aerosol therapy, chest physical therapy, IPPB, and incentive should be administered.

(Q) Which of the following bronchial hygiene procedures should be administered *first* to treat airways plugged with secretions?

a. postural drainage — 225 c
b. chest percussion — 225 B
c. aerosol therapy — 225 a

FRAME 134. ORAL AND NASOPHARYNGEAL AIRWAYS

Oral and nasopharyngeal airways are used to relieve obstruction caused when the tongue moves posteriorly and rests against the pharyngeal wall. Usually the airways are placed after unsuccessful attempts to relieve the obstruction by repositioning the head or by anterior displacement of the mandible. These airways are used to provide a means for ventilation until an endotracheal tube can be placed.

A wooden tongue blade may be used to move the tongue anteriorly when placing an oral airway. Some practitioners insert oral airways with the tip initially pointing toward the hard palate, and then advance the airway and simultaneously turn it 180 degrees so that the tip slides behind the tongue into the hypopharynx. When turning the oral airway, caution should be taken to prevent loose teeth from becoming dislodged. Also, oral airways should be used only in patients whose protective reflexes are obtunded, since the airway may stimulate gag reflexes and trigger vomiting.

A nasopharyngeal airway is much better tolerated by semicomatose and awake patients than an oropharyngeal airway. Suctioning of the pharynx is possible with a suction catheter that has been lubricated with viscous lidocaine or water-soluble gel and passed through the airway. The airway should also be lubricated before insertion and advanced gently into the naris with care taken not to traumatize the turbinates. If resistance is encountered, the other naris or a smaller airway should be used. To ensure that the nasopharyngeal airway does not slip into the esophagus or trachea it should have a ring or cone. Those airways without a cone or ring should have a pin passed through the proximal end to ensure the tube remains in position. The proper length airway may be estimated by measuring the distance from the tip of the nose to the tragus of the ear plus 1 in. The distal tip of the airway rests between the base of the tongue and posterior wall of the pharynx.

(Q) Which of the following would be best for a conscious patient whose tongue is obstructing his airway?

a. oropharyngeal airway 224 B
b. nasopharyngeal airway 225 A
c. oral endotracheal tube 224 a

FRAME 135. ENDOTRACHEAL TUBES

The endotracheal tube has an important role in airway care and tracheal intubation may be lifesaving. It provides a patent airway for mechanical ventilation and application of end-expiratory pressure while sealing off the lower airways from the danger of aspiration of gastric fluids. Careful examination of endotracheal tubes will reveal that a great deal of useful information is printed on the tube. The following can usually be found on tracheostomy and most endotracheal tubes: (1) the tube caliber in millimeters (both internal and external diameter) and (2) length in centimeters. The letters "IT" (implant tested) indicate that the tube has been tissue-tested and will not elicit a toxic response. Modern endotracheal tubes often have side ports and cuffs specifically designed to reduce the pressure applied to the tracheal wall. A large cuff volume allows a seal to be made using inflation pressure that is 25 mm Hg or less, which reduces mucosal ischemia and necrosis in the trachea. The side port and beveled tip allow ventilation to occur when the end of the tube is against the tracheal wall or when obstructed by a mucous plug. The recommended size for endotracheal tubes is 8.5 to 9.0 mm inside diameter (ID) for adult males and 8.0 to 8.5 mm ID for adult women. One size larger and one size smaller should be allowed for individual variations. (See Table 8–1.)

TABLE 8–1
RECOMMENDED SIZES FOR ENDOTRACHEAL TUBES AND SUCTION CATHETERS

Age	Internal Diameter (mm)	Suction Catheters (Fr)
Newborn	3.0	6
6 months	3.5	8
18 months	4.0	8
3 years	4.5	8
5 years	5.0	10
6 years	5.5	10
8 years	6.0	10
12 years	6.5	10
16 years	7.0	10
Adult (female)	75.–8.0*	12
Adult (male)	8.0–8.5*	14

*One size larger and one size smaller should be allowed for individual variations.
Source: American Heart Association: 1985 National Conference on Standards for Cardiopulmonary Resuscitation and Emergency Cardiac Care. JAMA 255:2962, 1986. Used with permission.

(Q) What size tube(s) would you select in preparing for endotracheal intubation of a 12-year-old male?
a. 6.5 mm OD (outside diameter) 224 C
b. 7.0, 8.0 mm OD 224 d
c. 6.0, 6.5., 7.0 mm ID 225 C
d. 6.5, 7.0., 7.5 mm ID 225 d

FRAME 136. CONFIRMING ENDOTRACHEAL TUBE POSITION

The most practical way to determine if an endotracheal tube is in the trachea is auscultation of the chest bilaterally in the axillary region, anterior chest wall, and the epigastrium. Esophageal intubation may cause a noticeable epigastric bulge, low-pitched gurgling sounds over the epigastrium, and minimal or no rise in the chest in response to ventilation. It is important to look for symmetrical chest expansion. Right main-stem intubation should be suspected in adults when the marking on the proximal end of the tube at the lips is greater than 23 cm, compliance is low, the chest moves asymmetrically, and breath sounds are unequal on auscultation.

The most reliable method of determining if the endotracheal tube is in the trachea is end-tidal CO_2 monitoring. End-tidal air reflects the concentration of CO_2 found in mixed venous blood and contains approximately 6% carbon dioxide. If the endotracheal tube is in the esophagus, the end-tidal CO_2 monitor will reflect the concentration of CO_2 found in room air (0.04%) and the carbon dioxide concentration will change little from breath to breath. Pulse oximetry can be very useful in detecting the hypoxemia caused by intubation of the esophagus or right main-stem bronchus. A chest x-ray should be routinely done after an endotracheal tube has been placed to determine its position in the trachea. Alternatively a fiberoptic bronchoscope may be used to determine the position of the tube in the trachea.

The improper placement of an endotracheal tube may cause the patient's condition to deteriorate quickly. Accordingly, the evaluation process immediately following endotracheal intubation should take only 20 to 30 seconds. If a patient becomes hypoxic or vital signs deteriorate immediately following intubation, then incorrect tube placement must be suspected. If auscultation of the chest and epigastrium area confirm esophageal intubation, the endotracheal tube must be removed and the patient ventilated with 100% oxygen.

(Q) If, immediately following endotracheal intubation, the end-tidal CO_2 monitor climbs to 6% after each tidal volume but the pulse oximeter indicates tachycardia and a decreasing arterial saturation, where is the endotracheal tube located?

a. trachea 224 D
b. right main-stem bronchus 225 D
c. esophagus 224 b

FRAME 137. TRACHEAL TUBE CUFF INFLATION

The goal of endotracheal intubation is to provide a patent airway for ventilation and to protect the upper airways from aspiration of gastric material or secretions from the upper airways. The tracheal tube cuff provides the seal that allows manual and mechanical ventilation to be delivered to the lungs and protects the lower airways from aspiration. Modern disposable endotracheal tubes have cuffs designed to provide a maximum seal with a minimum of pressure. Practitioners would like to have cuffs seal at pressures of 15 mm Hg (21 cm H_2O) or even as low as 5 mm Hg. This concern for low pressure stems from the assumption that arterial and venous blood flow would be present throughout the entire ventilatory cycle if inflation pressure does not exceed 15 mm Hg. Pressure below 5 mm Hg would allow normal lymphatic flow and avoid development of mucosal edema.

The cuff inflation method that provides the best compromise between an adequate seal and minimum inflation pressure is the minimal occluding volume (MOV) technique. The MOV technique calls for the cuff to be slowly inflated with an in-line pressure monitor until no air can be heard escaping past the cuff during a positive pressure inflation when listening with a stethoscope placed over the laryngeal area. Next the air in the cuff is slowly removed in ¼ to ½ mL increments until a small leak is heard at the point of peak inspiratory pressure. An in-line manometer is used to monitor the inflation pressure, which might be high if the endotracheal tube is too small and the cuff does not have enough surface area in contact with the tracheal wall. Except when peak airway pressures are very high, cuff pressure exceeding 25 mm Hg is considered unacceptable and requires the tube to be replaced with the next larger size. Periodic deflation of the cuff has not been shown to prevent tracheal damage and may result in the cuff being improperly reinflated. Hypoxemia (from loss of positive end-expiratory pressure) and hypoventilation (due to smaller tidal volumes) may occur during the deflation period.

(Q) Which of the following cuff inflation pressures would allow both arterial and venous blood flow to be present throughout the entire ventilatory cycle?

a. 30 mm Hg 224 c
b. 25 mm Hg 225 b
c. 15 mm Hg 224 A

224A (from page 223, frame 137)
Correct. A cuff pressue of 15 mm Hg or less is optimal because it will allow both arterial and venous blood flow to occur throughout the ventilatory cycle. Please continue on page 226, frame 138.

224B (from page 220, frame 134)
Wrong. Oral airways should be used only in patients whose protective reflexes are obtunded. The oral airway may cause a conscious patient to gag and vomit when it touches the posterior pharyngeal wall. Return to page 220, frame 134, and select another answer.

224C (from page 221, frame 135)
Wrong. Endotracheal tube sizes are based on the inside diameter in order to facilitate selection of the proper suction catheter, which must not be larger than one half the inside diameter of the tube. More than one tube should be prepared to allow for individual differences. Return to page 221, frame 135, and select another answer.

224D (from page 222, frame 136)
Wrong. If the endotracheal tube is in the trachea, why are clinical signs of moderate hypoxemia present? Return to page 222, frame 136, and select another answer.

224a (from page 220, frame 134)
Wrong. Endotracheal intubation may not be necessary and it will be difficult to intubate a conscious patient, since gag reflexes may be stimulated and cause the patient to vomit. Return to page 220, frame 134, and select another answer.

224b (from page 222, frame 136)
Wrong. If the tube is in the esophagus, the end-tidal CO_2 monitor would not climb to 6% CO_2 with each exhalation. Return to page 222, frame 136, and select another answer.

224c (from page 223, frame 137)
Wrong. A cuff pressure of 30 mm Hg will completely stop capillary blood flow. Return to page 223, frame 137, and select another answer.

224d (from page 221, frame 135)
Wrong. Endotracheal tube sizes are based on the inside diameter to facilitate selection of the proper size suction catheter, which must not be larger than one half the inside diameter of the tube. One size larger and one size smaller endotracheal tubes should be prepared to allow for individual differences. Return to page 221, frame 135, and try again.

225A (from page 220, frame 134)
Correct. A nasopharyngeal airway is much better tolerated by a conscious patient and will allow ventilation to occur. Please continue on page 221, frame 135.

225B (from page 219, frame 133)
Wrong. Until the secretions are rehydrated and made less viscous, you will have little success. Return to page 219, frame 133, and try again.

225C (from page 221, frame 135)
Correct. The correct tube size is 6.5 mm ID, and one size above and below that in order to deal with variation among individuals. Please continue on page 222, frame 136.

225D (from page 222, frame 136)
Correct. The end-tidal CO_2 monitor reveals that alveolar gas is passing through the endotracheal tube. However, the pulse oximeter indicates that a large right-to-left shunt is causing the patient to be moderately hypoxemic. Thus, it is likely that the tube has slipped into the right main-stem bronchus. Please continue on page 223, frame 137.

225a (from page 219, frame 133)
Correct. The first step would be to rehydrate the dry secretions to facilitate their removal from the airways. Postural drainage and chest percussion may be helpful in removing secretions after aerosol therapy has been administered. Please continue on page 220, frame 134.

225b (from page 223, frame 137)
Wrong. A cuff pressure of 25 mm Hg will allow some arterial capillary blood flow, but will cause venous flow obstruction. Return to page 223, frame 137, and select another answer.

225c (from page 219, frame 133)
Wrong. Until the secretions are rehydrated and made less viscous, you would have little success unless the patient had a chronic secretion problem. Return to page 219, frame 133, and select another answer.

225d (from page 221, frame 135)
Wrong. One of the tubes you selected is the wrong size for a 12-year-old, even allowing for variation among individuals. Return to page 221, frame 135, and select another answer.

FRAME 138. TRACHEAL SUCTIONING

Suctioning the aritifical airway is a necessary but dangerous procedure. The goal is to remove secretions from the trachea and main-stem bronchi that accumulate due to the patient's inability to cough effectively. The suction catheter used should not be larger than one half the inside diameter of the tracheal tube. Endotracheal tubes are marked with the inside diameter (mm), outside diameter (mm), and length. The size of tracheal tubes is designated using the ID. For example, a *size 8* endotracheal tube will have an *inside diameter* of 8 millimeters. Suction catheters are commonly labeled in French (Fr) dimensions using a system that uses catheters sized by circumference stated in millimeters. The conversion from French (circumference) to outside diameter in millimeters is based on the formula for calculating the circumference of a circle ($C = \pi D$, circumference $= 3.14 \times$ diameter). To ease the conversion, π is rounded to 3 and diameter = circumference ÷ 3. For example, a 12-Fr suction catheter has a 4-mm OD, and would be appropriate for use with a size 8 (8 mm ID) endotracheal tube.

Vacuum applied to a suction catheter should be limited to − 80 to − 120 mm Hg for adults and − 50 to − 80 mm Hg for infants. The vacuum should be applied for only 10 to 15 seconds and 10 seconds or less for infants. The patient should be ventilated with 100% oxygen before and after suctioning. A minimum of five large tidal volumes should be delivered and reoxygenation should continue until vital signs return to baseline before suctioning the trachea again.

The catheter should be inserted without suction until resistance is met and then pulled back 1 cm. Then the catheter should be removed while intermittent suctioning is applied. The catheter may stimulate a vagal reflex and cause bradycardia; removal of oxygen may cause hypoxemia, which usually manifests itself as tachycardia and occasionally as bradycardia. Accordingly, the electrocardiographic monitor should be observed during suctioning for cardiac dysrhythmias, such as tachycardia, bradycardia, or premature ventricular contractions. At the first sign of cardiac dysrhythmias or other types of patient distress, the procedure should be stopped immediately and the patient ventilated with 100% oxygen.

(Q) What size French catheter should be used to suction a patient with a size 8 endotracheal tube?

a. 12 Fr 232 A
b. 14 Fr 233 A
c. 16 Fr 233 b

FRAME 139. COUGH EVALUATION AND INSTRUCTION

The cough is a major defense mechanism against accumulation of secretions in the airways. Cough instruction is an important part of bronchial hygiene therapy, since it is one of two mechanisms that move secretions to the upper airways where they can be expectorated or swallowed. Teaching a patient with retained secretions to cough productively requires instruction and coaching. The following steps should be explained: (1) a deep breath (at least 15 mL/kg); (2) an inspiratory pause to allow time for peripheral distribution of the tidal volume and time for increasing intrathoracic pressure; (3) with the glottis closed, increased intrathoracic pressure occurs when the contraction of abdominal muscles pushes the diaphragm upward (intercostal muscles must contract to resist expansion of the chest wall); and (4) finally the patient must suddenly open the glottis and let the gas explode out of the lungs at a velocity that may be as high as 300 L/min.

Patients who cannot breath deeply will have weak coughs and may require aerosol therapy, incentive spirometry, IPPB, or chest physiotherapy to reinflate atelectatic areas, reverse bronchospasm and mucosal edema, and unplug totally obstructed airways. Attention should also be directed at discovering the cause of a weak cough, such as incisional pain, abdominal musculature limitations, neuromuscular diseases, and obstructive or restrictive pulmonary disease. Once identified, some of the causes of shallow breathing can be alleviated, such as reducing incisional pain by planning bronchial hygiene therapy to follow the administration of analgesics and by teaching the patient to support the incision when coughing.

(Q) Which of the following should be done first when administering bronchial hygiene therapy?

a. IPPB 233 e
b. aerosol therapy 233 B
c. postural drainage 232 a
d. cough instruction 232 b

FRAME 140. INDICATIONS FOR CHEST PHYSICAL THERAPY

The indications for chest physical therapy (CPT) are primarily related to the patient's inability to maintain normal bronchial hygiene. Prophylactic use of CPT is usually reserved for high-risk abdominal or thoracic surgery patients who have a high pack-year smoking history and abnormal pulmonary function preoperatively. Patients who cannot cough effectively or breathe deeply following surgery are given CPT to prevent secretion retention and airway plugging. Ventilator patients who are immobilized, are subjected to humidity deficits, and have trouble coughing with an endotracheal tube keeping the glottis open, have a tendency to retain secretions, and usually benefit from chest physiotherapy.

Therapeutic indications include atelectasis caused by secretions partially or totally plugging airways. Moving thick secretions in an important goal of CPT when a weak cough results in plugged airways. Patients with abnormal breathing patterns caused by primary or secondary dysfunction would usually be considered for prophylactic or therapeutic CPT. Patients with chronic obstructive pulmonary disease, decreased exercise tolerance, or pulmonary disease that causes chronic airway secretion problems (cystic fibrosis or bronchiectasis) will benefit from mobilization of retained secretions. Patients with a musculoskeletal deformity that prevents deep breathing and thus makes coughing ineffective usually benefit from postural drainage and other CPT procedures.

(Q) All of the following patients would benefit from CPT *except*

a. patients who have a vital capacity of 15 mL/kg. 232 C
b. ventilator patients. 233 D
c. preoperative chronic obstructive pulmonary disease (COPD) patients. 232 c

FRAME 141. CHEST PERCUSSION AND VIBRATION

Chest percussion is a technique done to loosen thick secretions in the airways. Air trapped between cupped hands and the chest produces sound waves that are transmitted through the chest wall to the airways. The percussion is applied over the surface landmarks of lung segments with retained secretions. Special care should be taken to avoid the clavicles, spine of the scapula, and spinal column. The cupped hands must strike the chest with wrists loose and flexible so that not too much force is delivered. Patients with osteoporosis, long-term steroid use, and cancer of the ribs may have brittle bones that may fracture if chest percussion is administered too aggressively or if the wrists are not kept loose and flexible. Percussion is done throughout inspiration and expiration with the patient in the appropriate bronchial drainage position. Aerosol therapy should precede the percussion to hydrate thick mucus or to deliver other bronchoactive aerosols such as mucolytics, decongestants, and bronchodilators. The procedure is contraindicated for patients with resectable tumors of the lung, fractured ribs, active tuberculosis, and empyema.

Chest vibration is done with the hands on the chest and arms held straight. A high-frequency motion, which begins just before the patient exhales and lasts throughout exhalation, is created through the arms from the shoulders. Some practitioners find mechanical vibrators more consistent, effective, and less tiring. The purpose of chest vibration is to loosen and move mucus plugs toward larger airways. The therapist's hands may be placed side by side or one hand can be placed on top of the other, with the fingers and palm flat on the chest. Typically, vibrations are done with 5 to 10 deep breaths in combination with chest percussion and postural drainage. Patients with artificial airways or those being mechanically ventilated should have a large tidal volume delivered with a manual resuscitator; vibrations should be delivered as the bag is released quickly so that exhalation is rapid.

(Q) The best sequence for delivering bronchial hygiene therapy is

a. percussion, vibrations, followed by postural drainage. 232 B
b. postural drainage, followed by percussion and vibrations. 233 a
c. postural drainage, percussion, and vibrations all concurrently. 232 d

FRAME 142. POSTURAL DRAINAGE POSITIONS

Mucus flow is facilitated by the effect of gravity. Placing the patient in gravity-dependent positions helps retained secretions to drain to larger airways. Chest percussion and vibration are more effective in moving retained secretions when the patient is placed in the appropriate postural drainage position.

A patient placed in a postural drainage position should be told to breathe normally and to cough as necessary. The postural drainage positions commonly used to drain specific lung segments are illustrated in Figures 8-1 and 8-2. Several of the lung segments require the patient to be placed in a Trendelenburg's position, which may be contraindicated immediately following intracranial surgery, esophageal anastomosis, tube feeding for spontaneously breathing patients, or for patients who have recently suffered an acute myocardial infarction or cerebral vascular accident. Blood pressure and other vital signs should be stable before extreme positioning is attempted. It may be necessary to modify the position when the patient is unable to tolerate the appropriate postural drainage position.

Gravity-dependent positions may affect diaphragmatic excursion with improvement seen when the patient is turned from supine to side lying. Restriction of diaphragmatic movement usually occurs when the patient is placed in a head-down position. The patient should remain in the appropriate postural drainage position for 5 to 10 minutes, but tolerance should be assessed carefully and the position modified or discontinued as necessary.

(Q) Which postural drainage position is best to drain secretions from the right lateral basal segment?

a. Fowler's position 232 D
b. prone Trendelenburg's 233 C
c. supine Trendelenburg's 233 c
d. left-side-down Trendelenburg's 233 d

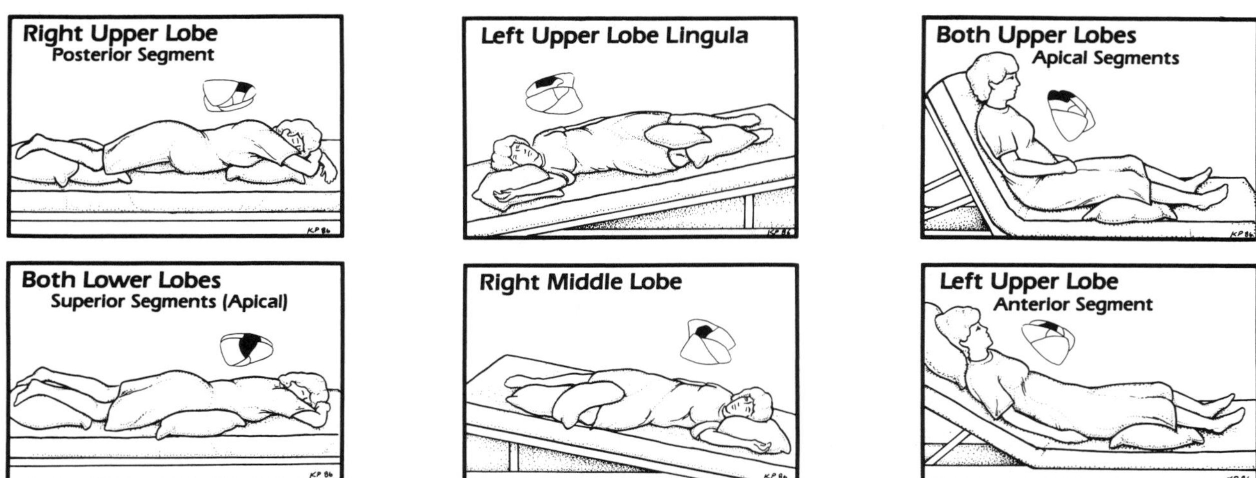

Figure 8–1 Postural drainage positions. (Source: Frownfelter, DL: Chest Physical Therapy and Pulmonary Rehabilitation: An Interdisciplinary Approach, ed 2. Year Book Medical Publishers, Chicago, 1987. Used with permission.)

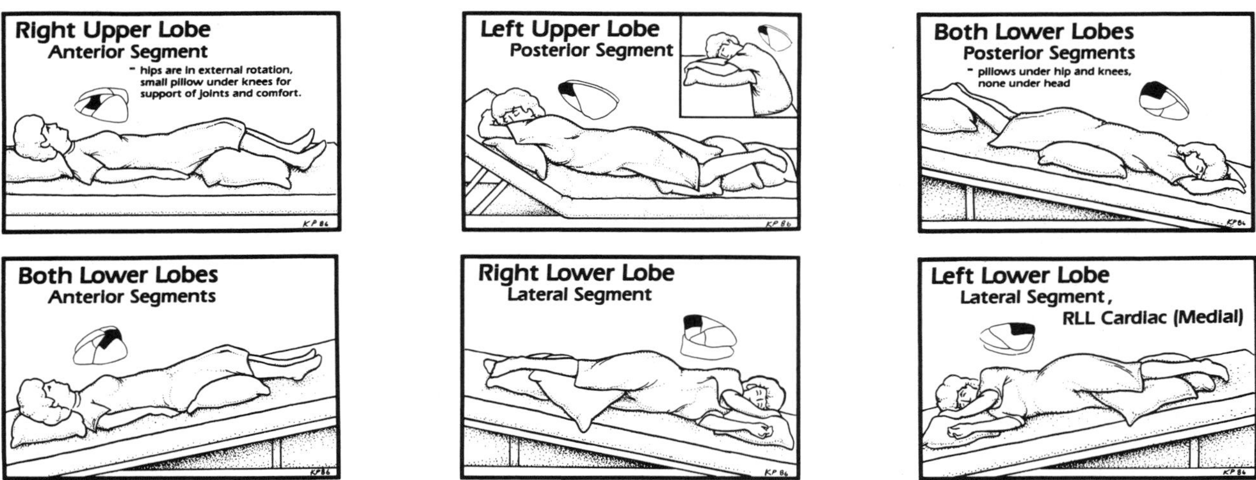

Figure 8–2 Postural drainage positions. (Source: Frownfelter, DL: Chest Physical Therapy and Pulmonary Rehabilitation: An Interdisciplinary Approach, ed 2. Year Book Medical Publishers, Chicago, 1987. Used with permission.)

232A (from page 226, frame 138)
Correct. A 12-Fr suction catheter has an OD of 4 mm, which does not exceed one half of the 8-mm ID of the size 8 endotracheal tube. Please continue on page 227, frame 139.

232B (from page 229, frame 141)
Wrong. You have neglected to put gravity to work to move secretions to larger airways. Return to page 229, frame 141, and select another answer.

232C (from page 228, frame 140)
Correct. IPPB and CPT treatments given QID have not proven as effective in preventing atelectasis or secretion retention as incentive spirometry every hour. Please continue on page 229, frame 141.

232D (from page 230, frame 142)
Wrong. The Fowler's position is used to drain the apical segments of both upper lobes. The semi-Fowler's position is used to drain the anterior segment of the left upper lobe. Return to page 230, frame 142, and select another answer.

232a (from page 227, frame 139)
Wrong. Except for patients with chronic secretion problems, aerosol therapy should be given before postural drainage in order to hydrate dried secretions or to deliver mucolytics to loosen retained secretions. If the patient's vital capacity is below 15 mL/kg, IPPB may be needed to improve distribution of ventilation and medications. However, cough instruction and evaluation should be provided before starting the aerosol therapy. Return to page 227, frame 139, and try again.

232b (from page 227, frame 139)
Correct. The patient's cough should be evaluated and cough instruction provided before other bronchial hygiene procedures are administered. Please continue on page 228, frame 140.

232c (from page 228, frame 140)
Wrong. Because of their chronic secretion problems and pulmonary dysfunction, COPD patients will benefit from CPT procedures such as postural drainage, chest percussion, and breathing exercises before surgery. Return to page 228, frame 140, and try again.

232d (from page 229, frame 141)
Correct. Postural drainage, percussion, and vibrations should be administered together. If the patient is receiving IPPB, all three chest physiotherapy procedures should be done along with the IPPB treatment. Please continue on page 230, frame 142.

233A (from page 226, frame 138)
Wrong. A 14-Fr suction catheter has a 14-mm circumference and a 4.67-mm OD which exceeds one half the 8-mm ID of a size 8 endotracheal tube. Remember, the conversion from the French (circumference value) to OD requires dividing the French size by 3. Return to page 226, frame 138, and try again.

233B (from page 227, frame 139)
Wrong. Aerosol therapy will help to restore and maintain the mucociliary escalator, and should be given before postural drainage and IPPB (if the patient has a vital capacity greater than 15 mL/kg). However, cough instruction and evaluation should be provided before starting the aerosol therapy. Return to page 227, frame 139, and select another answer.

233C (from page 230, frame 142)
Wrong. The prone Trendelenburg's position drains the posterior segments of both lower lobes. Return to page 230, frame 142, and try again.

233D (from page 228, frame 140)
Wrong. A ventilator patient will have secretion retention problems caused by immobility, humidity deficits, and inability to cough effectively. Return to page 228, frame 140, and select another answer.

233a (from page 229, frame 141)
Wrong. You have gravity working for you, but without the help of percussion and vibration to move secretions to larger airways. Return to page 229, frame 141, and select another answer.

233b (from page 226, frame 138)
Wrong. A 16-Fr suction catheter has a 16-mm circumference and a 5.33 OD, which exceeds one half the 8-mm ID of the size 8 endotracheal tube. Remember, the conversion from the French (circumference value) to OD requires dividing the French size by 3. Return to page 226, frame 138, and try again.

233c (from page 230, frame 142)
Wrong. The supine Trendelenburg's position drains the anterior basal segments. Return to page 230, frame 142, and select another answer.

233d (from page 230, frame 142)
Correct. The left-side-down Trendelenburg's position drains the right lateral basal segments. Please continue on page 234, frame 143.

233e (from page 227, frame 139)
Wrong. IPPB is appropriate only when the patient has a vital capacity of less than 15 mL/kg. A patient who cannot breathe deeply may benefit from IPPB, which may promote the cough mechanism. Also, improved distribution of ventilation and aerosol medication may occur with IPPB. However, evaluating the patient's ability to cough and cough instruction should be done first. Return to page 227, frame 139, and try again.

FRAME 143. COMPLICATIONS AND HAZARDS OF AIRWAY CARE

Administering bland aerosol therapy or mucolytic agents often leads to dyspnea, increased airway resistance, bronchospasm, and increased work of breathing. Hydrating the mucus blanket may cause the secretions to swell and decrease the caliber of the airway. Mucus plugs when broken by mucolytic will travel to larger airways and may impede ventilation. The aerosol particle itself may be irritating to airway mucosa and high-density aerosol generators such as ultrasonic nebulizers frequently cause bronchospasm. The patient should be assessed during aerosol therapy and chest percussion, vibration, and postural drainage should be given concurrently to move loosened secretions. A bronchodilator should be added to solutions delivered by ultrasonic nebulizer and when acetylcysteine (Mucomyst) is delivered by any type of nebulizer. The aerosol therapy should be temporarily stopped when dyspnea occurs and chest physiotherapy started to raise loosened secretions.

Dyspneic patients with a sudden decrease in sputum should be evaluated for retained secretions caused by airway obstruction or infection. If a generalized secretion problem has been resolved except for one area of the lung, then chest physical therapy should be directed to that region.

When patients become obtunded and lose their oropharyngeal reflexes a cuffed endotracheal tube should be placed to protect the lower airways from aspiration. Subglottic edema may develop where the cuff makes contact with the tracheal wall. A cuff pressure greater than 25 mm Hg may cause damage to the trachea which may result in a severe obstruction when the tube is removed. Cuff pressure, not cuff volume, is the key factor and should be kept as low as possible. If the peak inspiratory pressure of a ventilator patient drops substantially, the cuff should be reinflated. Patients should not be extubated until their upper airway reflexes are fully intact and they are able to ventilate adequately without ventilator support. The criteria used to wean patients from ventilators should be used to help make this decision. The vital capacity should be at least 15 mL/kg, maximum inspiratory pressure $\geq$ 20 cm H_2O, and blood gases should have returned to the patient's baseline. The patient should not be weaned if one or more systems are in failure.

Not all patients will be able to withstand the position changes required for postural drainage. The patient should be evaluated for recent intracranial surgery, myocardial infarction, or cerebral vascular accidents, and drainage positions modified if necessary. Aggressive chest percussion should be avoided with recent rib fractures or replaced with vibrations. Caution needs to be taken with patients who have osteoporosis (brittle bones). Osteoporosis is often encountered with chronic lung disease patients who receive steroids routinely over a long span. Untreated pulmonary tuberculosis and tumors of the chest are contraindications of chest percussion since the disease may be spread to other regions.

(Q) All of the following would be clinical signs that a patient is not tolerating aerosol therapy *except*

a. 40/min increase in pulse, unproductive coughing. 240 B
b. 15/min increase in pulse, anxiety. 241 A
c. active use of accessory muscles, unproductive coughing. 240 a

FRAME 144. INDICATIONS FOR IPPB

The primary indication for intermittent positive-pressure breathing (IPPB) treatments is to provide deep breathing to patients afflicted with a disease that limits the depth of tidal volumes. The control of the inspiratory-to-expiratory ratio along with a much larger tidal volume may improve (1) the coughing mechanism, (2) the distribution of ventilation, and (3) the delivery of aerosol medications to the lung periphery. IPPB can be used to facilitate coughing in acutely ill patients who are unable to produce a vital capacity of at least 15 mL/kg. A deep breath is a critical part of an effective cough and IPPB should be combined with other bronchial hygiene techniques when a deep breath cannot be taken spontaneously.

Patients with diminished inspiratory capacity or those with rapid and inefficient ventilatory patterns may have atelectasis reversed by IPPB therapy. However, IPPB must be administered correctly with large tidal volumes that require pressure of 30 cm H_2O or higher, and a 1 to 2 second inspiratory pause. The use of large tidal volumes, inspiratory pause, and adequate exhalation will limit the rate to 6 to 8 per minute. A major problem is that the IPPB therapy must be given frequently or the atelectasis will return when the patient returns to a rapid shallow breathing pattern.

IPPB therapy should only be used to deliver aerosol medications when a person has a limited ability to breathe deeply. Control of the inspiratory flow rate is an important variable which will affect aerosol deposition. Low flows of less than 30 L/min result in a greater peripheral deposition than high flows. Accordingly, IPPB therapy may improve particle deposition in the periphery for patients who breathe shallowly at fast rates.

(Q) How often should IPPB therapy be given to prevent or substantially reverse atelectasis?

a. every hour — 240 A
b. every 4 hours — 241 B
c. QID — 240 b

FRAME 145. RELATIVE CONTRAINDICATIONS AND HAZARDS OF IPPB

Dizziness and headaches during IPPB may be due to increased mean intrathoracic pressure, which restricts venous return, lowers cardiac output, and results in increased intracranial pressure. This should not be a problem if the IPPB treatment is administered properly and the patient is placed in the Fowler's position to facilitate venous drainage from the head. This problem usually occurs when the patient is allowed to trigger the IPPB machine at a high rate. Giving the IPPB therapy with rest periods and using rates of 6 to 8/min should prevent increased intracranial pressure from developing.

Dizziness during IPPB may also be caused by hyperventilation which lowers the CO_2 and results in less blood flow to the brain. Hyperventilation will occur if an anxious patient triggers the IPPB machine at fast rates without rest periods. Coaching the patient should minimize this problem but it is important to insist on slow deep breathing with rest periods.

The development of a pneumothorax during IPPB may occur as a result of better distribution of ventilation and high pressure that develops as a result of coughing that may occur during the treatment. If a pneumothorax is suspected, the IPPB therapy must be stopped immediately until the patient is evaluated. Any complaint of chest pain during or after coughing must be evaluated carefully to rule out pneumothorax. The high pressure generated by IPPB-induced coughing may cause bronchial venous bleeding which stops on its own. However, hemoptysis observed in the sputum during IPPB requires that the treatment be stopped and the patient's physician notified. The bleeding may be related to a tumor or left-sided heart failure and the therapist should not continue the treatment until the cause of the bleeding is determined.

Special care must be taken not to administer IPPB with high oxygen concentrations to patients with chronic CO_2 retention who breathe on a hypoxic drive. IPPB machines can be powered by central piped-air systems or by portable air compressors so that arterial oxygen tension does not rise to levels that would remove their respiratory drive. Gastric distention may be caused during IPPB if high-peak inspiratory pressure forces air into the stomach. This is most likely to occur if a mask is used or if the patient swallows. The distended stomach may impede diaphragmatic excursion and cause discomfort and pain. The most hazardous event would be vomiting with the chance that gastric contents with low pH might be aspirated into the lungs. If gastric insufflation occurs, the treatment should be discontinued and thought given to administering the IPPB at a lower pressure or discontinuing it all together.

Other hazards of IPPB include the chance of nosocomial infections being spread to a patient via his breathing circuit. Proper hand washing when moving between patients, replacing the circuit at regular intervals, and the use of bacterial filters on IPPB machines should prevent this hazard from occurring. Only small medication nebulizers should be used with IPPB machines and the nebulizer should always be left clean and dry.

(Q) Which of the following cycling rates should be used during IPPB?

a. 6 to 8/min with rest periods 240 C

b. 6 to 8/min with no rest periods 241 D

c. 10 to 14/min with no rest periods 241 b

FRAME 146. IPPB—PATIENT INSTRUCTION

The success of IPPB therapy relies heavily on how well instructed the patient is regarding the procedure and therapeutic goal. The importance of coughing correctly should be reviewed and the patient encouraged to stop the treatment to cough as necessary. The patient should be instructed to take slow, deep breaths, and hold inspiration for 1 to 2 seconds. The tidal volume delivered by the IPPB machine should be at least 100% of the patient's limited vital capacity. The patient should not be receiving IPPB therapy unless his vital capacity is less than 15 mL/kg. A primary therapeutic goal is to provide deep breathing to facilitate the cough mechanism so that retained secretions can be cleared from the peripheral airways. Accordingly, IPPB is given with chest percussion, vibrations, and postural drainage when the patient cannot cough effectively as a result of a limited vital capacity.

Patient cooperation is important and the person should be instructed to avoid premature termination of the inspiratory cycle by voluntarily splinting of the chest wall, closure of the epiglottis, or occluding the mouthpiece with his tongue. Exhaled volumes should be monitored and the cycling pressure increased as needed. The patient should be encouraged to relax and try to assist by taking slow deep breaths. The therapist should provide support with hands or towel over surgical incisions, fractures, or wounds. The rest periods of 1 to 2 minutes are a good time to review with the patient the importance of deep breaths, a slow inhalation time, the 1 to 2 second breath hold, and a slow cycling rate of 6 to 8/min with adequate time for exhalation. Patients should be encouraged to inform the therapist of chest pain, the need to cough, dizziness, headache, or a tingling sensation in their hands.

(Q) Which of the following tidal volumes should be used with IPPB therapy when the patient's limited vital capacity is 1000 mL?

a. 500 mL 240 D
b. 750 mL 241 a
c. 1000 mL 241 C

FRAME 147. MONITORING PATIENT RESPONSE TO IPPB

The monitoring of a patient receiving IPPB therapy begins before you enter the patient's room to administer the treatment. A careful review of the patient's chart helps the therapist formulate therapeutic objectives and understand why the patient is breathing with small tidal volumes. A quick review of the respiratory care or treatment section of the chart will provide information about how well the patient has tolerated previous IPPB and bronchial hygiene treatments. X-ray reports and the current respiratory care orders should be reviewed before treatment begins.

Before starting IPPB, vital signs should be checked to provide a point of reference for assessing the effect of the therapy. The vital signs should be measured before, during, and after the treatment to monitor for adverse reactions. Administering aerosolized bronchodilators with IPPB may cause tachycardia, and the treatment should be promptly terminated if an increase in heart rate of 20 or more over pretherapy levels is observed. A primary therapeutic goal of administering IPPB is to promote the cough mechanism of patients unable to cough adequately. The patient may generate high alveolar pressure during coughing, which may cause a pneumothorax. If the patient complains of chest pain, and/or suddenly exhibits signs of moderate hypoxemia, the treatment should be discontinued and the patient carefully evaluated for signs of pneumothorax.

The patient should be monitored carefully for complaints of dizziness, headache, and a tingling sensation in the fingers, which are signs of hyperventilation or increased intracranial pressure. This should not be a problem if the rate is held to 6 to 8 positive-pressure breaths per minute and 1 to 2 rest periods are provided every 20 breaths. Increased airway resistance may develop during IPPB from swollen secretions or bronchospasm if an ultrasonic nebulizer is placed in the circuit to deliver high density aerosols. Mucolytics aerosolized with IPPB may cause dyspnea as loosened mucus plugs move toward larger airways. Both mucolytics and high-density aerosols delivered with IPPB may cause bronchospasm. Thus, breath sounds should be monitored before, during, and after the treatment.

The record of therapy and patient response is charted after each treatment. This note should include (1) duration of therapy; (2) peak pressure used; (3) tidal volume achieved; (4) aerosol medication, dose, and amount delivered; (5) patient's response to therapy, including breath sounds, vital signs, ability to cough; (6) sputum production—volume, color, texture, and smell; (7) special equipment needed such as a face mask; (8) other bronchial hygiene procedures combined with IPPB, such as chest percussion and bronchial drainage.

(Q) Which of the following are signs that a patient cannot tolerate IPPB therapy?

a. dizziness 240 c
b. headache 241 c
c. chest pain 240 E

FRAME 148. CONTROL INTERACTION DURING IPPB

In order for IPPB to be effective, the machine-delivered tidal volume must be large and delivered at the appropriate inspiratory flow rate. Proper adjustment of controls on IPPB machines such as the Bird Mark 7 is critical to giving a successful treatment. Slow, deep breathing can be accomplished with a Mark 7 by eliciting patient cooperation, adjusting inspiratory flow and pressure cycling controls. The sensitivity control must be set so that the patient can trigger an assisted breath with less than 1 cm H_2O of subatmospheric pressure.

The inspiratory flow control should be set high enough so that the patient's inspiratory effort is not stifled by inadequate flow before the desired tidal volume is reached. The patient should be coached to inhale slowly so that the inspiratory flow control on the IPPB machine can be gradually decreased.

The delivery of large tidal volumes will require using a relatively high cycling pressure of 30 to 50 cm H_2O. Gas insufflation is uncommon in the alert and cooperative patient but may be a problem with the neurologically obtunded. The initial pressure should be 15 to 20 cm H_2O for a few breaths, thus allowing time for the patient to gradually increase his tidal volume to 100% of his limited vital capacity. Both the pressure and flow-rate controls will need to be increased as the tidal volume is increased. If only the pressure-limit control is increased on a Mark 7, the inspiratory time may become uncomfortable too long. Inspiration must be short enough to allow adequate time for exhalation. Limiting the rate to 6 to 8/min will reduce the impact of inspiratory time on the time available for exhalation. Another reason for limting rate is to reduce the increase in mean intrathoracic pressure that occurs with the combination of long inspiratory time, 1 to 2 second breath hold, and high cycling pressure. The principles discussed regarding control interaction with the Bird Mark 7 should be applied to other IPPB machines so that one ventilation parameter is not adjusted at the expense of another control of equal importance.

(Q) After gradually increasing the pressure limit on an IPPB machine to 30 cm H_2O, the patient appears to be breathing with difficulty and the pressure manometer lags behind the patient's inspiratory effort; what control needs to be adjusted?

a. decrease the pressure limit — 240 d
b. increase flow rate — 241 d
c. increase sensitivity — 241 E

240A (from page 235, frame 144)
Correct. IPPB treatments must be given every hour to be effective in preventing or reversing atelectasis. This makes using IPPB therapy to treat atelectasis financially impractical. Please continue on page 236, frame 145.

240B (from page 234, frame 143)
Wrong. You should temporarily discontinue the treatment and use chest percussion, vibrations, and postural drainage, if you have evidence that retained secretions are causing the dyspnea. Return to page 234, frame 143, and select another answer.

240C (from page 236, frame 145)
Correct. This will reduce the chance of increasing intracranial pressure and should prevent hyperventilation. Please continue on page 237, frame 146.

240D (from page 237, frame 146)
Wrong. The tidal volume should be 100% of the limited vital capacity. Return to page 237, frame 146, and select another answer.

240E (from page 238, frame 147)
Correct. The IPPB treatment should be stopped immediately if the patient complains of chest pain especially during coughing or following a cough. The patient should be evaluated for pneumothorax, which may become a tension pneumothorax if the IPPB therapy were allowed to continue. Please continue on page 239, frame 148.

240a (from page 234, frame 143)
Wrong. You should temporarily discontinue the treatment and use percussion, vibrations, and postural drainage if you have evidence that retained secretions are causing the dyspnea. Return to page 234, frame 143, and select another answer.

240b (from page 235, frame 144)
Wrong. IPPB treatments must be given every hour to be effective in preventing or reversing atelectasis. This makes using IPPB therapy to treat atelectasis financially impractical. Please continue on page 236, frame 145.

240c (from page 238, frame 147)
Wrong. This may be the result of hyperventilation caused by inadequate patient instruction. After a rest period, provided the dizziness is gone, IPPB should be tried again with the rate held to 6 to 8/min with rest periods every 20 breaths. Return to page 238, frame 147, and try again.

240d (from page 239, frame 148)
Wrong. This will shorten the inspiratory time and increase the inspiratory flow rate, which may make the patient more comfortable. However, IPPB therapy administered with small tidal volumes is of little value. Return to page 239, frame 148, and select another answer.

241A (from page 234, frame 143)
Correct. You should continue the aerosol therapy and monitor the heart rate and breath sounds. Please continue on page 235, frame 144.

241B (from page 235, frame 144)
Wrong. IPPB treatments must be given every hour to be effective in preventing or reversing atelectasis. This makes using IPPB therapy to treat atelectasis financially impractical. Please continue on page 236, frame 145.

241C (from page 237, frame 146)
Correct. The tidal volume should be 100% of the limited vital capacity. Please continue on page 238, frame 147.

241D (from page 236, frame 145)
Wrong. Rest periods are needed to reduce the chance of increasing intracranial pressure and to prevent hyperventilation. Return to page 236, frame 145, and try again.

241E (from page 239, frame 148)
Wrong. The sensitivity setting is not the problem. The difficulty the patient is exhibiting is related to another control that interacts with the pressure-limit control. You can assume the sensitivity control was readjusted after the pressure limit was increased. What other control might cause the manometer to lag behind the patient's own breathing? Return to page 239, frame 148, and select another answer.

241a (from page 237, frame 146)
Wrong. The tidal volume should be at least 100% of the limited vital capacity. Return to page 237, frame 146, and try again.

241b (from page 236, frame 145)
Wrong. A rate this high with large tidal volumes may subject the patient to high intracranial pressure and hyperventilation. Return to page 236, frame 145, and select another answer.

241c (from page 238, frame 147)
Wrong. This may be the result of increased intracranial pressure caused by restriction of venous return occurring because of inadequate patient instruction. After a rest period, provided the headache is gone, the IPPB should be tried again with the rate held to 6 to 8/min with rest periods every 20 breaths. Return to page 238, frame 147, and try again.

241d (from page 239, frame 148)
Correct. The increased flow rate will make the patient more comfortable. Increasing the pressure limit has lengthened the inspiratory time and this patient has increased the flow rate as he or she tries to breathe deeply, which decreases the inspiratory time. With coaching the patient can be taught to lengthen the inspiratory time at the higher cycling pressure and then the flow setting can be reduced. Please continue on page 242, frame 149.

FRAME 149. ETIOLOGY AND PATHOPHYSIOLOGY OF ATELECTASIS

Figure 8–3 illustrates the conditions and mechanisms contributing to the development of atelectasis. The diagram presents a summary of the etiological and pathological factors that place patients at risk for atelectasis. It is important for respiratory care practitioners to be familiar with these factors, since prophylactic and therapeutic bronchial hygiene attempts to prevent or reverse atelectasis.

(Q) In general, decreasing transpulmonary pressure leads to

a. alveolar inflation and expansion. 246 A

b. alveolar collapse. 246 c

c. increased alveolar pressure. 247 C

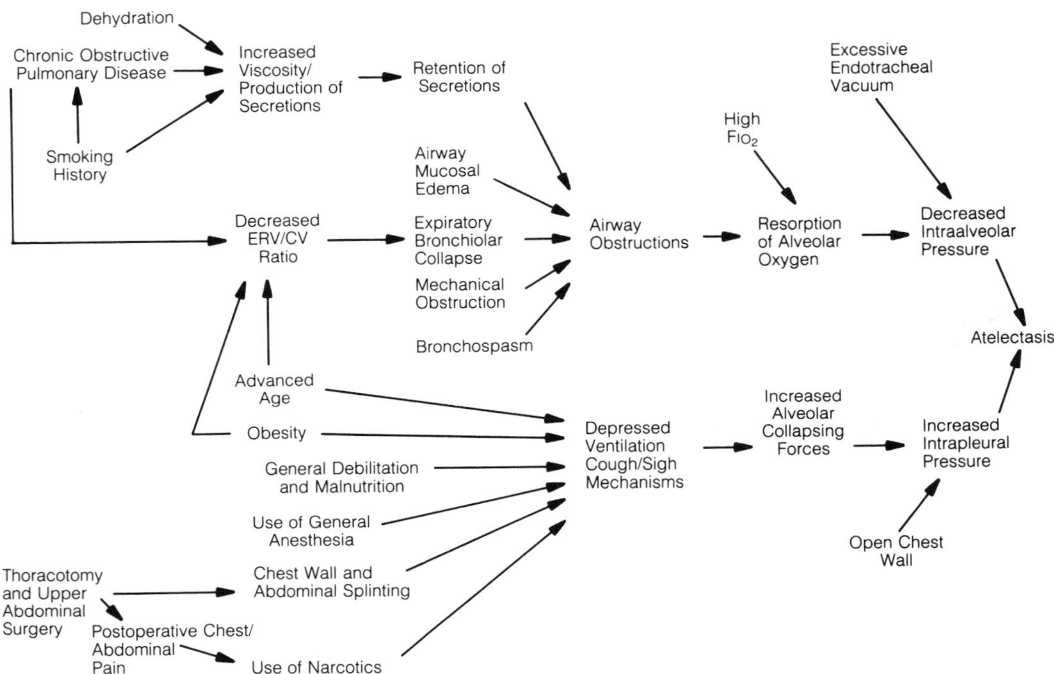

Figure 8–3 Conditions and mechanisms contributing to the development of atelectasis. (Source: Barnes, TA: Respiratory Care Practice. Year Book Medical Publishers, Chicago, 1988. Used with permission.)

FRAME 150. INDICATIONS FOR INCENTIVE SPIROMETRY

Incentive spirometry is a prophylactic mode of bronchial hygiene therapy that attempts to prevent alveolar collapse. Incentive spirometers are designed to encourage patients to breathe deeply and to sustain the inspiratory flow as long as possible. Candidates for incentive spirometry are those patients who are at risk for development of atelectasis. The patient must be cooperative and motivated since the incentive spirometer must be used each hour the patient is awake. Children 4 years old or younger are generally not good candidates because their ability to follow instructions and motivation to use the incentive device hourly are limited.

Incentive spirometry is prophylactic therapy; thus the lungs should be without retained secretions, substantial alveolar collapse, or infection. The patient at risk for atelectasis is likely to have a forced vital capacity (FVC) that is less than 50% of that predicted, but FVC should be at least 15 mL/kg. When postoperative inspiratory capacity (IC) is 50% to 80% of preoperative or predicted volume, incentive spirometry usually is used. Incentive spirometry is not indicated when postoperative IC is 80% of the preoperative or predicted value unless signs of atelectasis and pulmonary complications are present.

Maintaining and increasing the FVC should help patients cough more effectively. Thus the chance of atelectasis developing from retained secretions or plugged airways should be substantially reduced. A sudden decrease in the patient's ability to reach previously achieved incentive spirometry goals may signal the development of atelectasis and pneumonia. Therapeutic bronchial hygiene therapy would then be indicated and might include a combination of aerosol therapy, IPPB, and CPT.

(Q) Candidates for incentive spirometry should have a FVC of at least

a. 10 mL/kg. 246 C
b. 15 mL/kg. 247 A
c. 20 mL/kg. 247 a

FRAME 151. INCENTIVE SPIROMETRY—PATIENT INSTRUCTION

The goal of incentive spirometry is to have the patient create and hold for 2 to 3 seconds the largest transpulmonary pressure possible in order to inflate collapsed alveoli. The inspired volume is the clinical measure used by most incentive spirometers to indicate how much transpulmonary pressure has been created during inspiration. There are some incentive breathing exercisers that require a ball to be maintained at the top of a tube for 2 to 3 seconds to encourage the patient to continue the sustained maximum inspiratory effort as long as possible. Incentive spirometers that do not show inspired volume have various ways of displaying and adjusting the sustained inspiratory flow created by the patient.

The patient must fully understand how to use the incentive spirometer and why it needs to be used hourly. The benefit achieved by sustaining the maximum inspiratory flow for 2 to 3 seconds needs to be stressed. The patient should be taught to use the incentive spirometer sitting in a semi-Fowler's position. The advantages of relaxed deep breathing should be explained and the patient taught muscle relaxation exercises. For example, ask the patient to shrug his shoulders, and let them drop; or to make a fist and tighten his arms and chest, hold it, and then let it go. A higher tidal volume may be achieved if diaphragmatic breathing is reviewed with the patient.

The initial volume level should be set at twice the patient's measured tidal volume and the goal adjusted higher if appropriate. A patient who cannot reach the initial goal, may need more instruction or re-evaluation for the appropriateness of incentive spirometry. The patient should be instructed to do 5 to 10 sustained maximal inspirations (SMI) per waking hour. Only 5 SMIs should be done if the patient becomes exhausted doing 10 per hour. One SMI every 30 to 60 seconds should prevent the patient from hyperventilating and will provide rest periods.

The patient should be evaluated and observed doing incentive spirometry at least twice daily for the first 48 hours postoperatively and then daily. To meet quality assurance criteria, the goals of incentive spirometry and the results of initial and ongoing evaluations should be documented in the patient's chart. The following should be monitored: ability to inspire the preoperative inspiratory capacity, understanding and compliance with instructions, the need for setting new volume or sustained flow objectives, and assessment for evidence of atelectasis and pneumonia. When the patient has the ability to inspire 80% of the preoperative inspiratory capacity, the daily evaluations by the therapist can be discontinued. Disposable incentive breathing devices are commonly used and thus incentive spirometry often continues unsupervised through recovery.

(Q) How long should the maximum inspiratory effort last when a patient does incentive breathing therapy?

a. 1 second 246 B
b. 2 seconds 247 B
c. as long as possible 246 a

FRAME 152. BREATHING EXERCISES

Breathing exercises are an important part of chest physiotherapy and usually accompany postural drainage, percussion, vibration, and cough instruction. The four most commonly used breathing exercises are diaphragmatic breathing, pursed-lip breathing, segmental breathing, and lateral costal breathing. Breathing exercises are most successful when the patient is as relaxed as possible. The instruction is best done in a supine semi-Fowler's position with relaxation exercises leading to an awareness of the movements of breathing.

Diaphragmatic breathing involves focusing the patient's attention on his or her breathing pattern and depth of tidal volumes. The patient is taught to breathe against the pressure of his or her hand, which is placed on the upper abdomen. This exercise allows diaphragmatic excursion to be monitored by the patient, who is encouraged to do hourly self-checks to make sure that he or she is breathing properly.

A relaxed form of pursed-lip breathing will allow patients to create back pressure on the airways during exhalation, which reduces airway collapse and air trapping. Pursed-lip breathing by patients in respiratory distress who try to force air out may increase intrathoracic pressure to a level that may restrict venous return to the heart. However, the relaxed form of pursed-lip breathing may allow dyspneic patients to regain control of their breathing.

The therapist or patient's hand can be used to facilitate deeper ventilation in a specific area of the lungs. The pressure of the hand on the chest surface results in more air moving into the lung segments directly under the area where the pressure has been applied. This type of breathing exercise is called segmental breathing and is very useful in increasing ventilation to congested areas of the lung.

Lateral costal breathing exercises will increase ventilation to the lower lobes and facilitate diaphragmatic breathing. The therapist's hands are placed over the costal margins at the lower edge of the ribs, and as the patient exhales through pursed lips, the hands follow the contracting rib margins. Near the end of exhalation the therapist exerts a forceful squeeze and holds the pressure firmly. Pressure is gradually released as inhalation begins with some resistance to the expanding ribs maintained. Patients are told to focus on their waist and to inhale against the pressure of the therapist's hand pressure. Moving the hands higher up to the midaxillary area will increase ventilation to the middle lobes. Patients can be taught to apply the pressure to the costal margin with their own hands to facilitate diaphragmatic breathing without restricting the movement of the abdomen.

(Q) Who should apply the hand pressure used with diaphragmatic, segmental, and lateral costal breathing?

a. the therapist 246 b
b. the patient 247 b
c. either therapist or patient 247 c

246A (from page 242, frame 149)
Wrong. Decreased transpulmonary pressure can occur as a result of intra-alveolar pressure or increased intrapleural pressure. Return to page 242, frame 149, and select another answer.

246B (from page 244, frame 151)
Wrong. The goal of incentive breathing therapy is a sustained maximal inspiratory effort. Return to page 244, frame 151, and try again.

246C (from page 243, frame 150)
Wrong. Incentive spirometry is a prophylactic bronchial hygiene therapy. A FVC of 10 mL/kg is evidence of an acute pulmonary disease, such as pneumonia or atelectasis. Return to page 243, frame 150, and try again.

246a (from page 244, frame 151)
Correct. Healthy people can sustain a transpulmonary pressure gradient in excess of 40 cm H_2O for 5 to 15 seconds. Thus, patients should be encouraged to sustain the maximum inspiratory effort as long as possible. The patient should be encouraged to inspire slowly to sustain the inspiratory effort for a minimum of 3 to 5 seconds. Please continue on page 245, frame 152.

246b (from page 245, frame 152)
Wrong. The therapist will use his or her hands for the breathing exercises when treating the patient. However, what happens when the patient needs the breathing exercises and the therapist is not available? Return to page 245, frame 152, and select another answer.

246c (from page 242, frame 149)
Correct. Alveolar collapse will occur from decreased transpulmonary pressure caused by decreased alveolar and/or increased pleural pressure. Please continue on page 243, frame 150.

247A (from page 243, frame 150)
Correct. A FVC of 15 mL/kg or higher makes a patient a good candidate for incentive spirometry. The patient must be motivated and able to cooperate so that the incentive breathing device is used correctly every hour the patient is awake. Please continue on page 244, frame 151.

247B (from page 244, frame 151)
Almost. Two seconds may be all that some patients can sustain, but healthy people can sustain a transpulmonary pressure gradient in excess of 40 cm H_2O for 5 to 15 seconds. Thus, patients should be encouraged to sustain the maximum inspiratory effort as long as possible. The patient should be encouraged to inspire slowly and sustain the inspiratory effort for a minimum of 3 to 5 seconds. Please continue on page 245, frame 152.

247C (from page 242, frame 149)
Wrong. Decreased transpulmonary pressure can occur as a result of decreased alveolar pressure or increased pleural pressure. Return to page 242, frame 149, and study Figure 8–3; then try again.

247a (from page 243, frame 150)
Wrong. We are looking for *minimum* criteria for a patient to be a good candidate for incentive spirometry. Return to page 243, frame 150, and select another answer.

247b (from page 245, frame 152)
Wrong. This is not the best answer, there will be times especially at first where the therapist will be able to teach the breathing exercises better if the patient relaxes and concentrates on the pressure applied to the chest by the therapist. Later the patient will be taught to do the breathing exercises unassisted. Return to page 245, frame 152, and try again.

247c (from page 245, frame 152)
Correct. At first the patient is better off relaxing and focusing on the hand pressure applied to the chest by the therapist. Later the patient will be taught to do the breathing exercises unassisted. Please continue on page 248 and complete the chapter exercises.

EXERCISES

1. List three therapeutic goals for each of the following modalities of bronchial hygiene therapy: chest physiotherapy, IPPB therapy, and incentive spirometry.
2. Describe how to determine what length nasopharyngeal airway should be used.
3. List five ways to confirm the proper placement of an endotracheal tube.
4. Draw a diagram that shows how a manometer can be connected to the pilot tube and syringe used to inflate the cuff on an endotracheal tube.
5. Calculate the largest French-sized suction catheter that can be used with each of the following endotracheal tube sizes: 3, 4, 6, 7, 8, and 9.
6. List the steps necessary to generate a strong cough.
7. List the postural drainage positions for each of the lung segments.
8. Describe how to instruct a patient to breathe properly during an IPPB treatment.
9. List six colors that may be observed in the sputum of a patient produced by a strong cough and identify the significance of each color.
10. Compare and contrast the indications for incentive spirometry against indications for IPPB.

POSTTEST

This test is designed to evaluate what you have learned by completing chapter 8. Check your answers on page 251 and review the topics where your answer choice is incorrect.

1. Which of the following would be best to remove retained secretions?
   A. chest percussion
   B. chest vibrations
   C. aerosol therapy
   D. postural drainage
   E. combination of all of the above
2. Which of the following airways may use a safety pin through the proximal end to keep the tube in position?
   A. nasotracheal tube
   B. orotracheal tube
   C. nasopharyngeal tube
   D. oropharyngeal tube
   E. esophageal obturator
3. All of the following help to prevent obstruction of an endotracheal tube by a mucus plug *except*
   A. beveled tip on the distal end of the tube.
   B. use of high-volume cuffs.
   C. side holes on the distal end of the tube.
   D. adequate humidification.
   E. periodic suctioning of the tube.
4. Following tracheal intubation, the time taken to confirm proper placement of the tube should be less than
   A. 5 to 10 seconds.
   B. 10 to 20 seconds.
   C. 20 to 30 seconds.
   D. 30 to 60 seconds.
   E. 1 to 2 minutes.
5. The minimal occluding volume technique involves slowly inflating the cuff until air is
   A. *not* heard leaking throughout inspiration.
   B. *not* heard leaking throughout expiration.
   C. *not* heard leaking at end inspiration.
   D. heard leaking only at end inspiration.
   E. heard leaking starting at midinspiration.
6. Vacuum applied to a suction catheter of an infant should be limited to
   A. − 20 to − 50 mm Hg.
   B. − 50 to − 80 mm Hg.
   C. − 80 to − 120 mm Hg.
   D. − 120 to − 160 mm Hg.
   E. − 160 to − 200 mm Hg.

7. To produce a strong cough a deep breath should be at least
   A. 7 mL/kg.
   B. 12 mL/kg.
   C. 15 mL/kg.
   D. 20 mL/kg.
   E. 30 mL/kg.

8. Patients with a musculoskeletal deformity may need chest physiotherapy to mobilize retained secretions that occur as a result of
   I. hyperventilation.
   II. hypopnea.
   III. chronic CO_2 retention.
   IV. ineffective coughing.
   V. bradypnea.
   A. I only
   B. III only
   C. II and IV only
   D. I, III, and V only
   E. II, IV, and V only

9. Which postural drainage position would be best to drain the posterior basal segments of both lower lobes?
   A. prone Trendelenburg's
   B. supine Trendelenburg's
   C. modified sideways with left side down
   D. semi-Fowler's
   E. Fowler's

10. Which of the following chest physiotherapy procedures is done only during exhalation with hands held constantly on the patient's chest?
    A. percussion
    B. vibrations
    C. segmental breathing
    D. diaphragmatic breathing
    E. pursed-lip breathing

11. An endotracheal tube cuff should be deflated and reinflated
    A. every 2 hours.
    B. every 8 hours.
    C. every 24 hours.
    D. only when the peak inspiratory pressure changes.
    E. when a leak is heard at peak inspiration.

12. To deliver a tidal volume with an IPPB machine that is 100% of a patient's limited vital capacity may require a pressure that exceeds
    A. 10 cm H_2O.
    B. 15 cm H_2O.
    C. 20 cm H_2O.
    D. 30 cm H_2O.
    E. 50 cm H_2O.

13. Complaints of chest pain during or after coughing may be related to
    A. pneumothorax.
    B. bronchospasm.
    C. mucosal swelling.
    D. airway obstruction.
    E. loosening of retained secretions.

14. A primary reason for administering IPPB therapy is to
   A. reverse atelectasis.
   B. prevent atelectasis.
   C. facilitate the cough mechanism.
   D. lower arterial CO_2 tension.
   E. raise arterial O_2 tension.

15. The number of tidal volumes delivered during IPPB therapy should be limited to
   A. 2 to 4/min.
   B. 4 to 6/min.
   C. 6 to 8/min.
   D. 8 to 10/min.
   E. 10 to 12/min.

16. Which of the following changes in control settings may result in an IPPB machine delivering a larger tidal volume?
   A. increased flow
   B. decreased pressure
   C. increased sensitivity
   D. decreased flow
   E. increased apnea time

17. All of the following may depress ventilation and cough mechanisms *except*
   A. positive end-expiratory pressure.
   B. general anesthesia.
   C. narcotics.
   D. obesity.
   E. chest wall splinting.

18. A sudden decrease in the patient's ability to reach previously achieved incentive spirometry goals may signal
   A. a need to discontinue incentive spirometry.
   B. absence of retained secretions.
   C. atelectasis.
   D. a need for a replacement spirometer.
   E. a need for IPPB therapy.

19. A patient should be taught to use an incentive spirometer in which of the following positions?
   A. supine
   B. standing
   C. Fowler's
   D. semi-Fowler's
   E. alternate side lying

20. The breathing exercise that improves ventilation by creating back pressure in the bronchioles during exhalation is called
   A. segmental breathing.
   B. lateral costal breathing.
   C. pursed-lip breathing.
   D. diaphragmatic breathing.
   E. relaxation exercises.

ANSWERS TO POSTTEST

1. E (F133)
2. C (F134)
3. B (F135)
4. C (F136)
5. D (F137)
6. B (F138)
7. C (F139)
8. C (F140)
9. A (F142)
10. B (F141)
11. D (F143)
12. D (F144)
13. A (F145)
14. C (F147)
15. C (F146)
16. D (F148)
17. A (F149)
18. C (F150)
19. D (F151)
20. C (F152)

BIBLIOGRAPHY

Aloan, CA: Respiratory Care of the Newborn: A Clinical Manual. JB Lippincott, Philadelphia, 1987.

Barnes, TA: Respiratory Care Practice. Year Book Medical Publishers, Chicago, 1988.

Bell, CW, Blodgett, D, Goike, CA, Green, M, Kieffer, J, and Smith, M: Home Care and Rehabilitation in Respiratory Medicine. JB Lippincott, Philadelphia, 1984.

Burton, GG and Hodgkin, JE: Respiratory Care: A Guide to Clinical Practice, ed 2. JB Lippincott, Philadelphia, 1984.

Eubanks, DH and Bone, RC: Comprehensive Respiratory Care, ed 2. CV Mosby, St. Louis, 1990.

Finucane, BT and Santora, AH: Principles of Airway Management. FA Davis, Philadelphia, 1988.

Frownfelter, DL: Chest Physical Therapy and Pulmonary Rehabilitation, ed 2. Year Book Medical Publishers, Chicago, 1987.

Kacmarek, RM and Stoller, JK: Current Respiratory Care. BC Decker, Philadelphia, 1989.

Koff, PB, Eitzman, DV, and Neu, J: Neonatal and Pediatric Respiratory Care. CV Mosby, St. Louis, 1988.

Scanlon, CL, Spearman, CB, Sheldon, RL, and Egan, DF: Egan's Fundamentals of Respiratory Therapy, ed 5. CV Mosby, St. Louis, 1990.

Shapiro, BA, Harrison, RA, Kacmarek, RM, and Cane, RD: Clinical Application of Respiratory Care, ed 3. Year Book Medical Publishers, Chicago, 1985.

9

Mechanical Ventilation

PRETEST

This pretest is designed to measure what you already know about mechanical ventilation. Check your answers on page 256 and then continue on page 257, frame 153.

1. Which of the following maximum inspiratory pressure measurements indicate that ventilatory support may not be needed?
   A. 5 cm H_2O
   B. 10 cm H_2O
   C. 15 cm H_2O
   D. 20 cm H_2O
   E. 25 cm H_2O
2. Mechanical ventilation is required when spontaneous breathing cannot overcome which of the following?
   I. elastic forces
   II. flow resistive forces
   III. hypoxemia
   IV. hypercarbia
   A. I and II only
   B. II and IV only
   C. II and III only
   D. II, III, and IV only
   E. I, II, and IV only
3. Which of the following modes of ventilation will support a patient who suddenly becomes apneic?
   I. controlled
   II. assisted
   III. assist-control
   A. I only
   B. II only
   C. III only
   D. I and II only
   E. I and III only
4. Which mode of ventilation combines spontaneous breathing with mandatory machine delivered tidal volume?
   A. controlled
   B. synchronized intermittent mandatory ventilation
   C. assist-control
   D. assisted
   E. pressure support
5. Which mode of ventilation has an inspiratory flow rate that is high at first and then decreases in order to maintain a constant pressure as air flows into the lungs?
   A. controlled
   B. assist-control
   C. SIMV
   D. pressure-support
   E. continuous positive-airway pressure (CPAP)
6. All of the following are common physical findings of a tension pneumothorax *except*
   A. shift of trachea toward affected area.
   B. sharp pain over affected side.
   C. hypotension.
   D. hyperresonant percussion note over affected area.
   E. change in heart rate.

7. The *initial* tidal volume for mechanical ventilation should be
   A. 7 mL/kg.
   B. 10 mL/kg.
   C. 12 mL/kg.
   D. 15 mL/kg.
   E. 18 mL/kg.
8. Slight hyperventilation may benefit patients with
   A. third-degree burns.
   B. carbon monoxide poisoning.
   C. chronic hypercarbia.
   D. chest trauma.
   E. head trauma.
9. Pulmonary oxygen toxicity is more likely to occur when the FIO_2 exceeds
   A. 0.21.
   B. 0.30.
   C. 0.50.
   D. 0.70.
   E. 0.90.
10. Mechanical dead space should be added only with which mode of ventilation?
    A. control-mode ventilation (CMV)
    B. assist control-mode ventilation (AMV)
    C. synchronized intermittent mandatory ventilation (SIMV)
    D. intermittent mandatory ventilation (IMV)
    E. pressure-support ventilation (PSV)
11. The lowest mean thoracic pressure occurs with
    A. CMV 12/min.
    B. AMV 12/min.
    C. IMV 14/min.
    D. SIMV 12/min.
    E. assist-control mode 12/min.
12. When continuous positive-airway pressure (CPAP) is applied to a breathing circuit and no ventilator-delivered tidal volumes are provided, the result is called
    A. continuous positive-pressure ventilation (CPPV).
    B. positive end-expiratory pressure (PEEP).
    C. continuous positive-pressure breathing (CPPB).
    D. negative end-expiratory pressure (NEEP).
    E. intermittent positive-pressure breathing (IPPB).
13. The optimal level of PEEP should be limited to a duration of
    A. 1 hour.
    B. 2 hours.
    C. 4 hours.
    D. 6 hours.
    E. 24 hours.
14. When the patient is recovering, the PEEP level should be lowered in small decrements every
    A. hour
    B. 2 hours.
    C. 6 hours.
    D. 12 hours.
    E. 24 hours.

15. The alarm system least likely to be triggered on a volume-preset ventilator set on the CMV mode is the
    A. I:E ratio.
    B. low pressure.
    C. PEEP pressure.
    D. high pressure.
    E. exhaled volume.
16. When severe hypoxemia is anticipated because of an unstable cardiopulmonary status, the initial F_{IO_2} set on a ventilator should be
    A. 0.30.
    B. 0.50.
    C. 0.70.
    D. 0.90.
    E. 1.00.
17. If a ventilator patient has ventilation parameters of V_T 0.5 L, $\dot{V}$ 30 L/min, and CMV 20/min, the patient will have an inspiratory time of
    A. 1 second.
    B. 2 seconds.
    C. 3 seconds.
    D. 200 milliseconds.
    E. 500 milliseconds.
18. If a patient is breathing spontaneously with rate of 20/min, tidal volume of 300 mL, and an I:E ratio of 1:2, the minimum continuous flow provided to the breathing circuit in the IMV mode should be
    A. 6 L/min.
    B. 9 L/min.
    C. 12 L/min.
    D. 15 L/min.
    E. 20 L/min.
19. Monitoring changes in pulmonary compliance and airway resistance will require all of the following *except*
    A. peak inspiratory pressure.
    B. mean airway pressure.
    C. positive end-expiratory pressure.
    D. pleateau pressure.
    E. measured exhaled volume.
20. During weaning from mechanical ventilation the Pa_{O_2} should be held higher than 55 torr (mm Hg) using an F_{IO_2} in the range of
    A. 0.21 to 0.30.
    B. 0.25 to 0.35.
    C. 0.30 to 0.50.
    D. 0.40 to 0.60.
    E. 0.50 to 0.70.

ANSWERS TO PRETEST

1. D (F153)
2. E (F154)
3. E (F155)
4. B (F155)
5. D (F155)
6. A (F156)
7. B (F156)
8. E (F156)
9. C (F156)
10. A (F162)
11. D (F157)
12. C (F160)
13. D (F162)
14. B (F162)
15. A (F161)
16. E (F159)
17. A (F161)
18. E (F161)
19. B (F163)
20. C (F164)

FRAME 153. INDICATIONS FOR MECHANICAL VENTILATION

TABLE 9-1
CRITERIA FOR VENTILATORY SUPPORT OF ADULTS

Datum	Normal Range	Tracheal Intubation and Ventilation Indicated
Mechanics		
Respiratory rate, breaths/min	12–20	>30
Vital Capacity, mL/kg	65–75	<15
FEV_1, mL/kg	50–60	<10
Maximal inspiratory pressure, cm H_2O	75–100	<20
Oxygenation		
$Pa{O_2}$, on 40% O_2, mm Hg	75–100 (air)	<60
$P(A\text{-}a)O_2$ on 100% O_2, mm Hg*	<35	>350
a/A ratio	>0.75	<0.45
Ventilation		
$Pa{CO_2}$, mm Hg†	35–45	>55
V_D/V_T ratio	0.25–0.40	>0.60

*After 20 minutes of 100% oxygen.
†Except in patients with chronic hypercapnia.

The indications for mechanically ventilating a patient can be divided into three categories related to the functions of the lungs: (1) ventilation, (2) oxygenation, and (3) mechanics. Criteria for providing ventilatory support to adults with respiratory failure can be found in Table 9-1. A single criterion by itself is usually not sufficient to institute mechanical ventilation; instead a pattern formed by several abnormal indicators is required. Ventilatory support is appropriate when paralysis of ventilatory muscles is imminent, such as with myasthenia gravis, Guillain-Barré syndrome, and barbiturate poisoning. Mechanical ventilation with positive end-expiratory pressure (PEEP) can be used to stabilize the chest wall when paradoxical breathing occurs as a result of a blunt or penetrating trauma to the chest.

Severe respiratory insufficiency seen with infant or adult respiratory distress syndrome will cause severe hypoxemia and hypercarbia that may require mechanical ventilation until pulmonary function improves. Cardiac, upper abdominal, thoracic, or neurosurgical operations may lead to postoperative respiratory failure caused by anesthesia and narcotics that depress the respiratory centers. If postoperative pain is not adequately treated or the patient is exposed to long periods of hypoxemia during or after surgery, the pulmonary capillaries may leak, making the lungs stiff and difficult to ventilate. Mechanical ventilation becomes necessary when decreased pulmonary compliance leads to decreased functional residual capacity and vital capacity as alveolar units collapse.

(Q) Which of the following data indicates that mechanical ventilation is indicated?

	FVC	$Pa{CO_2}$	$P(A\text{-}a)O_2$ on 100% O_2	
a.	20 mL/kg	43 torr	200 torr	264 A
b.	12 mL/kg	45 torr	300 torr	265 B
c.	10 mL/kg	56 torr	450 torr	264 C

FRAME 154. THERAPEUTIC GOALS

Mechanical ventilation is begun when spontaneous breathing produces inadequate alveolar ventilation. Conditions causing respiratory failure range from paralysis of respiratory muscles to problems that increase the work of breathing to the point where the patient can no longer maintain adequate oxygen uptake and carbon dioxide clearance. A primary goal of mechanical ventilation is to provide the right volume of oxygen-enriched and CO_2-free gas to the alveoli. The best indicator of adequate ventilation is a normal arterial carbon dioxide tension. A direct relationship exists between $Paco_2$ and alveolar ventilation because (1) the partial pressure of CO_2 in alveolar gas is a function of the volume of gas being moved in and out of alveoli, and (2) there is an equilibrium for CO_2 found between alveolar gas and oxygenated blood leaving the pulmonary capillaries.

Loss of lung volume is a common finding of acute respiratory disease syndrome (ARDS). Clinical problems that cause acute hypoxemia and hypercapnia often result from decreased functional residual capacity (FRC) caused by increased extravascular lung water resulting from fluid and albumin leaking from pulmonary capillaries. The increased lung water compromises the patency of bronchioles, which leads to absorption atelectasis. ARDS may not respond to supplemental oxygen therapy and mechanical ventilation but usually improves when PEEP is added. The mechanical breath delivers enough pressure to expand the atelectatic area, and PEEP holds the alveoli and small airways open so that gas exchange can occur throughout the entire ventilatory cycle.

Mechanical ventilation is required when a normal $Paco_2$ and pH cannot be maintained. During inspiration, respiratory muscles must overcome two forces: (1) *elastic forces,* which result from movement of pulmonary and thoracic tissues, and (2) *flow resistive forces,* caused by gas moving in the airways. In ARDS the decreased compliance of the lung and increased airway resistance may increase the work of breathing to a level where the patient quickly becomes exhausted even with smaller tidal volumes. Smaller tidal volumes require a higher respiratory rate to maintain adequate gas exchange and lead to atelectasis and hypoxemia. Thus, mechanical ventilation is required to maintain normal arterial blood gases until pulmonary function is restored.

(Q) Which of the following is a goal of mechanical ventilation?

a. Maintain arterial blood gases at normal levels. 264 B

b. Improve pulmonary compliance. 265 A

c. Reduce airway resistance. 265 D

FRAME 155. MODES OF VENTILATION

The mechanisms that a ventilator has available for ending the expiratory phase and allowing inspiration to begin are called modes of ventilation. These modes include controlled cycling by the ventilator only, combined patient- and ventilator-triggered breaths, or a combination of ventilator-delivered breaths and spontaneous breathing. Some simple ventilation devices (such as pressure-cycled machines) provide only the *assist* mode (patient-triggered). Other ventilators have an *assist-control* mode (patient-triggered with machine triggering if necessary). The distinguishing feature is whether the patient triggers inspiration by generating a negative pressure or the ventilator automatically triggers the inspiratory phase after a preset interval. The assist-control mode (AMV/CMV) allows patients to cycle the ventilator at their own rate only if the control-mode ventilation (CMV) rate is exceeded. The advantage of the assist-control mode is that it protects the patient from periods of apnea and guarantees a life-sustaining baseline of ventilation.

When the patient can breathe spontaneously from the ventilator circuit and also receive machine-delivered tidal volumes at preset intervals, the mode of ventilation is called *intermittent mandatory ventilation* (IMV). The more the patient can breathe unassisted, the fewer ventilator-delivered tidal volumes will be needed. The intrathoracic pressure is lower with IMV than with control, assist, or assist-control modes of ventilation because of fewer positive-pressure waveforms. The use of IMV allows the patient to be weaned from the ventilator without T-tube trials off the ventilator. The number of IMV breaths delivered can be decreased as the patient's pulmonary function returns to normal. *Synchronized intermittent mandatory ventilation* (SIMV) is similar to IMV except that mandated breaths are synchronized with the patient's spontaneous breathing rate. The use of the SIMV mode prevents the ventilator from delivering tidal volumes on top of the patient's spontaneous inspiration.

Pressure-support ventilation (PSV) is a mode that allows a spontaneous breath to be assisted by a preset amount of constant pressure, which is added to the baseline pressure level and applied throughout the inspiratory phase. The inspiratory flow rate is high at first and then decreases in order to maintain the constant pressure as air flows into the lungs. In pressure-control ventilation (PCV) pressure support is applied throughout inspiration, but the rate, inspiratory time, and inspiratory hold are regulated. Pressure-control ventilation is similar to the assist-control mode in the way that inspiration is triggered. Some ventilators allow pressure support to be combined with modes of ventilation that allow the patient to breathe spontaneously (e.g., PSV combined with SIMV).

(Q) Which of the following modes of ventilation allow the patient to vary the number of ventilator-delivered tidal volumes?

a. SIMV 264 a
b. PCV 265 b
c. AMV/CMV 265 d

FRAME 156. COMPLICATIONS

The possibility of a pneumothorax developing as a result of high alveolar pressure is unlikely in patients with ARDS, since their lungs are noncompliant and filled with fluid. The high airway pressure needed to provide ventilation is balanced by all the forces that are trying to collapse alveoli and small airways. Once the patient's pulmonary function improves, the danger of alveolar rupture and air leaks into the pleural space increases. The incidence of pneumothorax even with high levels of PEEP and peak airway pressure is low when patients are supported with IMV. The pressure-limit control on most modern ventilators is designed to prevent high pressure from developing in the lungs and trigger an alarm if the limit is reached. The clinical signs of a pneumothorax should be reviewed and the patient monitored for this complication. Common physical findings of a tension pneumothorax include (1) absent or distant bilateral breath sounds, (2) hyperresonant percussion note, (3) shift of the trachea away from the side with the pneumothorax, (4) presence of subcutaneous emphysema, (5) decrease in arterial blood pressure, venous return, and cardiac output, (6) decrease in ventilation, (7) sharp pain over the pneumothorax, and (8) change in heart rate.

The manner in which a ventilator delivers gas to the lungs may have adverse effects on the systemic circulation. Ventilation parameters that increase mean intrathoracic pressure subsequently decrease venous return and cardiac output. Ventilators need to be adjusted so that adequate ventilation is provided with the lowest possible mean airway pressure. Parameters that can be changed include respiratory rate, tidal volume, I:E ratio, peak inspiratory flow and pattern, PEEP, and inspiratory pause time. Steps can be taken to lower mean intrathoracic pressure. For example, the use of SIMV will decrease the number of positive-pressure tidal volumes delivered to the lungs. Also, smaller tidal volumes (10 mL/kg) should be used when the patient is first connected to the ventilator to allow time for a compensatory rise in venous tone. The infusion of the correct amount of blood, electrolyte solutions, or plasma expanders to maintain blood volume slightly above normal should help to minimize the decrease in cardiac output. The use of higher levels of PEEP (>5 cm H_2O) and larger tidal volumes (12 to 15 mL/kg) should be attempted only after the cardiovascular system has been stabilized.

During mechanical ventilation there is the potential to provide too much alveolar ventilation and cause respiratory alkalosis. Modes of ventilation such as SIMV reduce the risk by allowing the patient to breathe spontaneously and thus reduce their risk of hyperventilation. The respiratory alkalosis that develops may lead to electrolyte changes, such as a decrease in serum potassium (hypokalemia), which may cause life-threatening arrhythmias. Another complication of the alkalosis is a shift of the oxyhemoglobin dissociation curve to the left, which results in less oxygen being released to the tissues. The cerebral arterioles respond to the decreased CO_2 tension by contracting and limiting cerebral blood flow to levels that may cause tetanic muscular contractions and seizures. If hyperventilation is severe, cerebral blood flow may be reduced to levels that may cause brain damage. The greatest danger is to patients with chronic obstructive pulmonary disease who may live in a constant state of compensated respiratory acidosis, with consistently elevated arterial CO_2 tensions. When a chronically hypercarbic patient is hyperventilated, the arterial CO_2 tension may decrease too quickly causing a sudden drop in cerebral blood flow, thereby depriving the brain of adequate amounts of oxygen. Conversely, a patient with an acute rise in arterial CO_2 tension should have it returned to the normal range (35 to 45 mm Hg) within one hour. Some neurosurgical patients with high intracranial pressure will benefit from being slightly hyperventilated, thus limiting cerebral blood and reducing the pressure within the cranium. Head trauma or lesions may cause abnormal breathing patterns which require the control mode of ventilation. Since all tidal volumes are delivered under positive pressure, there is a potential for hyperventilation. Some practitioners recommend adding mechanical dead space to the ventilator breathing circuit so that rebreathing exhaled CO_2 maintains arterial CO_2 tension in the normal range. This is a difficult technique to administer safely and requires increased monitoring and serial blood gases to assure that hypoxemia and hypercarbia do not occur. Mechanical dead space should only be added when respiratory alkalosis occurs in the control mode when a patient with neuromuscular or neurologic disease needs large tidal volumes to satisfy the need to feel ventilated.

Pulmonary oxygen toxicity may occur in ventilator patients who receive high oxygen concentrations. The duration of exposure and the level of FIO_2 determine the degree to which pathophysiological changes will occur. However, 100% oxygen may produce changes in pulmonary function within 6 to 12 hours. If the FIO_2 is held to 0.50 or lower, it is highly unlikely that any effects of oxygen toxic response will be seen even after several days of exposure have occurred. The initial symptoms seen with FIO_2 over 0.50, usually develop over several days, and include burning and retrosternal pain, decreased vital capacity, atelectasis, increased capillary permeability, interstitial edema, alveolar septal thickening, alveolar hemorrhage, inflammation, fibrin deposition, and hyaline membrane formation.

(Q) Which of the following modes of ventilation will cause the least increase in mean intrathoracic pressure?

	Mode	f/min	V_T (mL/kg)	PEEP (cm H_2O)	
a.	CMV	10	12	0	264 D
b.	AMV	14	10	0	264 d
c.	IMV	6	15	5	265 C
d.	SIMV	10	15	5	265 a

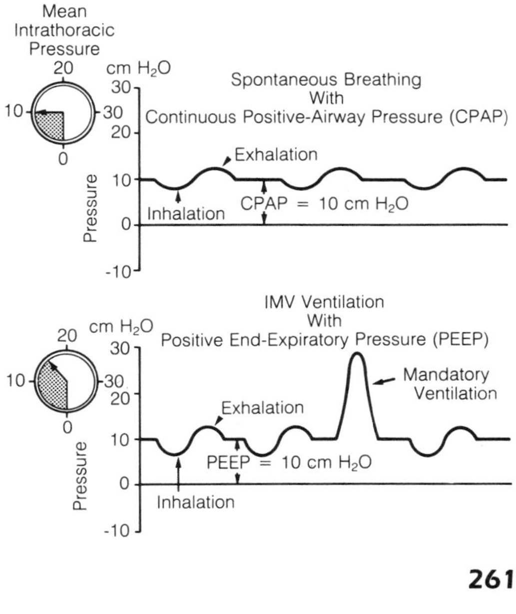

Figure 9–1 Continuous positive-pressure breathing (CPPB). (Source: Barnes, TA: Respiratory Care Practice. Year Book Medical Publishers, Chicago, 1988. Used with permission.)

FRAME 157. AIRWAY PRESSURE

The pressure waveforms in Figures 9–1, 9–2, and 9–3 should be studied and reviewed in order to appreciate the affect that various modes of ventilation have on airway pressure. Spontaneous breathing without positive pressure breaths or PEEP results in the lowest mean intrathoracic pressure. The control mode of ventilation with PEEP raises mean airway pressure throughout the entire ventilatory cycle and has the greatest impact on venous return and cardiac output. Modes of ventilation with spontaneous breathing supplement mandatory tidal volumes and allow optimal PEEP levels to be used to improve oxygenation. The peak pressure, plateau pressure, PEEP level, inspiratory time, inspiratory pause time, and expiratory resistance all impact the mean airway pressure. SIMV and IMV modes of ventilation at very high rates (>10/min) create mean airway pressures comparable to the control and assist modes at the same rate per minute, especially when the patient's spontaneous inspiratory efforts are weak. Also, care should be taken when using SIMV at high rates with pressure support since both mandatory and spontaneous breaths will be delivered with positive pressure.

(Q) Which of the following will lower mean airway pressure the most?

a. reducing the inspiratory pause from 1.0 to 0.5 seconds — 265 c
b. increasing the expiratory resistance — 264 b
c. suctioning the trachea to lower peak airway pressure — 264 c

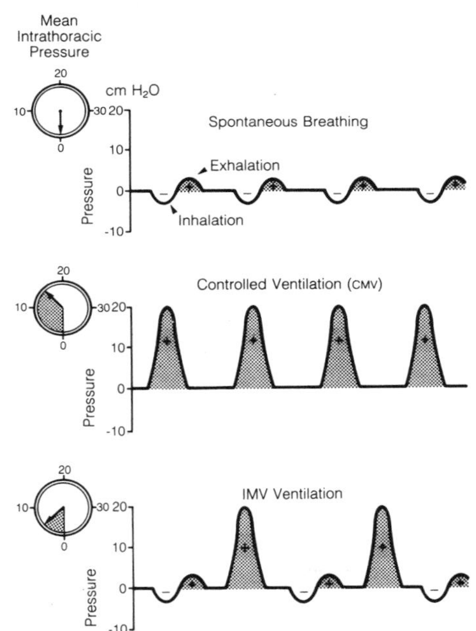

Figure 9–2

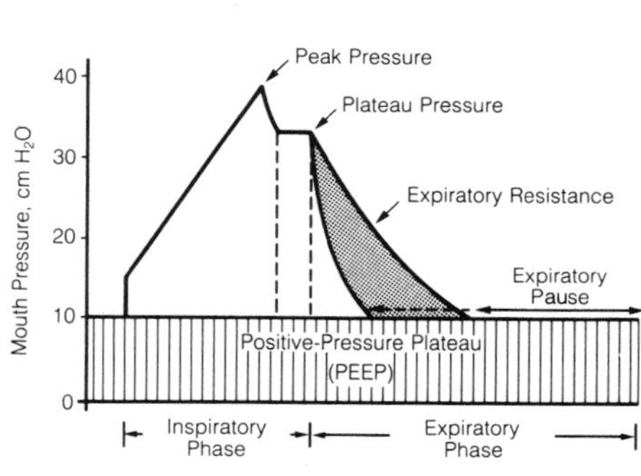

Figure 9–3

Figure 9–2 Intrathoracic pressure is lower with IMV than with controlled or assisted ventilations, since fewer positive-pressure waveforms are delivered. (Source: Barnes, TA: Respiratory Care Practice. Year Book Medical Publishers, Chicago, 1988. Used with permission.)

Figure 9–3 Pressure waveforms seen with and without apparatus resistance during expiration. (Source: Barnes, TA: Respiratory Care Practice. Year Book Medical Publishers, Chicago, 1988. Used with permission.)

FRAME 158. VENTILATOR SELECTION

The concept of an "ideal" ventilator provides a focal point for discussing the critical components that all ventilators should have and identifies related problems that need to be monitored. The one characteristic that all ventilators should have is reliability. They must run without failure for several days or weeks. It makes sense to use ventilators that have proved to be reliable after extensive field testing. The control panel, monitoring, and alarm systems must be designed with the patient's safety in mind. The proper labeling and grouping of controls is necessary so that no confusion occurs when changing ventilation or alarm parameters. Important monitoring data such as proximal airway pressure, inspired oxygen concentration, and delivered tidal volumes must be clearly displayed, connected to alarm systems, and easily read from a distance.

The gas delivered for mechanical and spontaneous breaths must be adequately humidified (100% relative humidity at 37°C). An in-line temperature probe should be placed in the breathing circuit close to the patient, since there is a danger of burning the patient's airways if the humidifier becomes empty and overheats. An ideal ventilator would monitor and display the temperature, sound an alarm, and shut off the humidifier if a high temperature occurs.

Volume-cycled ventilators should be used for long-term ventilation of adults and pressure-cycled ventilators reserved only for intermittent positive-pressure breathing (IPPB) treatments or short-term ventilation. The capability to provide ventilation and oxygenation often depends on adjusting parameters such as tidal volume, inspiratory flow rate, and waveform, F_{IO_2}, PEEP, mode of ventilation, pressure limit, inspiratory time, inspiratory hold, and rate. Not all patients will need to have pressure and flow waveforms modified. However, ventilators must have the capability to control basic ventilation parameters and should include critical alarm systems such as (1) high pressure, (2) low pressure, (3) loss of PEEP, (4) exhaled volume, and (5) F_{IO_2}.

(Q) Which of the following types of ventilators would be appropriate for a patient with adult respiratory distress syndrome (ARDS)?

a. flow-cycled 274 B
b. pressure-cycled 275 A
c. volume-cycled 275 d

264A (from page 257, frame 153)
Wrong. The vital capacity and $P(A\text{-}a)O_2$ on 100% O_2 are outside the normal range but not enough to indicate a need for mechanical ventilation. Also, the $PaCO_2$, a very sensitive indicator, is within the normal range. Return to page 257, review the guidelines in Table 9–1, and try again.

264B (from page 258, frame 154)
Correct. Mechanical ventilation is used to maintain normal arterial blood gases when increased work of spontaneous breathing results in hypercarbia and hypoxemia. Please continue on page 259, frame 155.

264C (from page 257, frame 153)
Correct. All three indicators provide support for instituting mechanical ventilation. Please continue on page 258, frame 154.

264D (from pages 260–261, frame 156)
Wrong. When using CMV, every tidal volume is a positive-pressure breath. The tidal volume is midway in the normal range of 10 to 15 mL/kg and the mean intrathoracic pressure will be high. Return to pages 260–261, frame 156, and select another answer.

264a (from page 259, frame 155)
Wrong. Synchronized intermittent mandatory ventilations will be delivered at a specific rate per minute. The ventilator will pause long enough to coordinate the mandatory tidal volume with the patient's own spontaneous inspiratory efforts. The SIMV mode does not allow the patient to change the mandatory rate. Return to page 259, frame 155, and try again.

264b (from page 262, frame 157)
Wrong. Increasing expiratory resistance will increase the mean airway by holding pressure in the chest during the longer exhalation time. Return to page 262, frame 157, review the pressure waveforms, and try again.

264c (from page 262, frame 157)
Wrong. Suctioning the endotracheal tube and trachea may lower peak pressure as airway resistance is decreased. However, it will not lower the plateau pressure or mean alveolar pressure. Return to page 262, frame 157, review the pressure waveforms, and try again.

264d (from page 260–261, frame 156)
Wrong. When using AMV every tidal volume is a positive-pressure breath. Although the tidal volume is small and at the low end of the normal range of 10 to 15 mL/kg, the mean airway pressure will be high. Return to pages 260–261, frame 156, and try again.

265A (from page 258, frame 154)
Wrong. Mechanical ventilation does reduce the work of breathing by varying degrees dependent upon the mode of ventilation that is selected but may not improve pulmonary compliance. Return to page 258, frame 154, and select another answer.

265B (from page 257, frame 153)
Wrong. The vital capacity meets the criteria for starting mechanical ventilation but the $Paco_2$ is within the normal range, and the $P(A\text{-}a)o_2$ on 100% O_2 is below the guideline of 350 mm Hg. Remember to look for a pattern among indicators. Return to page 257, frame 153, review the criteria in Table 9-1, and select another answer.

265C (from pages 260–261, frame 156)
Correct. The use of IMV limits the number of positive pressure to 6/min. The use of 5 cm H_2O of PEEP will increase mean intrathoracic pressure but not as much as that caused by higher numbers of positive-pressure breaths. Please continue on page 262, frame 157.

265D (from page 258, frame 154)
Wrong. Mechanical ventilation does reduce the work of breathing by varying degrees dependent upon the mode of ventilation that is selected but may not reduce the airway resistance. Return to page 258, frame 154, and select another answer.

265a (from pages 260–261, frame 156)
Wrong. When the SIMV mode is used at high rates, the number of positive-pressure breaths increases. The mean intrathoracic pressure will increase to a level similar to that of the CMV and AMV modes of ventilation. Also, the PEEP level will increase the mean airway pressure by 5 cm H_2O. The tidal volume is large and at the high end of the normal range of 10 to 15 mL/kg. Larger tidal volumes require higher peak airway pressure and will increase mean intrathoracic pressure. Return to pages 260–261, frame 156, and select another answer.

265b (from page 259, frame 155)
Wrong. The number of breaths per minute is automatic with PCV and the patient cannot breathe spontaneously from the circuit. Return to page 230, frame 156, and select another answer.

265c (from page 262, frame 157)
Correct. Lowering the inspiratory pause time by 0.5 second will substantially lower the mean airway pressure. Please continue on page 263, frame 158.

265d (from page 259, frame 155)
Correct. The assist-control mode of ventilation (AMV/CMV) allows the patient to trigger the ventilator to deliver a positive pressure breath at variable rates as it exceeds the CMV backup rate. Please continue on pages 260–261, frame 156.

FRAME 159. INITIAL VENTILATION PARAMETERS

The ventilation parameters will be affected by the way a ventilator initiates the inspiratory phase. The AMV has the advantage of allowing a patient to determine the ventilator cycle rate. However, a lesion of the respiratory centers, pain, anxiety, or medication may cause the patient to hyperventilate or hypoventilate to dangerous levels. Use of the control mode may require that the patient be heavily sedated and/or paralyzed which leaves the patient totally dependent upon the ventilator. The control mode has the potential for providing too much or too little ventilation, especially when there is a sudden change in the patient's condition or a mechanical malfunction occurs. Both the CMV and AMV modes have the disadvantage of creating more positive pressure in the thorax than other modes of ventilation. The use of IMV or SIMV modes of ventilation will allow a patient to breathe spontaneously and thus lower the number of positive-pressure breaths per minute. The net effect will be to lower the mean intrathoracic pressure and allow higher levels of PEEP to be used.

When first mechanically ventilated, many patients have unstable cardiovascular systems that might be adversely affected by the CMV or AMV mode of ventilation. A low SIMV rate should be used, if possible, since a high SIMV rate differs very little from CMV in terms of the impact on venous return to the heart. In cases such as flail chest where strong inspiratory efforts destabilize the chest wall, CMV may be the mode of choice. However, use of the CMV mode concurrent with depression of spontaneous breathing by heavy sedation and/or muscle paralysis may place the patient in a life-threatening circumstance if the ventilator malfunctions or the patient becomes accidently disconnected from the ventilator. Thus, whenever possible, ventilator patients should be allowed to breathe spontaneously from the circuit.

The use of small tidal volumes (<10 mL/kg) to mechanically ventilate adult patients seriously affects the efficiency of oxygenation by promoting gradual alveolar and small airway closure. For adults, the accepted norm for ventilator-delivered tidal volumes is 10 to 15 mL/kg of ideal body weight. It is important to calculate the tidal volume needed using ideal body weight, since substantial errors can be made when using the actual weight of obese patients. The initial tidal volume should be 10 mL/kg to minimize the impact of increased intrathoracic pressure on cardiac output. Once the cardiovascular system is stabilized, the tidal volume should be increased to 12 ml/kg and eventually to 15 mL/kg.

The initial respiratory rate for adults is usually set at 10 to 12/min until an arterial blood-gas study can be done to evaluate the adequacy of ventilation. Then the rate is adjusted based on the arterial CO_2 tension. In patients who are hypoventilated with a mechanical rate of 8/min or higher, the practitioner should first assure that the tidal volume is appropriate. If the tidal volume is low, it should be increased before changes in cycle rate are made. If the tidal volume is set appropriately, the rate should be increased.

The F_{IO_2} delivered by a ventilator should be directed at reversing arterial hypoxemia. A Pa_{O_2} below 60 to 70 mm Hg in most critically ill patients is unacceptable since the saturation of hemoglobin with oxygen may be less than 90%. The long-term use of high oxygen concentrations should always be discouraged because it increases intrapulmonary shunt and elicits a toxic response from lung parenchyma. However, 100% oxygen should be used initially in the presence of cardiopulmonary instability when hypoxemia is anticipated. Once stability has been achieved, the F_{IO_2} should be lowered below 0.50 by using PEEP and large tidal volumes (15 mL/kg).

The inspiratory flow for ventilator-delivered tidal volumes and spontaneous breathing should at a minimum match the patient's peak inspiratory flow. A peak inspiratory flow of 30 L/min usually provides a laminar flow that comes close to matching that seen during quiet spontaneous breathing. Patients with moderate hypoxemia, pain, severe airway obstruction, or other sequelae may need a higher inspiratory flow. Some ventilators regulate inspiratory flow by adjusting inspiratory time. Inspiratory flow rate can be calculated by dividing the tidal volume by the inspiratory time in seconds and multiplying by 60, for example, $(V_T \div t_{insp}) \times (60\ s) = \dot{V}$. To assure adequate expiratory time for patients with severe obstructive lung disease, inspiratory flow may need to be increased to shorten inspiratory time.

(Q) A patient with an ideal body weight of 132 lb (60 kg) is brought to the emergency room with a complaint of chest pain and dyspnea. There is no history or physical signs of chronic pulmonary disease. While being examined the patient has a cardiac arrest and is successfully resuscitated. However, cardiogenic pulmonary edema has left the patient in need of mechanical ventilation. Which initial set of ventilation parameters would be most appropriate if the following data is available?

Heart rate 120/min	Pa_{O_2} 48 torr
Blood pressure 90/40 torr	Pa_{CO_2} 55 torr
Spontaneous respiratory rate 30/min	pH 7.30

	V_T	Mode of Ventilation	Cycle Rate	F_{IO_2}	
a.	900 mL	CMV	12/min	1.00	274 C
b.	600 mL	SIMV	10/min	1.00	274 b
c.	800 mL	AMV	. . .	0.50	276 c
d.	500 mL	CMV	12/min	0.80	275 b

FRAME 160. INDICATIONS FOR PEEP

Providing greater than ambient pressure to the airways during both inspiratory and expiratory phases of breathing helps to reverse small airway and alveolar collapse. The term *continuous positive-airway pressure* (CPAP) is used when above-ambient pressure is applied to a breathing circuit when no ventilator-delivered tidal volumes are provided, for example, during spontaneous breathing. When CPAP and mechanical ventilation are applied together, the increased baseline pressure is called PEEP. When PEEP is used the result is called *continuous positive-pressure ventilation* (CPPV). *Continuous positive-pressure breathing* (CPPB) occurs with CPAP. Both PEEP and CPAP increase functional residual capacity and splint the lung in a position of function. Increased interstitial hydrostatic pressure and other causes of alveolar instability may result in significant loss of alveolar volume during the expiratory phase. Given these conditions, the mechanically delivered tidal volume provides enough pressure to expand the involved areas, and PEEP assures continued expansion and gas exchange throughout the ventilatory cycle. The level of PEEP will need to be slightly above the mean alveolar closing pressure. The ventilator needs to be adjusted to deliver the *optimal* level of PEEP to improve ventilation-perfusion ratios and to allow a lower inspired oxygen concentration to be used. The safe way to arrive at the optimal level is to start with a baseline of zero and add PEEP in 3 to 5 cm H_2O increments while monitoring the criteria used to determine the greatest improvement in oxygen transport.

Optimal PEEP is the level of end-expiratory pressure that results in the lowering of intrapulmonary shunt, significant improvement in arterial oxygenation, and results in a small change in cardiac output, arteriovenous oxygen content difference, or mixed venous-oxygen tension. The use of the SIMV mode of ventilation, cardiovascular monitoring, and interventions to improve cardiovascular function allow the concept of optimal PEEP to be used safely. The improvements in arterial oxygen tension and decreases in intrapulmonary shunt should occur within 10 minutes. Since PEEP increases peak inspiratory pressure, some practitioners limit the duration of the optimal level of PEEP to approximately 6 hours. Commonly, PEEP is reduced by 3 to 5 cm H_2O decrements every 2 to 3 hours provided arterial oxygenation does not deteriorate. Arterial blood-gas studies should be done 10 to 15 minutes after the PEEP level is reduced. A minimum of 5 cm H_2O of PEEP usually is indicated during mechanical ventilation since tracheal intubation holds the larynx and glottis constantly open which leads to reduction in functional residual capacity caused by alveolar collapse.

(Q) All of the following are indications for PEEP *except*

a. toxic oxygen concentrations. 274 A
b. arterial oxygen tension less than 60 mm Hg. 274 d
c. above normal functional residual capacity with crushed chest injuries. 275 B
d. reduced intrapulmonary shunt. 275 c

FRAME 161. MONITORING THE PATIENT VENTILATOR SYSTEM

Compliance and airway resistance should be periodically evaluated in all ventilated patients to follow the course of pathological changes. The peak inspiratory pressure represents the amount of pressure required to overcome both total system elastic resistance to ventilation and nonelastic resistance to ventilation. The elastic resistance to ventilation (static compliance) is determined by dividing the exhaled tidal volume by the plateau pressure minus PEEP level. The plateau pressure is obtained by creating an inspiratory hold and measuring the proximal airway pressure with no airflow. The exhaled tidal volume should be corrected for compressible volume loss since the same type of ventilator circuit may not always be used on a particular patient. The difference between peak pressure and plateau pressure represents the nonelastic resistance to ventilation (airway resistance). The airway resistance can be estimated by dividing the difference between peak and plateau pressure by the inspiratory flow.

Five important independent variables associated with mechanical ventilation are (1) the rate of breathing (breaths per minute), (2) the size of each breath (tidal volume), (3) how fast each breath is given (inspiratory time, inspiratory flow rate), (4) the mixture of gas used (F_{IO_2}), and (5) the pressure in the system at end expiration (PEEP). The I:E ratio (inspiratory to expiratory) is determined by calculating the inspiratory time by dividing the volume by the flow rate, for example, $t_I = V_T \div \dot{V}$. Once the inspiratory time is calculated, the expiratory time can be determined by subtracting the inspiratory time from the total cycle time. Although the I:E must be carefully set initially it is the least likely alarm parameter on adult ventilators to be triggered.

(Q) Given the following ventilation parameters, what is the I:E ratio?
V_T 500 mL, $\dot{V}$ 30 L/min, f 20/min

a. 1:1 — 276 D
b. 1:2 — 275 C
c. 1:3 — 275 a

FRAME 162. ADJUSTMENT OF OXYGENATION AND VENTILATION

Alteration in the level of oxygenation will involve adjustment of F_{IO_2} or PEEP. Adjusting other ventilator controls to improve alveolar ventilation does reduce to some extent the hypoxemic effects of shunting and venous admixture. However, Pa_{O_2} is directly affected by adjustment of F_{IO_2} and PEEP. If the F_{IO_2} is below 0.40, and the hypoxemia is not a result of increased intrapulmonary shunting, the F_{IO_2} is normally the first variable to be increased. PEEP should be increased first when the F_{IO_2} is greater than 0.40 and the hypoxemia is caused by diffuse intrapulmonary shunting. If the F_{IO_2} is greater than 0.40 and the problem is the result of localized disease, the F_{IO_2} should be increased first and PEEP increased only if the problem does not respond to a higher F_{IO_2}. PEEP should be increased in increments of 3 to 5 cm H_2O until the optimal level is reached. This will require the patient to be carefully monitored for changes in cardiac output that may occur as the PEEP level is increased. F_{IO_2} is usually increased in increments of 0.05 to 0.10 but severe hypoxemia will require a larger increase or use of 100% oxygen. The ventilator should be set to deliver 100% oxygen when cardiovascular instability threatens to produce severe hypoxemia. Once the cardiovascular system is stable the F_{IO_2} should be lowered to a level that maintains Pa_{O_2} at a minimum of 60 to 70 mm Hg which should produce 90% saturation of hemoglobin with oxygen if the pH is normal. Adjusting PEEP to an optimal level, when diffuse intrapulmonary shunting exists, will allow a lower F_{IO_2} to be used and thus reduce the toxic effects of oxygen on lung parenchyma.

Overly corrected hypoxemia ($Pa_{O_2} > 100$ mm Hg) will require lowering either F_{IO_2} or PEEP. If the F_{IO_2} is over 0.50, it should be lowered before PEEP is reduced to decrease the possibility of a toxic response to high oxygen concentrations. PEEP should be reduced within 6 hours of reaching the "optimal" level but not until F_{IO_2} is below 0.50. The PEEP should be lowered in 3 to 5 cm H_2O decrements every 2 to 3 hours provided the Pa_{O_2} is maintained at a minimum of 60 to 70 mm Hg. Since venous return may increase substantially as intrathoracic pressure decreases the cardiovascular system and urine output should be carefully monitored. Blood-gas determinations should be made within 10 to 15 minutes of changing F_{IO_2} or PEEP.

Changing the minute volume delivered by the ventilator to correct for hyperventilation requires the rate or tidal volume to be lowered. The adjustment should be made to assure adequate alveolar ventilation (Pa_{CO_2} of 35 to 45 mm Hg) with a view toward holding the mean intrathoracic pressure as low as possible. Lowering the rate will usually have more of an affect on mean pressure than a decrease in tidal volume. Accordingly, the rate, instead of tidal volume, is usually lowered unless the volume is above 15 mL/kg of ideal body weight. If respiratory alkalosis is caused by a patient in the assist-control, IMV, or SIMV modes, an attempt should first be made to find and correct the cause of the hyperventilation. It may be caused by hypoxemia, or central nervous system lesions, metabolic acidosis, pain, or anxiety. If hyperventilation continues the IMV or SIMV rate should be lowered. Lowering the CMV rate in the assist-control mode will do little to solve the problem. Mechanical dead space should only be used in control-mode ventilation with paralysis and sedation. It is usually added only when large tidal volume is required to satisfy the needs of a patient with a neuromuscular or neurologic disease (adding mechanical dead space, even in the control mode is usually not indicated).

Lowering a high arterial CO_2 tension in ventilator patients should be done with concern for the consequent increase in intrathoracic pressure. An increase in tidal volume of 100 to 200 mL normally does not cause as great an increase in intrathoracic pressure as a 1 to 2/min increase in rate. If the rate is 8/min or higher, the tidal volume should be checked to make sure it is appropriate (12 to 15 mL/kg of ideal body weight). If the tidal volume is appropriate, the rate should be increased first. If the rate is less than 8/min, increase the rate first then increase tidal volume.

(Q) Given the data below, what changes should be made for a ventilator patient on the assist-control mode triggering at 12/min?

$P(A\text{-}a)O_2$ on 100% O_2 450 torr
F_{IO_2} 0.70
Pa_{O_2} 44 torr
Pa_{CO_2} 41 torr
pH 7.37

a. add PEEP 274 a
b. increase F_{IO_2} to 1.0 274 c
c. increase the tidal volume 274 D

FRAME 163. TROUBLESHOOTING USING SYSTEM PRESSURE

Monitoring the patient-ventilator system using changes in pressure that occur during the ventilatory cycle can provide a wealth of information. Static compliance can be calculated by measuring the end-inspiratory plateau pressure, end-expiratory pressure, and exhaled tidal volume. Changes in the static compliance will provide useful information about optimal PEEP levels and restoration of functional residual capacity. The difference between peak inspiratory pressure and plateau pressure provides an estimate of the amount of work done to overcome airway resistance. Airway resistance increases when the caliber of airways is reduced by mucosal edema, partial airway obstruction, or bronchospasm. Thus, decongestants, bronchial hygiene therapy, or aerosolized bronchodilators may be indicated.

System pressure can be used to check the integrity of the breathing circuit and ventilator for leaks by (1) setting the high-pressure alarm at maximum, (2) setting tidal volume at 1.0 L, (3) occluding the patient wye and preventing exhalation, and (4) delivering the tidal volume. The circuit should hold pressure at 80 cm H_2O for 2 to 4 seconds. A rapid drop in peak pressure with the patient connection and exhalation valve occluded means a leak is present.

A sudden drop in peak inspiratory pressure usually signals a loss of tidal volume from a leak in the breathing circuit or around the cuff of the tracheal tube. Conversely a sudden increase in pressure may be the result of right main-stem bronchus intubation or a tension pneumothorax. A drop in peak inspiratory pressure may also coincide with a loss of PEEP.

Monitoring the PEEP level itself is important and arterial oxygen tension may fall quickly if it is lost. Observing deflections below baseline pressure will also provide information regarding how much work the patient has to do to trigger a breath when in AMV/CMV. Equally as important, it will indicate whether the flow provided in the SIMV mode is high enough to match the patient's spontaneous peak inspiratory flow.

When peak inspiratory pressure drops as PEEP is decreased, compliance increases, or airway resistance decreases; the endotracheal tube cuff should be reinflated. Reinflating the cuff will take advantage of the lower pressure required to create a seal with the lower peak inspiratory pressure.

(Q) A ventilator patient in the assist-control mode of a Bennett MA-1 ventilator, has 5 cm H_2O of PEEP instituted and suddenly requires inspiratory pressure of 6 cm H_2O below the baseline to trigger an assisted breath. Which of the following ventilator controls needs to be adjusted?

a. peak inspiratory flow 276 d
b. sensitivity 276 B
c. PEEP 276 a

FRAME 164. WEANING FROM MECHANICAL VENTILATION

More important than the techniques used to wean patients from mechanical ventilation is the reversal of the pathophysiologic condition that necessitated ventilatory support. Before extubation the patient should have adequate ventilatory reserve and be capable of breathing spontaneously with minimal PEEP or CPAP (5 cm H_2O or less). The spontaneous rate should be less than 30/min, and tidal volumes should be at least 2 to 3 mL/kg. The vital capacity should be greater than 10 to 15 mL/kg of ideal body weight. Maximum inspiratory pressure (MIP) provides data about ventilatory reserve and is easier to obtain on intubated patients than a vital capacity. The MIP should be at >20 cm H_2O within 20 seconds before the patient is extubated or removed from a ventilator.

A $Pa{O_2}$ greater than 55 mm Hg, when the $F{IO_2}$ is held between 0.3 and 0.5, provides evidence of adequate oxygenation. The arterial pH and $Pa{CO_2}$ should be held within the normal range of 7.35 to 7.45, and 35 to 45 torr, respectively. Chronic CO_2 retainers will have a different baseline and may have a $Pa{CO_2}$ as high as 50 to 60 torr. In the absence of knowledge about previous ventilatory status, pH may be used as a primary guide to the adequacy of ventilation. Intrapulmonary shunting should be at an acceptable level as indicated by a $P(A\text{-}a)O_2$ on 100% O_2 of $\leq$300 mm Hg or an a/A ratio >0.75.

None of the weaning techniques commonly used will be successful if the patient still needs ventilatory support. However, the following protocol that relies on the SIMV mode and PEEP may facilitate weaning when the patient is physiologically ready to be weaned. The SIMV rate is reduced independently from $F{IO_2}$ or PEEP.

The initial SIMV rate seldom exceeds 6 to 8 breaths per minute and is decreased 1 to 2 breaths per minute as long as the arterial pH is maintained above 7.30 and the spontaneous rate is less than 30/min. A minimal SIMV rate of 2 breaths per minute is recommended to prevent a fall in $Pa{O_2}$. The addition of 2 positive-pressure breaths per minute appears to recruit and expand unstable alveoli. The goal of weaning is adequate gas exchange at 5 cm H_2O or less of PEEP.

Removal of the endotracheal tube is dependent on the following: $F{IO_2}$, arterial blood-gas tensions, pH, SIMV rate, and PEEP or CPAP level. Also, the patient must have the ability to maintain a patent airway as exhibited by intact pharyngeal and laryngeal reflexes. The patient should have acceptable cardiovascular reserves since the increased work of spontaneous breathing may stress the heart.

(Q) Which of the following indicate that a patient's ventilatory reserve is adequate to sustain the stress of weaning from mechanical ventilation?

a. spontaneous rate ≤35/min 276 C

b. spontaneous tidal volume ≥ 7 to 9 mL/kg 276 b

c. maximum inspiratory pressure ≥ 20 cm H_2O in 20 seconds 276 A

274A (from page 268, frame 160)
Wrong. Lowering F_{IO_2} to 0.50 or less while maintaining the Pa_{O_2} at a minimum of 60 to 70 mm Hg is an important indiction of PEEP. It is important to use optimal PEEP so that exposure to toxic concentrations can be limited. Return to page 268, frame 160, and select anther answer.

274B (from page 263, frame 158)
Wrong. Flow-cycled ventilators will terminate inspiration when flow drops to a predetermined level regardless of the tidal volume delivered. Changes in pulmonary compliance and airway resistance affect the time it takes for flow to drop to the cycle threshold and tidal volume will vary. Thus the danger of hyperventilation or hypoventilation makes flow-cycled ventilators poor choices for long-term ventilation. Return to page 263, frame 158, and select another answer.

274C (from pages 266–267, frame 159)
Wrong. Until the cardiopulmonary system is stabilized the tidal volume should not be this large. Since the patient has a spontaneous respiratory rate of 30/min, CMV is not the best mode of ventilation. Return to pages 266–267, frame 159, and select another answer.

274D (from pages 270–271, frame 162)
Wrong. The Pa_{CO_2} indicates that the alveolar ventilation is adequate. Increasing the tidal volume is not the correct way to improve oxygenation. Return to pages 270–271, frame 162, and select another answer.

274a (from pages 270–271, frame 162)
Correct. PEEP should be added or increased first when the F_{IO_2} is greater than 0.40, except when the problem is localized in one area of the lung. Please continue on page 272, frame 163.

274b (from pages 266–267, frame 159)
Correct. The initial tidal volume should be 10 mL/kg or 600 mL. SIMV mode will allow the patient to continue to breathe spontaneously in addition to 10-ventilator delivered breaths per minute which should lower the mean intrathoracic pressure. Also, 100% oxygen should be given until the cardiopulmonary system is stabilized. Please continue on page 268, frame 160.

274c (from pages 270–271, frame 162)
Wrong. The F_{IO_2} is greater than 0.40 and the problem is not localized in one area of the lung. Return to pages 270–271, frame 162, and try again.

274d (from page 268, frame 160)
Wrong. Increasing the arterial oxygen tension to at least 60 to 70 mm Hg is a primary indication for using PEEP. If the pH is normal, a Pa_{O_2} of 60 to 70 mm Hg will result in 90% saturation of hemoglobin with oxygen. Return to page 268, frame 160, and select another answer.

275A (from page 263, frame 158)
Wrong. Pressure-cycled ventilators will terminate inspiration when peak inspiratory pressure (PIP) reaches a predetermined level regardless of the tidal volume delivered. Changes in pulmonary compliance and airway resistance affect the time it takes for PIP to reach the cycle threshold and tidal volume will vary. Thus, the danger of hyperventilation or hypoventilation make pressure-cycled ventilators poor choices for long-term ventilation. Return to page 263, frame 158, and select another answer.

275B (from page 268, frame 160)
Correct. PEEP is used to increase FRC, and internally stabilize the chest wall and to maintain mean airway pressure above the alveolar closing pressure. The FRC is already above normal. Please continue on page 269, frame 161.

275C (from page 269, frame 161)
Correct. First determine the inspiratory time (t_I) by dividing the tidal volume (500 mL) by the flow rate (30 L/min or 500 mL/s), for example, 500 mL ÷ 500 mL/s = t_I = 1 second. Next determine the total cycle time by dividing 60 seconds by the rate per minute (20), for example, 60 ÷ 20 = total cycle time = 3 seconds. Determine the expiratory time (t_E) by subtracting inspiratory time (t_I) from the total cycle time (t_{cycle}), for example, $t_E = t_{cycle} - t_I$, $t_E = 3 - 1$, $t_E = 2$. Therefore, the I:E ratio is 1:2. Please continue on pages 270–271, frame 162.

275a (from page 269, frame 161)
Wrong. First determine the inspiratory time (t_I) by dividing the tidal volume (500 mL) by the flow rate (30 L/min or 500 mL/s), for example, 500 mL ÷ 500 mL/s = t_I = 1 second. Next determine the total cycle time by dividing 60 seconds by the rate per minute (20), for example 60 ÷ 20 = total cycle time = 3 seconds. Determine the expiratory time (t_E) by subtracting inspiratory time (t_I) from the total cycle time (t_{cycle}), for example, $t_E = t_{cycle} - t_I$, $t_E = 3 - 1$, $t_E = 2$. Therefore, the I:E ratio is 1:2. Please continue on pages 270–271, frame 162.

275b (from pages 266–267, frame 159)
Wrong. The initial tidal volume should be larger. The oxygen concentration should be higher until the cardiopulmonary system is stabilized. The CMV mode is not the best mode of ventilation since it will result in high intrathoracic pressure and does not accommodate the patient's spontaneous rate of 30/min. Return to pages 266–267, frame 159, and try again.

275c (from page 268, frame 160)
Wrong. The use of PEEP to assure continued expansion of alveoli during the expiratory phase will improve ventilation-perfusion ratios and decrease the intrapulmonary shunt. Return to page 268, frame 160, and select another answer.

275d (from page 263, frame 158)
Correct. Volume-cycled ventilators will deliver preset tidal volume regardless of whether changes occur in pulmonary compliance or airway resistance. Thus, there is a reduced danger of hyperventilation or hypoventilation. Please continue on pages 266–267, frame 159.

276A (from page 273, frame 164)
Correct. The ventilatory reserve most likely is adequate when the maximum inspiratory pressure is >20 cm H_2O in 20 seconds, the spontaneous tidal volume is >2 to 3 mL/kg, and the spontaneous rate is < 30/min. Please continue on page 277 and complete the chapter exercises.

276B (from page 272, frame 163)
Correct. The MA-1 ventilator is not PEEP compensated. You need to readjust the threshold of the sensitivity control so that the patient will trigger an assisted breath when the system pressure is dropped to + 5 cm H_2O. Please continue on page 273, frame 164.

276C (from page 273, frame 164)
Wrong. The spontaneous breathing rate should be less than 30/min for weaning to begin. Return to page 273, frame 164, and try again.

276D (from page 269, frame 161)
Wrong. First determine the inspiratory time (t_I) by dividing the tidal volume (500 mL) by the flow rate (30 L/min or 500 mL/s), for example, 500 mL ÷ 500 mL/s = t_I = 1 second. Next determine the total cycle time by dividing 60 seconds by the rate per minute (20), for example, 60 ÷ 20 = total cycle time = 3 seconds. Determine the expiratory time (t_E) by subtracting inspiratory time (t_I) from the total cycle time (t_{cycle}), for example, $t_E = t_{cycle} - t_I$, $t_E = 3 - 1$, $t_E = 2$. Therefore, the I:E ratio is 1:2. Please continue on pages 270–271, frame 162.

276a (from page 272, frame 163)
Wrong. Lowering the PEEP level would reduce the work required to trigger an assisted breath but the PEEP of 5 cm H_2O is necessary to increase the FRC and reinflate collapsed alveoli. Return to page 272, frame 163, and select another answer.

276b (from page 273, frame 164)
Wrong. The spontaneous tidal volume only needs to be 2 to 3 mL/kg in order for the weaning process to begin. A spontaneous tidal volume of 7 to 9 mL/kg is larger than found with most healthy people. Return to page 273, frame 164, and select another answer.

276c (from pages 266–267, frame 159)
Wrong. Until the cardiovascular system is stabilized the tidal volume should not be this large. The oxygen concentration should be higher until the patient is reoxygenated and the Pao_2 is >60 torr. Assisted ventilation may result in high intrathoracic pressure and hyperventilation. Return to pages 266–267, frame 159, and try again.

276d (from page 272, frame 163)
Wrong. Adjusting the peak inspiratory flow will change the inspiratory time and the peak pressure but does not solve the problem. Return to page 272, frame 163, and select another answer.

EXERCISES

1. List the normal ranges and thresholds of six indicators that provide evidence that ventilatory support is needed.
2. Describe the goal of mechanical ventilation in terms of restoring pulmonary compliance and airway resistance to normal levels.
3. Identify two ventilators whose capabilities include the following modes of ventilation: CMV, AMV, AMV/CMV, IMV, SIMV, PSV, and PCV.
4. Describe how adjustment of ventilator controls can reduce the incidence of the following complications of mechanical ventilation: pneumothorax, hyperventilation, hypoventilation, restriction of venous return, oxygen toxicity, and cerebral hypoxemia.
5. Draw the pressure waveforms that illustrate CPPB and CPPV.
6. Explain how the optimal level of PEEP is determined.
7. Design an "ideal ventilator" by describing the ventilation parameters that would be controlled and the alarm systems.
8. Outline the recommended initial ventilator control settings used before the first blood-gas report is received.
9. Calculate the tidal volume given a CMV rate of 10/min, I:E ratio of 1:2, and an inspiratory flow of 30 L/min.
10. List the ventilation parameter that would indicate that there is a leak in the ventilator patient system?

POSTTEST

This test is designed to evaluate what you have learned by completing Chapter 9. Check your answers on page 280 and review the topics where your answer is incorrect.

1. Patients requiring mechanical ventilation often have a V_D/V_T greater than
   A. 0.25.
   B. 0.33.
   C. 0.40.
   D. 0.50.
   E. 0.60.
2. The best indicator of adequate ventilation is a normal
   A. maximum inspiratory pressure.
   B. spontaneous tidal volume.
   C. arterial CO_2 tension.
   D. vital capacity.
   E. inspiratory capacity.
3. Which of the following allow the triggering of positive-pressure tidal volumes at a rate determined by the patient?
   I. CMV
   II. AMV
   III. AMV/CMV
   IV. PSV
   V. PCV
   VI. SIMV
   A. I, V, and VI only
   B. II, IV, and V only
   C. III, IV, and VI only
   D. II, III, and IV only
   E. II, III, IV, and V only
4. All of the following modes of ventilation deliver *only* positive pressure breaths *except*
   A. CMV.
   B. AMV.
   C. AMV/CMV.
   D. SIMV.
   E. PSV.
5. Which of the following statements about hyperventilation are true?
   I. A very high Pa_{CO_2} should be lowered slowly if the patient is chronically hypercarbic.
   II. Patients with high intracranial pressure may benefit from being slightly hyperventilated.
   III. Patients with acute hypercarbia should have their Pa_{CO_2} lowered to normal within one hour.
   A. I only
   B. II only
   C. III only
   D. II and III only
   E. I, II, and III
6. Symptoms of oxygen toxic response to high F_{IO_2} include all of the following *except*
   A. retrosternal pain and burning.
   B. increased capillary permeability.
   C. alveolar septal thickening.
   D. air trapping and increased FRC.
   E. hyaline membrane formation.

7. All of the following changes to ventilation parameters will increase mean intrathoracic pressure *except*
   A. increasing tidal volume.
   B. adding an inspiratory hold.
   C. increasing inspiratory flow rate.
   D. increasing expiratory resistance.
   E. increasing PEEP.
8. If the optimal PEEP level is exceeded, which of the following may occur?
   A. Arteriovenous oxygen content difference will increase.
   B. Mixed venous-oxygen tension will be higher.
   C. Cardiac output will remain constant.
   D. Arterial oxygen tension will continue to rise.
   E. Intrapulmonary shunting will continue to decrease.
9. Which of the following statements about an "ideal" ventilator humidification system are true?
   I. A thermal or servocontrolled switch should turn off the humidifier if it overheats.
   II. Inspired gas temperature should be displayed.
   III. An alarm should sound if a high inspired-gas temperature occurs.
   A. I only
   B. II only
   C. III only
   D. I and II only
   E. I, II, and III
10. The reliability of mechanical ventilators can be determined by
    A. practitioners' reports.
    B. patient feedback.
    C. manufacturer's literature.
    D. field testing.
    E. design specifications.
11. Four hours after mechanical ventilation is initiated the patient's delivered tidal volumes should be set at
    A. 7 mL/kg.
    B. 10 mL/kg.
    C. 13 mL/kg.
    D. 17 mL/kg.
    E. 20 mL/kg.
12. The initial rate for ventilator-delivered breaths that is set while waiting for a blood-gas study should be
    A. 6/min.
    B. 8/min.
    C. 10/min.
    D. 12/min.
    E. 14/min.
13. The inspiratory flow needed when the ventilation parameters are CMV 12/min, I:E ratio 1:4, V_T 0.5 L is
    A. 20 L/min.
    B. 25 L/min.
    C. 30 L/min.
    D. 40 L/min.
    E. 50 L/min.

14. The initial PEEP setting for a ventilator patient should be
   A. 5 cm H_2O.
   B. 8 cm H_2O.
   C. 10 cm H_2O.
   D. 12 cm H_2O.
   E. 15 cm H_2O.

15. Ventilator control settings should be adjusted so that arterial oxygen tension is maintained at a minimum of
   A. 40 to 50 mm Hg.
   B. 50 to 60 mm Hg.
   C. 60 to 70 mm Hg.
   D. 70 to 80 mm Hg.
   E. 80 to 90 mm Hg.

16. Compressible volume loss should be monitored and subtracted from measured exhaled tidal volumes because
   I. the water level in the humidifier may affect the tidal volume delivered to the patient.
   II. compressible volume loss may change after a breathing circuit is replaced.
   III. some ventilators automatically increase tidal volume delivered to the patient ventilator system to correct for compressible volume loss and others do not.
   A. I only
   B. II only
   C. III only
   D. I and II only
   E. I, II, and III

17. The PEEP level should be increased during mechanical ventilation to the optimal level in increments of
   A. 1 to 2 cm H_2O.
   B. 3 to 5 cm H_2O.
   C. 5 to 8 cm H_2O.
   D. 8 to 10 cm H_2O.
   E. 10 to 15 cm H_2O.

18. Which of the following changes in ventilation parameters would be appropriate to increase the arterial CO_2 tension of a 60-kg patient on a CMV rate of 10/min and a tidal volume of 900 mL?
   A. Decrease V_T to 720 mL.
   B. Decrease V_T to 600 mL.
   C. Decrease CMV rate to 8/min.
   D. Increase CMV rate to 12/min.
   E. Increase V_T to 1000 mL.

19. A leak in the ventilator patient system would be indicated by a decrease in all of the following *except*
   A. peak inspiratory pressure.
   B. plateau pressure.
   C. PEEP level.
   D. measured exhaled tidal volume.
   E. inspired oxygen concentration.

20. During weaning from mechanical ventilation the arterial pH should be maintained *above*
   A. 7.25.
   B. 7.30.
   C. 7.35.
   D. 7.40.
   E. 7.45.

ANSWERS TO POSTTEST

1. E (F153)
2. C (F154)
3. D (F155)
4. D (F155)
5. E (F156)
6. D (F156)
7. C (F157)
8. A (F160)
9. E (F158)
10. D (F158)
11. C (F159)
12. C (F159)
13. C (F159)
14. A (F160)
15. C (F162)
16. E (F161)
17. B (F160)
18. C (F162)
19. E (F163)
20. B (F164)

BIBLIOGRAPHY

Barnes, TA: Respiratory Care Practice. Year Book Medical Publishers, Chicago, 1988.

Burton, GG and Hodgkin, JE: Respiratory Care: A Guide to Clinical Practice, ed 2. JB Lippincott, Philadelphia, 1984.

Eubanks, DH and Bone, RC: Comprehensive Respiratory Care, ed 2. CV Mosby, St. Louis, 1990.

Kacmarek, RM and Stoller, JK: Current Respiratory Care. BC Decker, Philadelphia, 1989.

Kirby, RR, Smith, RA, and Desautels, DA: Mechanical Ventilation. Churchill-Livingstone, New York, 1985.

Pilbeam, SP and Youtsey, JW. Mechanical Ventilation. CV Mosby, St. Louis, 1986.

Scanlon, CL, Spearman, CB, Sheldon, RL, and Egan, DF: Egan's Fundamentals of Respiratory Therapy, ed 5. CV Mosby, St. Louis, 1990.

Shapiro, BA, Harrison, RA, Kacmarek, RM, and Cane, RD: Clinical Application of Respiratory Care, ed 3. Year Book Medical Publishers, Chicago, 1985.

10

Cardiopulmonary Resuscitation

PRETEST

This pretest is designed to measure what you already know about CPR. Check your answers on page 285 and then continue on page 286, frame 165.

1. When encountering a patient lying on the floor and unresponsive to verbal stimuli or shaking, the next action should be to
   A. open the airway.
   B. check for breathing.
   C. give two initial breaths.
   D. check for pulse.
   E. call for help.

2. Rescue breathing should have an inspiratory time of
   A. 0.50 second.
   B. 0.75 second.
   C. 1.00 seconds.
   D. 2.00 seconds.
   E. 3.00 seconds.

3. Which maneuver will clear a foreign object from the upper airway?
   A. head-tilt/chin-lift maneuver
   B. modified jaw-thrust maneuver
   C. triple airway maneuver
   D. Heimlich maneuver
   E. mandibular-displacement maneuver

4. The *triple airway maneuver* combines which of the following to open the airway?
   I. mandibular displacement
   II. head tilt
   III. jaw thrust
   IV. chin lift
   V. retraction of the lower lip
   A. I, III, and IV only
   B. II, III, and IV only
   C. II, III, and V only
   D. III, IV, and V only
   E. I, II, and III only

5. Which airway maneuver(s) should be used with a cervical spine injury?
   I. modified jaw-thrust maneuver
   II. triple airway maneuver
   III. head-tilt/chin-lift maneuver
   A. I only
   B. II only
   C. III only
   D. II and III only
   E. I, II, and III

6. Which of the following maneuvers to open the airway may be dangerous to the practitioner if the patient has teeth?
   A. triple airway maneuver
   B. head-tilt/chin-lift maneuver
   C. modified jaw-thrust maneuver
   D. mandibular-displacement maneuver
   E. retraction of the lower lip

7. Without equipment which of the following would be best to ventilate an infant?
   A. mouth-to-mouth breathing
   B. mouth-to-nose breathing
   C. mouth-to-mouth and nose breathing
   D. modified jaw thrust
   E. triple airway maneuver

8. If the abdomen rises during rescue breathing, what should be done?
   I. Deliver larger tidal volumes.
   II. Reposition the head.
   III. Shorten the inspiratory time.
   A. I only
   B. II only
   C. III only
   D. I and III only
   E. I, II, and III
9. Correctly done chest compressions produce what proportion of normal cardiac output?
   A. 10%
   B. 30%
   C. 50%
   D. 75%
   E. 100%
10. In two-rescuer CPR the ratio of chest compressions to ventilations is
   A. 5:1.
   B. 5:2.
   C. 15:1.
   D. 15:2.
   E. 20:3.
11. The protocol for single-rescuer adult CPR calls for how many breaths to be delivered before chest compressions are started?
   A. 1
   B. 2
   C. 3
   D. 4
   E. 5
12. What is the ratio of chest compressions to ventilation for single-rescuer adult CPR?
   A. 5:1
   B. 5:2
   C. 15:1
   D. 15:2
   E. 20:3
13. When a second person arrives at the scene to help with CPR, that person should *first*
   A. get ready to do chest compressions.
   B. get ready to ventilate.
   C. palpate carotid artery without chest compressions for 5 seconds.
   D. listen for breath sounds without chest compressions for 5 seconds.
   E. palpate carotid artery while the other person continues chest compressions.
14. During two-rescuer CPR, the first thing done after switching positions by the person who has just moved to the head is to
   A. reposition the head.
   B. palpate carotid artery without chest compressions for 5 seconds.
   C. listen for breath sounds without chest compressions for 5 seconds.
   D. use the phone to call for more help.
   E. suction the upper airways.

15. The best way to improve manual ventilation of a patient intubated with an endotracheal tube during CPR is
    A. one-hand compression of the bag.
    B. two-hand compression of the bag.
    C. unrestricted refill of bag during expiratory phase.
    D. to shorten inspiratory time to 0.5 second.
    E. O_2 flow at flush without reservoir attached.
16. The oxygen concentration delivered by a manual resuscitator without an oxygen reservoir with oxygen flow of 15 L/min is
    A. 20 to 30%.
    B. 30 to 40%.
    C. 40 to 60%.
    D. 60 to 80%.
    E. 90 to 100%.
17. Mouth-to-mouth ventilation will deliver an oxygen concentration of approximately
    A. 10 to 15%.
    B. 15 to 18%.
    C. 18 to 21%.
    D. 21 to 30%.
    E. 30 to 40%.
18. A conscious patient without COPD who is in moderate hypoxemia and has a normal inspiratory flow rate, tidal volume, and rate should receive oxygen by
    A. nasal cannula at 2 L/min.
    B. nasal cannula at 6 L/min.
    C. 50% Venturi mask.
    D. rebreathing mask at 10 L/min.
    E. non-rebreathing mask at 8 L/min.
19. Delivering tidal volumes in <1 second may result in
    A. distention of the stomach.
    B. increase in cardiac output.
    C. increase in ventilation.
    D. increase in tidal volume.
    E. lower airway pressure.
20. Chest compression during CPR may have all of the following complications *except*
    A. formation of fat emboli.
    B. pneumothorax.
    C. hemothorax.
    D. laceration of the kidneys.
    E. laceration of the gastroesophageal junction.

ANSWERS TO PRETEST

1. E (F165)
2. C (F168)
3. D (F166)
4. C (F167)
5. A (F167)
6. D (F167)
7. C (F168)
8. B (F168)
9. B (F169)
10. A (F169)
11. B (F170)
12. D (F170)
13. C (F171)
14. B (F171)
15. B (F172)
16. C (F172)
17. B (F173)
18. E (F173)
19. A (F174)
20. D (F174)

FRAME 165. ESTABLISHING A NEED FOR RESUSCITATION

Upon encountering a patient who appears to be unconscious, for example, slumped over or lying on the floor, you should gently tap or shake the patient, and ask, "Are you all right?" If a response is received, the following questions should be asked: (1) Do you have neck pain? (2) Do you have a loss of feeling in your hands or feet? and (3) Can you move your arms and legs? If no response is observed, then the rescuer should shout for help and ask someone at the scene to activate the emergency medical system. A cardiopulmonary arrest is established by determining (1) that the patient is unconscious as described above, (2) that there is an absence of breathing by observing the chest for motion and by listening and feeling at the patient's mouth and nose for no air movement (respiratory arrest; see Fig. 10–1), and (3) that there is no carotid pulse (cardiac arrest).

The "ABCs" of resuscitation—airway, breathe, and circulate—should immediately be started by opening the airway, checking again for breathing, and looking for any sign of airway obstruction. Next breathe for the patient, giving two initial breaths, each delivered slowly in 1 to 1½ seconds and watch for chest excursion. If pulse is still absent, cardiac arrest has occurred and chest compressions should be started immediately. A patient who is found on the floor unconscious and in cardiopulmonary arrest should be resuscitated on the floor, since a hard surface is needed for chest compressions to be effective and time will be lost by moving the patient to a bed and locating a board to slip under the back.

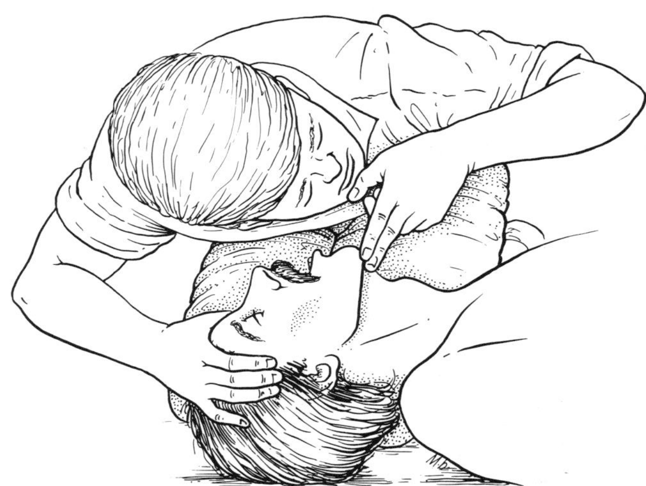

Figure 10–1 Listening and feeling at the patient's mouth and nose for no air movement. (Source: Finucane, BT and Santora, AH: Principles of Airway Management. FA Davis, Philadelphia, 1988. Used with permission.)

(Q) Which of the following should be done *first* when a patient is found slumped over in bed?

a. Check for absence of breathing. 292 A

b. Check for absence of pulse. 293 A

c. Establish level of consciousness. 293 D

FRAME 166. COMPLETE AIRWAY OBSTRUCTION

Foreign-body airway obstruction may be the cause of acute respiratory arrest when the patient cannot be ventilated regardless of the position of the head. Witnessed foreign-body airway obstruction should be suspected when the victim is eating and suddenly stops breathing, becomes cyanotic, and loses consciousness. Attempts to establish a patent airway and initiate mouth-to-mask or bag-mask ventilation may prove to be ineffective. It is important to know the clinical signs of complete obstruction: (1) victim cannot speak, cough, or breathe; (2) victim grips the throat between thumb and fingers; (3) chest wall retractions can be observed. The Heimlich maneuver which is described in Chapter 5 may expel the obstruction from the airway. Increased intrathoracic pressure occurs when the diaphragm rises as a result of thrusts applied to the abdomen (see Figure 10–2). Unconscious patients should first be placed on a hard surface with the heel of one hand placed between the xiphoid process and the umbilicus, and quick thrusts applied inward and upward. Care must be taken *not* to apply pressure to the ribs or xiphoid process.

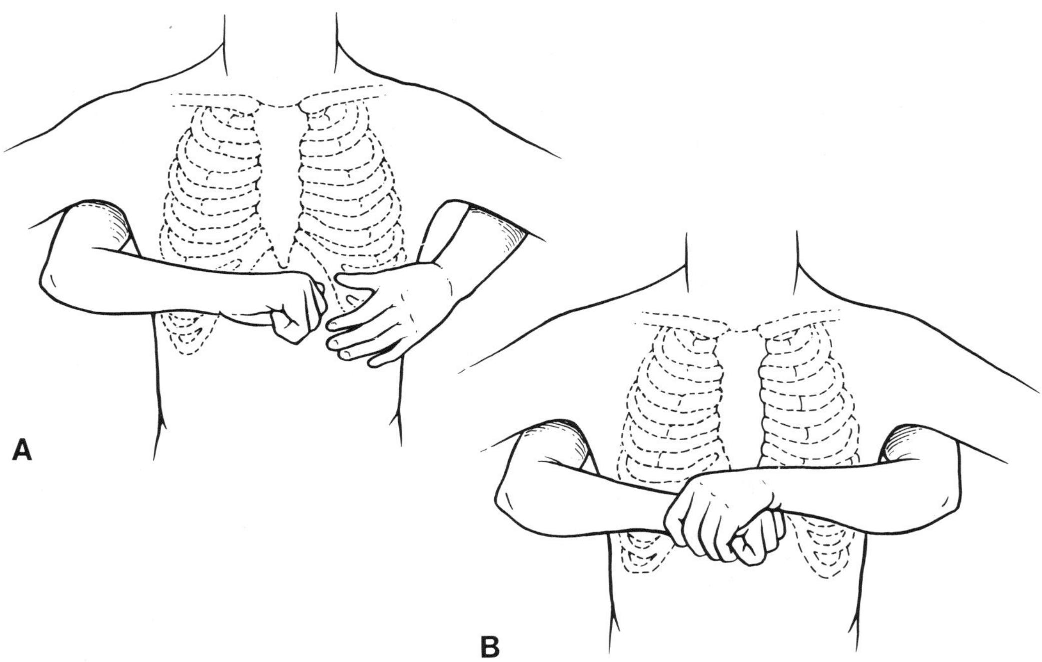

Figure 10–2 Heimlich maneuver. (Source: Finucane, BT and Santora, AH: Principles of Airway Management. FA Davis, Philadelphia, 1988. Used with permission.)

(Q) Which of the following is a sign of complete airway obstruction?

a. inspiratory strider 292 B

b. chest wall retractions 293 B

c. nasal flaring 293 a

FRAME 167. MANEUVERS FOR OPENING THE AIRWAY

The *head-tilt/chin-lift maneuver* is recommended by the American Heart Association as the most effective and safest method for opening the airway of an unconscious patient (Fig. 10–5). The airway is opened by placing one hand on the victim's forehead and tilting the head backward. The fingers of the other hand are placed firmly beneath the bony portion of the victim's chin, lifting it upward. The *head-tilt/neck-lift maneuver*, is less effective and may cause or exacerbate injury to the cervical spine.

When a cervical spine injury is suspected, the *modified jaw-thrust maneuver* will be safer than the head-tilt/chin-lift method for opening the airway. The jaw-thrust maneuver is performed by gripping the angles of the mandible with both hands from one side and pulling forward, while at the same time the head is tilted backward. When a cervical spine injury is suspected, the jaw-thrust maneuver is modified by deleting the head tilt. It is the method of choice for opening the airway since it does not involve extension of the neck.

Two other methods for opening the airway are the *triple airway maneuver* and *mandibular displacement.* The *triple airway maneuver* simply adds a third component to the head-tilt/jaw-thrust maneuver (Fig. 10–3). The third component opens the mouth by retracting the lower lip with the thumb. *Mandibular displacement* involves placing the thumb in the victim's mouth, the fingers beneath chin, and then pulling. This procedure can be quite effective but is dangerous for the rescuer when the victim has teeth (Fig. 10–4).

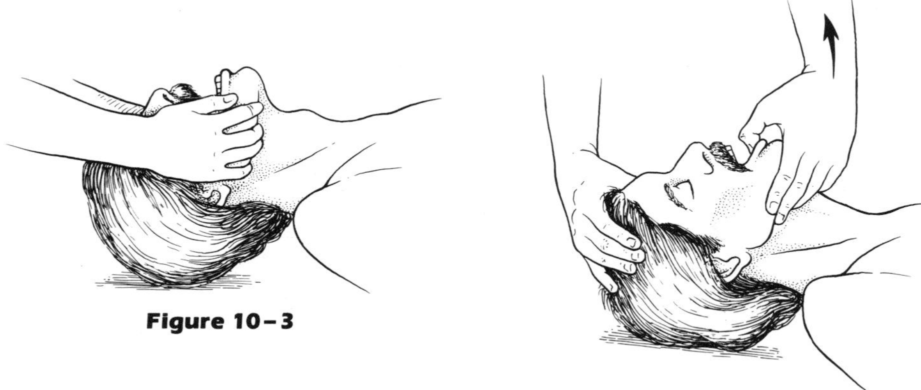

Figure 10–3

Figure 10–4

Figure 10–3 Triple airway maneuver. (Source: Finucane, BT and Santora, AH: Principles of Airway Management. FA Davis, Philadelphia, 1988. Used with permission.)

Figure 10–4 Mandibular displacement. (Source: Finucane, BT and Santora, AH: Principles of Airway Management. FA Davis, Philadelphia, 1988. Used with permission.)

(Q) Which of the following maneuvers would be best for a patient with an obstructed upper airway and an injury to his cervical spine?

a. triple airway maneuver 292 C
b. head-tilt/chin-lift maneuver 292 d
c. modified jaw-thrust maneuver 293 C
d. mandibular-displacement maneuver 293 d

FRAME 168. RESCUE BREATHING

After clearing and opening the airway, give the victim two breaths before beginning chest compressions. Each breath should be large enough to make the chest rise and fall and be given in 1 to 1½ seconds. A breath delivered with the correct inspiratory time reduces the risk of gastric distention, regurgitation, and pulmonary aspiration. Observe the rise and fall of the chest as the breath is delivered. If the airway is obstructed, reposition the head and ventilate again. In two-rescuer adult CPR, breathing should continue every 5 seconds, which results in 12/min. The ventilation rate for small children and infants is 20/min and 40/min, respectively.

Mouth-to-mouth and mouth-to-nose breathing (for infants) are commonly described, but the rescuer working in a hospital or other public setting should use mouth-to-mask or bag-valve-mask breathing to reduce the risk of exposure to the human immunodeficiency virus (HIV). To date, no cases have been reported in which AIDS was transmitted by saliva or airborne droplets of respiratory secretions. However, disposable mouth-to-mask, manual resuscitators, and airway equipment should be used instead of mouth-to-mouth breathing. Gloves, gown, and eye protection should be worn when exposed to blood or secretions.

Mouth-to-mask breathing (Fig. 10–6) allows the mask to be held with the same hand used to perform the chin-lift maneuver. Take care with a small child or infant not to deliver tidal volumes large enough to cause barotrauma to the lungs and gastric distention. If the abdomen rises during inspiration, reposition the airway and deliver smaller tidal volumes. If regurgitation occurs, turn the victim's head to one side, and suction the airway or wipe clear with a finger if suction equipment is not available. Intubation with a cuffed endotracheal tube lessens the risk of gastric distention and pulmonary aspiration and facilitates ventilation.

(Q) The rate for manual ventilation of an apneic infant is one breath every
- a. 3 seconds. 292 a
- b. 4 seconds. 292 D
- c. 5 seconds. 293 c

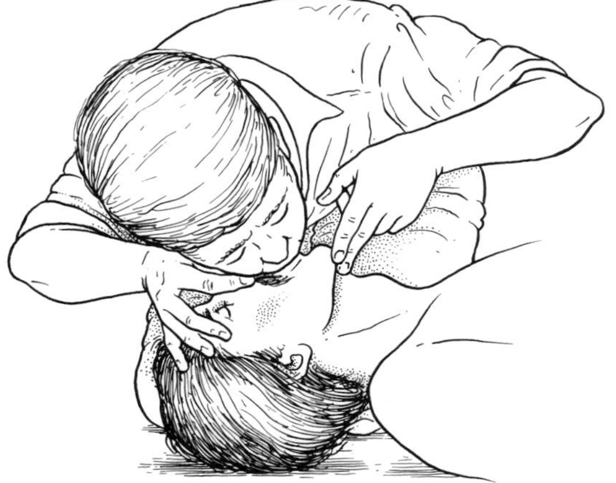

Figure 10–5 Mouth-to-mouth breathing using the head-tilt/chin-lift maneuver. (Source: Finucane, BT and Santora, AH: Principles of Airway Management. FA Davis, Philadelphia, 1988. Used with permission.)

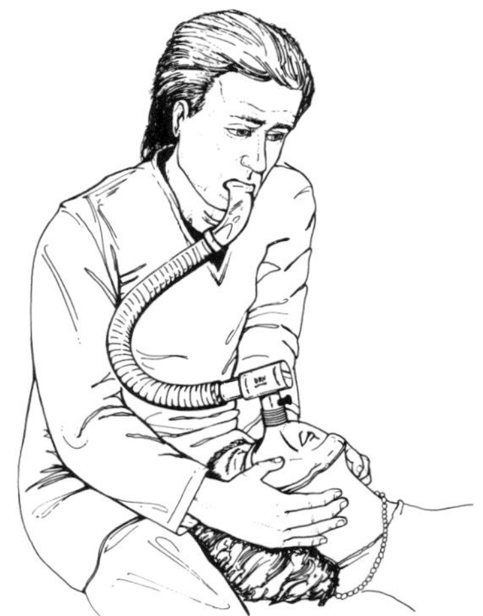

Figure 10–6 Mouth-to-mask breathing.

FRAME 169. CHEST COMPRESSIONS

The absence of a pulse requires that chest compressions be started immediately. The carotid artery in adults is the most accessible spot for checking the pulse. The femoral artery is a good alternative for establishing circulatory inadequacy. The apical pulse is auscultated to determine the heart rate of infants and small children.

The patient needs to be placed on a hard surface for chest compressions to be effective. The patient should be positioned supine to allow maximum blood flow to the brain during chest compressions. If the head is elevated, blood flow to the brain will not be adequate since, even when chest compressions are done properly, cardiac output is reduced to approximately 25 to 30% of normal.

To perform chest compressions, the rescuer places one hand on the lower half of the adult sternum 1½ in above the xiphoid process (Fig. 10–7). The other hand is placed on the top of the first and the fingers are interlocked. The arms are kept straight, with the shoulders directly over the sternum (Fig. 10–8). For an adult, pressure is directed downward to depress the sternum 1½ to 2 in at a rate of 80 to 100/min. When resuscitating alone, the rescuer delivers 15 compressions and then two breaths. With two rescuers, the ratio of compressions to ventilations is 5 : 1 for adults, children, and infants. However, remember that children and infants are ventilated at a faster rate. Thus an infant will receive five chest compressions within 3 seconds and a child will receive the same number within 4 seconds. If the effort is generating some cardiac output, the practitioner providing ventilation should be able to palpate a carotid pulse with each chest compression.

The chest compression technique with small children is similar to adults except that the heel of only one hand is placed over the midsternum and the sternum is depressed only 1 to 1½ in dependent upon the size of the child. Only the tips of the middle and index fingers are used to compress the midsternum of an infant ½ to 1 in (Fig. 10–9). The rate should be 100/min with a breath given every five compressions.

Rib fractures and costochrondral separation may occur if the compressions deviate from midline or if pressure is applied with fingers on the rib cage. Interlocking the fingers of both hands and keeping the heel of the hand constantly on the chest will help to prevent these complications. Also, it is important not to apply pressure on the xiphoid process, which extends downward over the upper abdomen, since laceration of the liver can lead to severe internal bleeding. For adults, palpating the xiphoid process with one hand and then placing the other hand so that it is 1½ in higher should reduce the risk. Laceration by the xiphoid process as a result of applying chest compressions too low on the sternum is equally important with children and infants, and may be the most common complication.

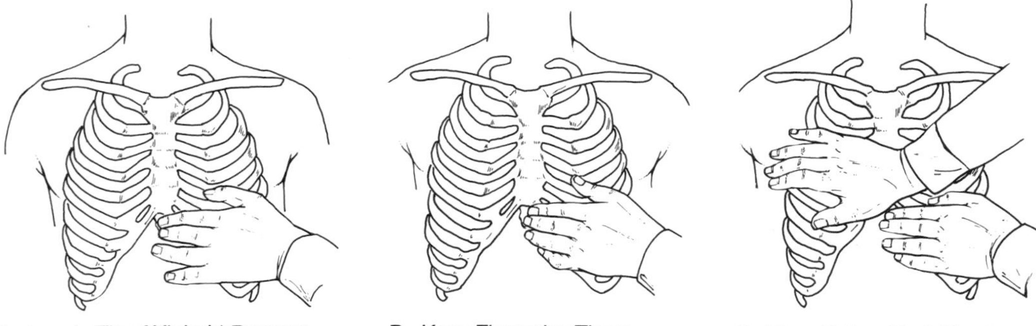

Figure 10–7 Hand positions for cardiac compressions.

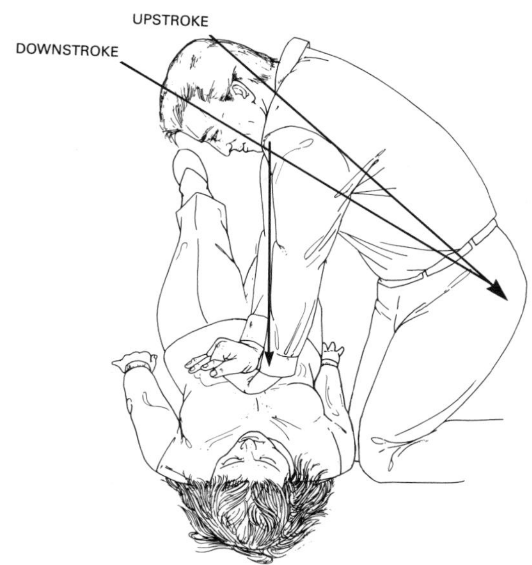

Figure 10–8 Arm positions for cardiac compressions.

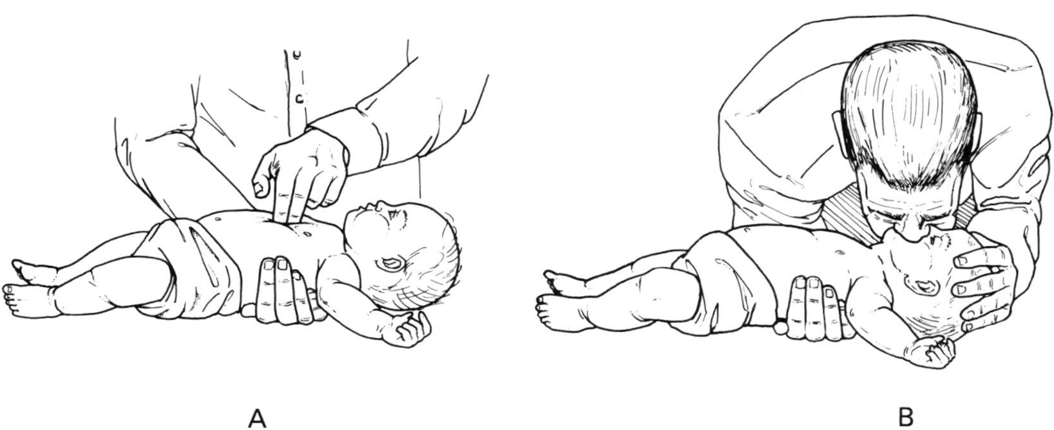

Figure 10–9 CPR for infants.

(Q) When applying chest compressions to children and infants, the hand or fingers apply pressure to the

a. xiphoid process. 292 b
b. midsternum. 292 c
c. lower half of the sternum. 293 b

292A (from page 286, frame 165)
Wrong. Sleeping patients normally breathe more slowly and shallowly than when awake. What action can be taken to check if the patient is asleep? Return to page 286, frame 165, and select another answer.

292B (from page 287, frame 166)
Wrong. Inspiratory strider may occur with partial airway obstructions, but not when the obstruction is complete. Remember, there is no airflow with a complete airway obstruction. Return to page 287, frame 166, and select another answer.

292C (from page 288, frame 167)
Wrong. The triple airway maneuver includes a head-tilt component which may exacerbate the spinal injury. Return to page 288, frame 167, and select another answer.

292D (from page 289, frame 168)
Wrong. This would result in a respiratory rate of 15/min which is the rate for children. Return to page 289, frame 168, and select another answer.

292a (from page 289, frame 168)
Correct. This would result in a respiratory rate of 20/min (every 3 seconds) and can be compared with the rate for adults of 12/min (every 5 seconds). Please continue on page 290, frame 169.

292b (from pages 290–291, frame 169)
Wrong. Compressing the xiphoid process may lacerate the liver, spleen, or stomach and cause severe bleeding. Return to pages 290–291, frame 169, and select another answer.

292c (from pages 290–291, frame 169)
Correct. Performing chest compressions over the midsternum will assure that the xiphoid process does not lacerate the liver, spleen, or stomach. Please continue on page 294, frame 170.

292d (from page 288, frame 167)
Wrong. The head-tilt component of this maneuver may exacerbate the spinal cord injury. Return to page 288, frame 167, and select another answer.

293A (from page 286, frame 165)
Wrong. Two other observations would be made before checking the pulse. Return to page 286, frame 165, and select another answer.

293B (from page 287, frame 166)
Correct. Chest wall retractions will occur as vigorous inspiratory efforts lower the interpleural pressure and pull the intercostal spaces inward. Please continue on page 288, frame 167.

293C (from page 288, frame 167)
Correct. The modified jaw-thrust maneuver eliminates the head-tilt component and thus is much safer for a victim suspected of having a cervical spine injury. Please continue on page 289, frame 168.

293D (from page 286, frame 165)
Correct. The level of consciousness must be determined first. Sleeping patients can easily be mistaken for patients in respiratory arrest. Please continue on page 287, frame 166.

293a (from page 287, frame 166)
Wrong. Nasal flaring only occurs with a partial upper airway obstruction, but not when the obstruction is complete. Return to page 287, frame 166, and select another answer.

293b (from pages 290–291, frame 169)
Wrong. Chest compressions are applied to the lower half of the sternum of adults, with care taken to be at least 1½ in above the xiphoid process. Hand placement is different for children and infants. Return to pages 290–291, frame 169, and select another answer.

293c (from page 289, frame 168)
Wrong. This would result in a respiratory rate of 12/min which would be appropriate for adults. Return to page 289, frame 168, and try again.

293d (from page 288, frame 167)
Wrong. Unless this patient has no teeth, the maneuver would be too dangerous for the rescuer to attempt. Return to page 288, frame 167, and select another answer.

FRAME 170. SINGLE-RESCUER ADULT CPR PROTOCOL

Respiratory care practitioners often find themselves alone with patients especially when working the night shift. Consequently, the full responsibility for providing CPR during the first few critical minutes rests with them. Appropriate action, taken quickly, and in the correct sequence is the key to successful resuscitation of the victim. The following protocol includes several actions which can form the basis for dealing with cardiopulmonary arrests in hospitals. The protocol includes actions recommended by the American Heart Association and other sources listed in the bibliography. Experienced respiratory care practitioners may be capable of doing some of the steps simultaneously. However, errors of omission are important since they may exacerbate the original problem.

Protocol for Basic Single-Rescuer Adult CPR

1. Establish unresponsiveness, observe pupillary response, and note time.
2. Call for help (do not leave the scene).
3. Place patient in a supine position on a hard surface.
4. Open the airway with head-tilt/chin-lift maneuver (except in suspected cervical spine injuries, where the modified jaw-thrust maneuver is recommended).
5. Confirm respiratory arrest and establish breathlessness.
6. Place an oropharyngeal airway (if available).
7. Deliver two breaths (use a mouth-to-mask device or manual resuscitator).
8. If ventilation attempts are unsuccessful, reposition head and try again.
9. If ventilation is still poor, check for foreign-body airway obstruction, remove obstruction using Heimlich maneuver or finger sweeps, and try to ventilate again.
10. Establish absence of pulse by palpating the carotid or femoral artery.
11. If a pulse is present, ventilate at a rate of 12/min.
12. If a pulse is absent, begin chest compressions at a rate of 80 to 100/min.
13. Alternate giving 15 compressions and two ventilations.
14. Assess the patient for return of pulse and breathing after four cycles and every few minutes thereafter. CPR should not be interrupted for more than 5 seconds to assess pulse and breathing.

(Q) What is the best way to notify other hospital personnel that you are initiating CPR?

a. Use phone in patient's room to call for help. 300 b
b. Shout for help. 301 b
c. Run quickly down to nursing station. 301 A

FRAME 171. TWO-RESCUER ADULT CPR PROTOCOL

If one person is alone at a CPR scene and a second person arrives to help, that person should first confirm the diagnosis by palpating the carotid or femoral artery. When the artery is palpated, the chest compressions are stopped for 5 seconds and the pulse is checked. If the pulse is absent, two-man CPR is begun with a breath delivered after every five compressions. The person ventilating the victim monitors the effectiveness of chest compressions by palpating the carotid artery for a pulse that should be felt simultaneously with chest compressions. The person compressing the chest needs to remember to pause after five compressions for 1 to 1½ seconds so that a tidal volume of approximately 800 mL can be delivered. When the two rescuers are ready to switch responsibilities, they must do so without interrupting the 5 : 1 compression-to-ventilation ratio. The person compressing the chest initiates the change by indicating that the switch will occur at the next 5 : 1 cycle. After giving the breath, the person performing the ventilations moves into position to give compressions. The person giving compressions moves to the head and checks the pulse after giving the fifth compression. If there is no pulse, the ventilator gives one breath and CPR is continued.

(Q) How long a pause in chest compression should occur to allow a breath to be delivered during resuscitation of an adult?

a. No pause is necessary. 300 C
b. 1 to 1½ seconds. 301 B
c. 3 to 5 seconds. 300 A

FRAME 172. MANUAL RESUSCITATORS

A manual resuscitator is frequently used to ventilate patients during cardiopulmonary resuscitation. It provides several advantages over mouth-to-mask ventilation including the capability of delivering high oxygen concentrations. An oxygen reservoir needs to be attached to the resuscitator bag proximal to the gas inlet valve in order for the device to deliver oxygen concentrations of 85% to 100% (Fig. 10–10). The oxygen flow to the resuscitator should be 15 L/min and always higher than the minute volume being delivered. Increasing oxygen flow from 15 to 20 L/min usually does not increase the delivered oxygen concentration (F_{DO_2}), and increasing oxygen flow to the highest possible setting may impede the normal operation of the patient valve. Prolonging the time it takes for the bag to refill will increase the F_{DO_2}.

A two-hand compression of the bag can increase the delivered tidal volume by 33%, for example, from 600 to 800 mL. Manual resuscitators without oxygen reservoirs typically deliver 40% to 45% oxygen with oxygen flow set at 15 L/min. Thus, forgetting to attach the oxygen reservoir to the gas intake valve is a serious error of omission which lowers F_{DO_2} to an unacceptable level. Increasing the cycle rate and/or stroke volume can increase the minute volume delivered by a manual resuscitator. If tidal volumes are delivered after five chest compressions, then a two-hand squeeze that delivers a large tidal volume would be best to increase minute volume since the cycle rate will be fixed at the approximately 12/min.

If the patient vomits into the non-rebreathing valve an attempt should be made to clear the valve by removing the resuscitator, squeezing the bag briskly, and shaking out any remaining material. If the valve of the resuscitator cannot be cleared in a few seconds (<10 seconds), then a mouth-to-mask device should be used to provide ventilation until another manual resuscitator can be located by someone not directly involved in the resuscitation effort.

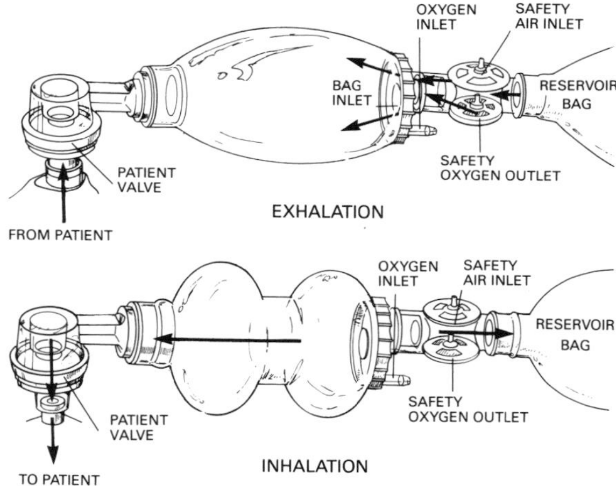

Figure 10–10 *Laerdal silicone adult resuscitator.*

(Q) Which of the following is the best way to increase the F_{DO_2} delivered by a manual resuscitator that does not have an oxygen reservoir attached?

a. Retard the inflation of the bag. 300 C
b. Cycle the resuscitator at a higher rate. 300 B
c. Decrease the minute volume being delivered. 301 d

FRAME 173. ADMINISTERING OXYGEN IN EMERGENCY SETTINGS

A primary goal of airway management is to provide a patent path to the lungs for oxygenation and ventilation. Attempts to establish a pulse and to restore spontaneous breathing will fail if severe hypoxemia is not reversed. Mouth-to-mask ventilation will deliver exhaled air from the rescuer containing only 15% to 18% oxygen unless an oxygen enrichment device is attached to the mask. Thus, the best method for ventilating an apneic patient will be the one that allows the highest oxygen concentration to be delivered. For example, it is always important to have a flow of oxygen to the gas intake valve of a manual resuscitator. The delivered oxygen concentration (FDO_2) will be limited to less than 70% even with retardation of bag refill unless an oxygen reservoir is added proximal to the gas intake valve. A properly designed oxygen reservoir will increase FDO_2 to 100% at O_2 flow of 15 L/min.

A conscious patient in the emergency room who is breathing spontaneously but suffers from moderate to severe hypoxemia should receive oxygen therapy at a FDO_2 as close to 100% as possible (except for chronic CO_2 retainers). Oxygen should be administered using a non-rebreathing mask at 10 L/min when the patient's ventilatory pattern (inspiratory flow rate, tidal volume, and respiratory rate) are close to normal. If the patient is extremely dyspneic and breathing rapidly, a Venturi mask (high-flow and fixed-performance) should be used to flood the nose and mouth with a total gas flow that matches or exceeds the patient's inspiratory flow.

Modern manual resuscitators have low-resistance non-rebreathing valves and can be used to provide 100% oxygen for spontaneous breathing provided (1) the oxygen reservoir is attached, (2) the oxygen flow to the unit is 15 L/min, and (3) the patient's inspiratory flow rate is not too high.

During CPR, ventilation should continue when chest compressions are stopped to check for a pulse or to evaluate an electrocardiogram strip. Ventilation with 100% oxygen should resume without delay immediately following an attempt to defibrillate the heart since hypoxemia, acidosis, and hypercarbia may work against attempts to reverse ventricular fibrillation.

(Q) How often should tidal volumes be delivered to an adult when chest compressions are stopped to check for a pulse or a sinus rhythm on the ECG monitor?

a. The patient should not be ventilated during this time. 301 C
b. Ventilation should occur at the rate of 12/min. 300 D
c. Ventilation should occur at the rate of 24/min. 301 a

FRAME 174. COMPLICATIONS OF CPR

Improper placement of the hands on the chest when attempting to do chest compressions can result in rib fractures and costochondral separation. Also, compression of the xiphoid process can cause laceration of the liver, aorta, stomach, spleen, or gastroesophageal junction, which can lead to severe internal bleeding. Pneumothorax, hemothorax, pericardial tamponade, and myocardial contusions are all complications of chest compressions that may occur even when CPR is done correctly. However, when time is taken to locate the correct hand position and when chest compressions are smooth, regular, and uninterrupted, the incidence of injury is reduced. Another complication of chest compressions is the formation of fat emboli. Compressing the bones of the rib cage and sternum may cause fat emboli to enter the venous circulation from the bone marrow, and may be a cause of postarrest mental deterioration.

Aspiration of gastric contents may occur during CPR as a result of regurgitation. If regurgitation occurs, the head should be turned to the side and the airway suctioned. A cuffed endotracheal tube will seal off the airway and help to prevent aspiration. If the stomach is observed to rise as the patient is ventilated, the head should be repositioned so that there is a minimal angle between the pharynx and trachea. Distention of the stomach may cause a decrease in venous return and cardiac output, and decrease ventilation by compressing the lungs.

Chest compressions must be continuous and interruptions limited to under 5 seconds. No longer than 5 seconds should be taken to check for a carotid or femoral pulse. Attempts to place an endotracheal tube in the trachea should not interrupt CPR for more than 15 to 30 seconds at which time, if the tube is not in the trachea, the procedure should be stopped, and CPR continued. Once the patient is reoxygenated another attempt to intubate may be initiated.

In cases where the victim and rescuers are in a location where they are at risk, such as a burning building, CPR can be interrupted for intervals of up to 30 seconds to move to a safer place where CPR is continued until another move is planned.

(Q) Which of the following actions should be taken to confirm that a tension pneumothorax has occurred during CPR?

a. Order a stat x-ray. 301 D

b. Use a large bore needle to check for air in the pleural space. 300 a

c. Check to see if manual ventilation is more difficult. 301 c

EXERCISES

1. Prepare a list of questions you would ask a patient who is found, confused but conscious on the floor of his room.
2. Describe the differences in applying the Heimlich maneuver to a conscious victim, an unconscious victim, a small child, an infant, or yourself.
3. List five different maneuvers for opening an obstructed upper airway. Explain how each maneuver is done, and include the advantages and disadvantages to each maneuver.
4. Explain why it is important to deliver tidal volumes with an inspiratory time of 1 to 1½ seconds during rescue breathing.
5. List three steps that can be taken to reduce the incidence of fractured ribs during chest compressions.
6. Outline the steps in the protocol for basic single-rescuer CPR. Then ask a peer to observe your performance during a simulation of single-rescuer CPR, and review your errors of omission and commission.
7. Practice switching positions with a friend during a simulation of two-rescuer CPR. Give special attention to chest compression-to-ventilation ratios, time elapsed while switching, and the responsibilities of each rescuer.
8. Obtain three different brands of manual resuscitators and locate the patient valve (non-rebreathing valve), bag refill valve, oxygen reservoir, and oxygen inlet nipple. Ventilate a lung analog with each resuscitator and measure the tidal volume delivered with one hand versus two hands at different compliance and airway resistance settings. Vary the oxygen flow to the resuscitator while holding the ventilation pattern constant, and measure the delivered oxygen concentration (F_{DO_2}). Determine the F_{DO_2} when the resuscitators are used without an oxygen reservoir.
9. List three clinical situations where you might want a patient to breathe spontaneously from a manual resuscitator.
10. List the complications that might occur from distention of the stomach caused by ventilating a patient during CPR with tidal volumes that are too large ($>$ 800 mL) and delivered too quickly ($<$1 second).

300A (from page 295, frame 171)
Wrong. A pause will be necessary so that a ventilation lasting 1 to 1½ seconds can occur after every five compressions. A chest compression rate of 80 to 100/min will not allow enough time for breath to be delivered without a slight pause in compressions. Return to page 295, frame 171, and select another answer.

300B (from page 296, frame 172)
Wrong. Increasing the cycle rate will increase minute volume and lower the F_{DO_2} further. Return to page 296, frame 172, and try again.

300C (from page 296, frame 172)
Correct. Retarding the inflation of the bag until just before the next tidal volume will allow less air to be mixed with oxygen from the reservoir. Increasing the cycle rate will increase minute volume and lower F_{DO_2} further. Please continue on page 297, frame 173.

300D (from page 297, frame 173)
Correct. Ventilation should continue at a rate of 12/min. Please continue on page 298, frame 174.

300a (from page 298, frame 174)
Wrong. The use of a large bore needle to decompress a tension pneumothorax is a treatment not a diagnostic test. Return to page 298, frame 174, and select another answer.

300b (from page 294, frame 170)
Wrong. Trying to call for help will delay beginning CPR. Return to page 294, frame 170, and select another answer.

300c (from page 295, frame 171)
Wrong. A breath should be delivered with an inspiratory time of 1 to 1½ seconds. If external heart compressions are delivered at a rate of 80 to 100/min, a pause to deliver a breath after every five compressions must occur. Return to page 295, frame 171, and select another answer.

301A (from page 294, frame 170)
Wrong. You should not leave the victim. Traveling to the nursing station is a serious error because it delays starting CPR. Return to page 294, frame 170, and select another answer.

301B (from page 295, frame 171)
Correct. A pause will be necessary so that a ventilation lasting to 1 to 1½ seconds can be given every 5 compressions. Please continue on page 296, frame 172.

301C (from page 297, frame 173)
Wrong. Hypoxemia, acidosis, and hypercarbia all decrease the chances of a normal sinus rhythm being restored. Return to page 297, frame 173, and select another answer.

301D (from page 298, frame 174)
Wrong. A chest x-ray would confirm the problem but would not be appropriate during CPR. Return to page 298, frame 174, and try again.

301a (from page 297, frame 173)
Wrong. Ventilation should not be given at a rate of 24/min. It will increase the mean intrathoracic pressure since positive-pressure breaths occur at twice the normal rate. The higher intrathoracic pressure may impede venous return to the heart. Return to page 297, frame 173, and select another answer.

301b (from page 294, frame 170)
Correct. This will allow you to begin CPR immediately. You may be able to send someone else to activate the hospital's CPR team. Please continue on page 295, frame 171.

301c (from page 298, frame 174)
Correct. A pneumothorax or hemothorax will make ventilation progressively more difficult and ineffective. A large bore needle or chest tube can be used to remove air from the pleural space. Please continue on page 299 and complete the chapter exercises.

301d (from page 296, frame 172)
Wrong. Decreasing the minute volume will increase F_{DO_2}, but this is not the best way since the patient may be hypoventilated. Return to page 296, frame 172, and select another answer.

POSTTEST

This test is designed to evaluate what you have learned from completing Chapter 10. Check your answers on page 304 and review the topics where your answer is incorrect.

1. On entering a room, you find a patient on the floor and apparently unconscious, what should you do next?
   A. Call for help.
   B. Lift the patient back into bed.
   C. Ask the patient if he or she is all right, tap or gently shake patient.
   D. Open the airway.
   E. Give two mouth-to-mask ventilations.

2. After opening the airway of an unresponsive patient which of the following actions should be taken?
   A. Deliver a precordial thump.
   B. Give two mouth-to-mask ventilations.
   C. Establish breathlessness.
   D. Call for help.
   E. Give 15 chest compressions.

3. Which of the following are signs of complete airway obstruction?
   I. victim cannot speak
   II. victim cannot cough
   III. chest wall retractions
   IV. nasal flaring
   A. I only
   B. I and II only
   C. II, III, and IV only
   D. I, II, and III only
   E. I, II, III, and IV

4. The Heimlich maneuver requires that thrusts be delivered to the
   A. midsternum.
   B. xiphoid process.
   C. abdomen.
   D. below the scapulae.
   E. costal angle.

5. The maneuver recommended by the American Heart Association as the most effective and safest method for opening the airway of an unconscious patient (who does not have an injury to the cervical spine) is the
   A. head-tilt/chin-lift maneuver.
   B. triple airway maneuver.
   C. modified jaw-thrust maneuver.
   D. head-tilt/neck-lift maneuver.
   E. mandibular-displacement maneuver.

6. Which of the following maneuvers to open the airway can be accomplished without head tilt?
   I. triple airway
   II. jaw-thrust
   III. modified jaw-thrust
   IV. mandibular-displacement
   A. I and II only
   B. II and III only
   C. III and IV only
   D. II, III, and IV only
   E. I, II, III, and IV

7. Mouth-to-mask rescue breathing for an adult with two practitioners administering CPR should be done at a rate of
   A. 6/min.
   B. 12/min.
   C. 15/min.
   D. 20/min.
   E. 24/min.
8. When ventilating an adult victim during CPR with a manual resuscitator, the minimum tidal volume delivered should be
   A. 450 mL.
   B. 600 mL.
   C. 800 mL.
   D. 900 mL.
   E. 1000 mL.
9. Chest compressions during CPR for an adult should be delivered at a rate of
   A. 40 to 50/min.
   B. 50 to 60/min.
   C. 60 to 70/min.
   D. 60 to 80/min.
   E. 80 to 100/min.
10. During CPR of an adult, chest compressions should move the sternum downward a distance of
    A. ½ to 1 in.
    B. 1 to 1½ in.
    C. 1½ to 2 in.
    D. 2 to 2½ in.
    E. 2½ to 3 in.
11. A single rescuer should not interrupt CPR to check for a pulse for longer than
    A. 1 second.
    B. 2 seconds.
    C. 5 seconds.
    D. 30 seconds.
    E. 60 seconds.
12. A single rescuer administering CPR should call for help after
    A. establishing unresponsiveness.
    B. opening the airway.
    C. establishing breathlessness.
    D. giving two ventilations.
    E. checking for a pulse.
13. The protocol for two-rescuer CPR calls for a ratio of chest compressions to ventilations of
    A. 5:1.
    B. 5:2.
    C. 15:1.
    D. 15:2.
    E. 20:3.
14. When a switch is announced by the rescuer doing chest compressions, the *other rescuer* providing ventilations does which of the following?
    A. Starts giving two ventilations after five compressions.
    B. Leaves room to call for help.
    C. Moves into position to give compressions.
    D. Waits for five compressions and gives a breath before moving.
    E. Waits for five compressions and checks pulse before moving.

15. During CPR a manual resuscitator becomes jammed with vomitus. After the airway is cleared, the resuscitator can be cleared by
   A. turning oxygen flow to the bag to flush.
   B. using the resuscitator without the oxygen reservoir.
   C. squeezing the bag briskly and shaking.
   D. disassembling the patient valve and rinsing with water.
   E. no attempt should be made to clear resuscitator.

16. The oxygen concentration delivered by a manual resuscitator may decrease if
   A. minute volume exceeds oxygen flow.
   B. inspiratory time exceeds 1 second.
   C. the oxygen reservoir is made larger.
   D. tidal volume is decreased.
   E. two hands are used to squeeze the bag.

17. An emergency room patient with no history of chronic obstructive pulmonary disease (COPD) complains of dyspnea and has a respiratory rate of 32/min. Which of the following types of oxygen therapy would be indicated?
   A. nasal cannula at 2 L/min
   B. nasal cannula at 6 L/min
   C. 40% Venturi mask
   D. rebreathing mask at 10 L/min
   E. non-rebreathing mask at 8 L/min

18. A patient receiving CPR has his pulse re-established and begins to breathe spontaneously. Which of the following should be done during transfer to the operating room?
   A. Administer oxygen by T-tube.
   B. Allow the patient to breathe spontaneously from the resuscitator.
   C. Provide controlled ventilation with the resuscitator.
   D. Connect a portable intermittent positive-pressure breathing (IPPB) machine using assist-control mode.
   E. Connect to a portable volume ventilator using an intermittent mandatory ventilation (IMV) mode.

19. Which of the following may reduce the incidence of rib fractures that are caused by chest compressions?
   A. Interlocking fingers of both hands.
   B. Lifting hands off the chest after each compression.
   C. Compressing the chest of adults only 1 to 1½ in.
   D. Applying pressure only on the xiphoid process.
   E. Bending arms when compressing the chest.

20. How long should chest compressions be interrupted so that an endotracheal tube can be placed?
   A. 5 to 10 seconds
   B. 10 to 15 seconds
   C. 15 to 30 seconds
   D. 30 to 60 seconds
   E. 1 to 2 minutes

ANSWERS TO POSTTEST

1. C (F165)
2. B (F168)
3. D (F166)
4. C (F166)
5. A (F167)
6. C (F167)
7. B (F168)
8. C (F172)
9. E (F169)
10. C (F169)
11. C (F174)
12. A (F170)
13. A (F171)
14. D (F171)
15. C (F172)
16. A (F172)
17. C (F173)
18. B (F173)
19. A (F169)
20. C (F174)

BIBLIOGRAPHY

American Heart Association: Standards and guidelines for cardiopulmonary resuscitation and emergency cardiac care. JAMA 255:21, 1986.

American Heart Association: Heart Saver Manual: A Student Handbook for Cardiopulmonary Resuscitation and First Aid for Choking. American Heart Association, Dallas, 1987.

Barnes, TA: Respiratory Care Practice. Year Book Medical Publishers, Chicago, 1988.

Burton, GG and Hodgkin, JE: Respiratory Care: A Guide to Clinical Practice, ed 2. JB Lippincott, Philadelphia, 1984.

Eubanks, DH and Bone, RC: Comprehensive Respiratory Care, ed 2. CV Mosby, St. Louis, 1990.

Finucane, BT and Santora, AH: Principles of Airway Management. FA Davis, Philadelphia, 1988.

Koff, PB, Eitzman, DV, and Neu, J: Neonatal and Pediatric Respiratory Care. CV Mosby, St. Louis, 1988.

11

Monitoring Patient Response

175. Collecting an arterial blood sample
176. Arterial blood-gas interpretation
177. Noninvasive assessment of oxygenation
178. Tracheal tube cuff pressure
179. Airway resistance and compliance
180. Intermittent positive-pressure breathing
181. Aerosol therapy
182. Bronchial hygiene therapy
183. CPAP/PEEP
184. Mechanical ventilation

PRETEST

This pretest is designed to measure what you already know about monitoring a patient's response to respiratory care. Check your answers on page 309 and then continue on page 310, frame 175.

1. What is the minimum amount of time a puncture site must be compressed after obtaining a radial artery sample?
   A. 30 to 60 seconds
   B. 1 to 2 minutes
   C. 2 to 5 minutes
   D. 5 to 10 minutes
   E. 10 to 15 minutes
2. Which of the following complications is likely to occur if strong continuous aspirating force is applied while collecting a sample from the radial artery?
   A. hematoma
   B. venous admixture
   C. spasm of the artery
   D. pulmonary emboli
   E. air dilution
3. What is the acid-base balance and oxygenation of a 60-year-old patient with the following blood-gas data: F_{IO_2} 0.21, pH 7.15, Pa_{CO_2} 50 torr (mm Hg), Pa_{O_2} 39 torr, HCO_3^- 17 mEq/L?
   A. partially compensated respiratory acidosis, severe hypoxemia
   B. partially compensated metabolic acidosis, severe hypoxemia
   C. metabolic alkalosis and respiratory acidosis, moderate hypoxemia
   D. metabolic acidosis and respiratory alkalosis, moderate hypoxemia
   E. respiratory and metabolic acidosis, severe hypoxemia
4. What is the acid-base balance and oxygenation of a 3-year-old patient with the following blood-gas data: F_{IO_2} 0.21, pH 7.26, Pa_{CO_2} 26 torr (mm Hg), Pa_{O_2} 85 torr, HCO_3^- 12 mEq/L?
   A. partially compensated respiratory acidosis, mild hypoxemia
   B. partially compensated metabolic acidosis, normal oxygenation
   C. metabolic and respiratory alkalosis, mild hypoxemia
   D. partially compensated respiratory alkalosis, normal oxygenation
   E. uncompensated metabolic acidosis, normal oxygenation
5. All of the following will affect the accuracy of a pulse oximetry *except*
   A. bilirubin of 12 mg/mL.
   B. poor perfusion at probe site.
   C. low cardiac output.
   D. hyperthermia.
   E. peripheral shunting.
6. Patients should have oxygenation supported to maintain a minimum pulse oximeter reading of
   A. 60%.
   B. 70%.
   C. 80%.
   D. 90%.
   E. 100%.
7. What volume is normally held by low-pressure tracheal tube cuffs?
   A. 3 mL
   B. 5 mL
   C. 7 mL
   D. 10 mL
   E. 12 mL

8. When inflating a tracheal tube cuff using the minimal leak technique for a patient receiving continuous positive-airway pressure (CPAP), a small leak should be heard at
   A. early inspiration.
   B. midinspiration.
   C. end inspiration.
   D. midexhalation.
   E. end exhalation.

9. Which of the following will occur if PEEP is increased by 5 cm H_2O?
   I. Peak pressure increases.
   II. Plateau pressure increases.
   III. Airway resistance increases.
   IV. Cardiac output increases.
   A. I only
   B. II only
   C. I and II only
   D. I, III, and IV only
   E. I, II, III, and IV
   E. I, II, III, and IV

10. If the difference between peak and plateau pressure decreases for a patient being mechanically ventilated, all of the following are true *except*
    A. Compliance is decreasing.
    B. Airway resistance is decreasing.
    C. Airway resistance is increasing.
    D. Compliance is increasing.
    E. The patient ventilator system has a leak.

11. All of the following clinical signs indicate that a patient receiving intermittent positive-pressure breathing (IPPB) is hyperventilating *except*
    A. dizziness
    B. sharp chest pain
    C. tingling of the extremities
    D. numbness of the extremities
    E. tremors of the hands

12. When aerosol medications are delivered, what is the maximum increase in heart rate allowed before the treatment is terminated?
    A. 10/min
    B. 15/min
    C. 20/min
    D. 30/min
    E. 50/min

13. If the initial FEV_1 is 1000 mL, which of the following posttreatment FEV_1 values indicates a bronchodilator treatment was effective?
    A. 900 mL
    B. 1000 mL
    C. 1050 mL
    D. 1100 mL
    E. 1150 mL

14. Which of the following may occur when an ultrasonic nebulizer delivers a bland solution to a patient with thick, dry secretions?
    I. decrease in compliance
    II. increase in compliance
    III. increase in airway resistance
    IV. dyspnea
    V. respiratory distress
    A. I only
    B. II and III only
    C. III, IV, and V only
    D. I, III and IV only
    E. II, III, IV, and V only

15. When sputum is yellow, the patient should be evaluated for
   A. *Pseudomonas aeruginosa.*
   B. bronchial asthma.
   C. infectious process.
   D. pulmonary edema.
   E. bronchial venous bleeding.

16. When sputum is green and has a musty odor, the patient should be evaluated for
   A. *Pseudomonas aeruginosa.*
   B. bronchial asthma.
   C. pulmonary edema.
   D. Klebsiella pneumonia.
   E. cystic fibrosis.

17. If blood pressure readings are not available, which of the following will be the best indicator the optimal PEEP level has been exceeded?
   A. increase in plateau pressure
   B. increase in peak airway pressure
   C. decrease in urinary output
   D. flushing of the extremities
   E. increase in arterial CO_2 tension

18. If a flow-directed (Swan-Ganz) catheter is in place, which of the following will help to determine the optimal PEEP level?
   I. hemoglobin concentration
   II. a-v O_2 content difference
   III. pulmonary artery pressure
   IV. mixed venous O_2 tension
   V. cardiac output
   A. I and III only
   B. II and V only
   C. I, II, and IV only
   D. II, IV, and V only
   E. II, III, IV, and V only

19. Low-pressure alarms for mechanical ventilators should be set at a threshold that is
   A. 2 to 5 cm H_2O below peak pressure.
   B. 5 to 10 cm H_2O below peak pressure.
   C. 10 to 20 cm H_2O below peak pressure.
   D. 5 to 10 cm H_2O above PEEP.
   E. 10 to 20 cm H_2O above PEEP.

20. Which of these may occur with endobronchial intubation during mechanical ventilation?
   I. increase in peak pressure
   II. increase in plateau pressure
   III. auto PEEP
   IV. loss of PEEP
   V. pneumothorax
   A. I and III only
   B. II and III only
   C. I, II, and IV only
   D. III, IV, and V only
   E. I, II, and V only

ANSWERS TO PRETEST

1. C (F175)
2. C (F175)
3. E (F176)
4. B (F176)
5. D (F177)
6. D (F177)
7. E (F178)
8. D (F178)
9. C (F183)
10. B (F179)
11. E (F180)
12. C (F180)
13. E (F181)
14. C (F181)
15. C (F182)
16. A (F182)
17. C (F183)
18. D (F183)
19. B (F184)
20. E (F184)

FRAME 175. COLLECTING AN ARTERIAL BLOOD SAMPLE

The radial artery is the most frequently used site for arterial puncture because it meets the criteria of (1) collateral blood flow, (2) vessel accessibility, (3) being surrounded by tissue relatively insensitive to pain, and (4) separation from adjacent veins. The modified Allen test should be done to assess collateral circulation via the ulnar artery. The Allen test is accomplished by having the patient make a fist several times to force as much blood from the hand as possible and then compressing both the radial artery and ulnar artery simultaneously while the fist is tight. Then ask the patient to relax the fist and remove the pressure from the ulnar artery while the fingers, thumb, and palm are observed to see if the ulnar artery alone is capable of perfusing the entire hand. Obviously it is critical to make this observation with the radial artery compressed. The restoration of a pink color within 15 seconds provides evidence that obstruction of the radial artery will not result in a loss of blood flow to the hand. If the Allen test is negative (the hand does not flush pink when the ulnar artery is released) you should not draw the radial sample and notify the physician of the problem.

The process and need for the arterial puncture is explained to the patient, the radial artery is palpated, Allen test completed, and then the skin at the puncture site is cleansed with alcohol swabs. Since it is impossible to reliably identify all patients infected with human immunodeficiency virus (HIV) or other blood-borne infections, gloves and eye protection should be worn when the sample is taken from the radial artery. A small-gauge (25-gauge) needle is often used to puncture the radial artery. A small-gauge needle has the advantage of causing less discomfort to the subject but may restrict the flow of blood into the syringe and is more susceptible to clotting. Larger gauge needles (20 to 23-gauge) make collection of the sample easier but are more likely to cause the subject discomfort. The injection of a local anesthetic through a 25-gauge needle under the skin in the area to be punctured is controversial. The Xylocaine injection may be painful and the procedure is time-consuming. Many practitioners can draw a sample with one arterial puncture that causes very little pain. The needle should be inserted into the artery at as small an angle as possible. Using a needle with a clear hub makes it easier to see when an artery is punctured. A glass syringe fills more readily, and arterial pulsations make it easier to tell when the artery is punctured and remove the need to aspirate blood into the syringe. Beginning practitioners should use glass syringes to help them identify the moment the needle punctures the artery. Air bubbles may be more difficult to expel from plastic syringes. Plastic syringes are preferred in some institutions because they are readily available. The incidence of sample loss due to glass syringe breakage or plunger slippage may be reduced by the use of plastic syringes. The size of the syringe should be the smallest that will contain the amount of blood required for analysis in order to minimize the amount of anticoagulant required to fill the dead space of the needle and syringe.

The skin should be punctured quickly and the needle advanced slowly toward the point where the artery lies under the fingers. The patient's pulse pressure should cause blood to flow freely into the syringe. If the needle goes completely through the artery, it should be slowly withdrawn while the plunger is intermittently and gently pulled backward. The practitioner should never apply strong or continuous aspirating force while withdrawing the needle since it may trigger spasm of the vessel. Once the sample is obtained (usually 2 to 4 mL), the needle should be withdrawn quickly, with care to prevent the plunger from slipping backward. The first action after the needle is withdrawn is compression of the puncture site. Firm pressure, using a sterile gauze pad, should be applied for a minimum of 2 minutes, longer if the patient is receiving anticoagulant therapy. Failure to compress the puncture site with firm pressure for 2 to 5 minutes or longer may cause a hematoma (periarterial accumulation).

The sample should be properly handled, which includes (1) expelling air bubbles; (2) sealing the syringe; (3) rolling the syringe between the hands to mix the anticoagulant throughout the sample; (4) placing the sample on ice; and (5) properly labeling the sample including whether or not the patient is receiving supplemental oxygen, mechanical ventilation, PEEP and other ventilation parameters, patient's name, temperature, and time of collection.

(Q) How much *anticoagulant* should be drawn into the syringe used to collect an arterial blood sample?

a. ½ mL 318 A

b. 1 ml 319 B

c. enough to fill the dead space of the needle and syringe 318 c

FRAME 176. ARTERIAL BLOOD-GAS INTERPRETATION

Arterial blood-gas studies provide information that can be interpreted to assess a patient's acid-base status and the lungs' ability to oxygenate blood and remove excess carbon dioxide. Changes in the level of CO_2 in blood plasma will affect the pH and is regulated by alveolar ventilation. The plasma HCO_3^- concentration is regulated primarily by the kidneys. The acid-base state is determined by the pH, $Paco_2$, and HCO_3^- concentration. The degree of compensation is determined by the pH. Compensation of primary respiratory disturbances comes from the metabolic system. Conversely, compensation of primary metabolic disturbances comes from the respiratory system. When compensation returns arterial pH to the normal range (7.35 to 7.45), the primary disturbance to the acid-base state is interpreted as fully compensated. A primary disturbance is partially compensated when pH is not restored to the normal range. Substantial metabolic compensation for a primary respiratory disturbance requires 24 to 48 hours. Compensation by the respiratory system for a primary metabolic disturbance can occur within minutes since $Paco_2$ is rapidly altered by changes in ventilation.

When two primary acid-base abnormalities (respiratory and metabolic) occur simultaneously, a mixed acid-base disturbance results. When both components (HCO_3^- and $Paco_2$) change from the normal range and move in the opposite direction to cause acidosis or alkalosis, the interpretation is easier since there is no compensation. HCO_3^- and $Paco_2$ move in the same direction when primary disturbances occur simultaneously to both systems and the pH may be in the normal range. For example, a mixed metabolic acidosis and respiratory alkalosis may result in a pH elevated slightly above 7.40 and may give the appearance of compensated metabolic acidosis. Conversely, this incorrect interpretation may be given to a patient with primary respiratory alkalosis when the decrease of plasma (HCO_3^-) exceeds the predicted amount. Table 11-1 shows expected compensation for acute and chronic acid-base disorders and can be used to determine if compensation for a primary disorder is appropriate. If the compensation exceeds the predicted amount, a mixed disturbance should be suspected.

Age, Fio_2, and barometric pressure will all affect the judgment regarding whether the arterial oxygen tension is in the normal range. The amount of oxygen carried by hemoglobin and delivered to the tissues is the critical factor of adequate oxygenation. The arterial oxygen tension should be maintained in a minimum range of 60 to 70 torr (mm Hg) or higher to ensure an arterial oxygen saturation of 90% in the upper plateau area of the oxyhemoglobin dissociation curve. Also, the amount of functional hemoglobin and the actual arterial oxygen content (Cao_2) is very important. The acceptable range of Pao_2 for patients with chronic obstructive pulmonary disease may be only 50 to 60 torr when CO_2 retention is a chronic problem. A large increase in alveolar-arterial oxygen tension, $P(A\text{-}a)o_2$ on 100% O_2, indicates shunt, ventilation to perfusion mismatching, or a diffusion defect.

TABLE 11-1
EXPECTED COMPENSATION FOR ACUTE AND CHRONIC ACID-BASE DISORDERS

Primary Disorder	Expected Compensation
Acute respiratory acidosis	For a 15 mm Hg increase in $Paco_2$, the HCO_3^- increases 1 mEq/L; significant compensation takes from 24 to 48 hours
Chronic respiratory acidosis	For every 10 mm Hg increase in $Paco_2$, HCO_3^- increases 4 mEq/L
Acute respiratory alkalosis	For every 5 mm Hg decrease in $Paco_2$, HCO_3^- decreases 1 mEq/L; significant compensation requires 24 to 48 hours
Chronic respiratory alkalosis	HCO_3^- falls 5 mEq/L for every 10 mm Hg decrease in $Paco_2$
Metabolic acidosis	$Paco_2$ = last two digits of pH $Paco_2 = (1.5 \times HCO_3^-) + 8 \pm 2$
Metabolic alkalosis	$Paco_2$ change is variable $Paco_2$ usually does not rise above 50–55 torr $Paco_2$ increases 0.6 mm Hg for each mEq/L increase in HCO_3^-

(Source: Wilkins, RL, Sheldon, RL, and Krider SJ: Clinical Assessment in Respiratory Care. CV Mosby, St. Louis, 1985.)

Tissue oxygenation will be dependent on oxygen transport, which will be determined by both Cao_2 and cardiac output. The mixed venous oxygen tension ($P\bar{v}o_2$) can be used to assess tissue oxygenation, and $P\bar{v}o_2$ should be in the normal range of 38 to 42 torr when Cao_2 and cardiac output are adequate.

(Q) Which of the following describe the acid-base balance and oxygenation of a 50-year-old patient breathing room air, given the following blood-gas data: pH 7.32, $Paco_2$ 32 torr, HCO_3^- 16 mEq/L, Pao_2 50 torr?
a. acute metabolic acidosis, severe hypoxemia 318 B
b. partially compensated respiratory alkalosis, moderate hypoxemia 318 d
c. partially compensated metabolic acidosis, moderate hypoxemia 319 A

FRAME 177. NONINVASIVE ASSESSMENT OF OXYGENATION

Pulse oximetry is a noninvasive technique that measures the oxygen saturation of hemoglobin by absorption of light of a particular wavelength. The amount of light passing through the ear or digit and on to a detector determines the oxyhemoglobin saturation. Pulse oximeters used in critical care have proven to be relatively precise (± 2%), as long as saturation values are above 80%. Pulse oximetry is most useful for detecting changes of saturation over time, and less acceptable for single determinations. The use of oximetry for *spot checks* often does not reduce the need for blood-gas analysis.

Two factors that affect the accuracy of pulse oximeters are perfusion at the probe site and the amount of dysfunctional hemoglobin. An elevated bilirubin concentration, smoke inhalation, and heavy cigarette smoking may independently increase carboxyhemoglobin levels. The pulse oximeter ignores the amount of dysfunctional hemoglobin and measures only the oxyhemoglobin and deoxygenated hemoglobin portion of the total. The pulse oximeter will not be accurate in the presence of an extremely low cardiac output, peripheral shunting, and hypothermia. One indicator of adequate perfusion and hence a reliable %Hbo_2 display is the degree of agreement between the actual heart rate and the displayed heart rate.

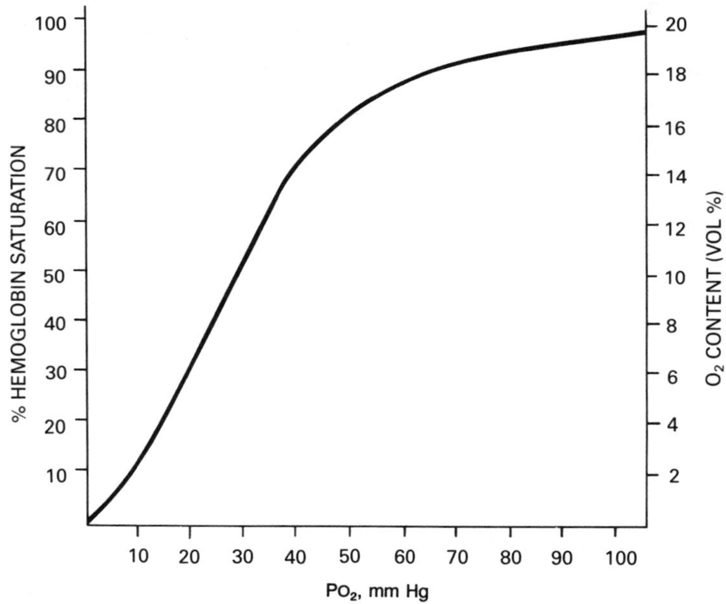

Figure 11-1 Oxyhemoglobin dissociation curve describing the relationship between oxygen tension, percent hemoglobin saturation, and oxygen content.

(Q) In order to remain on the flat portion of the oxyhemoglobin dissociation curve and to maintain the oxygen tension no lower than 60 torr the saturation on a pulse oximeter should read

a. 70%. 318 C

b. 80%. 319 a

c. 90%. 319 c

FRAME 178. TRACHEAL TUBE CUFF PRESSURE

Tracheostomy and endotracheal tube cuffs should be checked for pressure and volume every 8 hours or whenever the peak inspiratory pressure changes substantially for patients being mechanically ventilated. Tubes that have high-volume (floppy) cuffs should be used since they seal the airway at low inflation pressure. These low-pressure cuffs, out of the airway, have an unstretched volume of 12 mL. If the tube is the right size, the intracuff pressure necessary for no-leak ventilation will not exceed 20 mm Hg when measured during exhalation. Floppy, low-pressure cuffs are designed to contact a larger surface area of the tracheal wall with the cuff material having wrinkles and not fully distended. Expansion of some of the wrinkles allow increases in cuff volume to be accompanied by only small changes in pressure. The cuff-to-tracheal wall pressure will rise sharply to unacceptable levels (>25 mm Hg) if volume is added to the cuff until it is stretched tight and free of all wrinkles.

The minimal leak technique (minimal occluding volume) is the safest method to use to inflate low-pressure cuffs. This technique is accomplished by listening for a small leak past the cuff at the point in the ventilatory cycle where the trachea has the largest diameter. The stethescope should be placed over the trachea and the cuff inflated until an air leak can no longer be heard. For patients being mechanically ventilated, the air in the cuff is reduced in small increments until a small leak is heard at the point of peak inspiratory pressure. Patients breathing spontaneously should have small increments of gas removed from the cuff until a small leak is heard in early or midexhalation. It is important to record the volume needed to inflate tracheal tube cuffs to assure that they are not fully distended. Intracuff pressure is very important and should also be monitored as volume is added using a pressure manometer connected to the pilot tube of the cuff. Once the cuff is inflated using the minimal leak technique, the intracuff pressure should be measured during the expiratory phase and recorded along with the volume necessary to inflate the cuff.

High intracuff pressure (>25 mm Hg) will completely stop arterial capillary blood flow where the cuff makes contact with the tracheal wall and will cause tissue ischemia. Cuff pressure higher than 18 mm Hg will obstruct venous blood flow and cause congestion. Lymphatic flow obstruction and edema will occur if the cuff pressure is higher than 5 mm Hg.

(Q) Which of the following is the most important precaution that should be taken to reduce the incidence of tracheal stenosis?

a. Monitor cuff volume. 319 D
b. Minimize cuff pressure on the tracheal wall. 318 b
c. Minimize trauma during intubation. 319 b

FRAME 179. AIRWAY RESISTANCE AND COMPLIANCE

Total system resistance and compliance include factors from the lungs and ventilator circuit. It is often referred to as *static compliance* since plateau pressure is measured after the tidal volume has been delivered and inspiratory flow is close to zero. The plateau pressure is a reasonable estimate of static pressure resulting from system elasticity. Static compliance is determined by dividing the exhaled tidal volume by the difference between plateau pressure and baseline pressure (PEEP). When compressible volume loss in the ventilator circuit is significant and variable, many practitioners correct exhaled tidal volume for the volume lost to the circuit. A decrease in static compliance indicates that the system is stiffer and occurs with (1) endobronchial intubation, (2) total airway obstruction, (3) atelectasis, (4) consolidation, (5) ARDS, and (6) pneumothorax. Trends in static compliance can be used to evaluate the patient for improvement in the conditions that originally caused a decrease in compliance.

Nonelastic resistance to ventilation or system resistance focuses on airway resistance (RA) which can be estimated by dividing the pressure difference between peak pressure and plateau pressure by inspiratory flow. Since the plateau pressure represents the amount of work required to overcome the elastic forces of the system, it is reasonable to assume that the pressure difference between peak and plateau pressure is the work required to overcome the resistance to gas flow at the instant just before inspiration ends. Although inspiratory flow is not frequently measured on standard ventilators, it can be estimated when the flow waveform is square (constant flow pattern). Even with nonconstant flow patterns the estimated inspiratory flow can be used to indicate changes in airway resistance. For example, if the inspiratory flow is held constant, an increase in the difference between peak and plateau pressure will indicate increased airway resistance. Increases in airway resistance result from a decrease in airway caliber caused by (1) edema, (2) bronchospasm, or (3) partial airway obstruction.

(Q) What is the static compliance given a tidal volume of 1.2 L, plateau pressure of 40 cm H_2O, PEEP of 10 cm H_2O, peak pressure of 50 cm H_2O?

a. 0.024 L/cm H_2O 318 D
b. 0.030 L/cm H_2O 319 C
c. 0.040 L/cm H_2O 318 a

FRAME 180. INTERMITTENT POSITIVE-PRESSURE BREATHING

Intermittent positive-pressure breathing (IPPB) is justified only when the patient's ability to inspire adequately is limited. Commonly stated goals for IPPB include (1) improved cough, (2) mobilized secretions, (3) improved distribution of and deposition of aerosols, and (4) treatment of pulmonary edema. IPPB is indicated when the vital capacity is less than 15 mL/kg and should improve the patient's limited vital capacity by 100%. Pathology that may decrease vital capacity to a point where IPPB may be indicated include (1) pain following abdominal or thoracic surgery, (2) abdominal distention and pain, (3) nervous system and neuromuscular disease, and (4) restrictive and obstructive pulmonary disease.

Hazards associated with the administration of IPPB include (1) hyperventilation and respiratory alkalosis, (2) increased intrathoracic pressure, (3) pneumothorax, (4) hemoptysis, (5) effects on hypoxic drive of chronic obstructive pulmonary disease (COPD) patients, (6) increased intracranial pressure, (7) gastric insufflation, and (8) nosocomial infection. Vital signs should be measured before, during, and after IPPB therapy to monitor the impact of increased intrathoracic pressure. Persistent tachycardia may result when bronchoactive drugs are administered with IPPB. An increase in heart rate of 20/min or more should prompt the practitioner to terminate the treatment and to discuss the tachycardia with the patient's physician.

The emphasis of the IPPB therapy should be on delivering large tidal volumes to produce productive coughing. The number of large tidal volumes should be limited to 6 to 8/min with rest periods every 2 to 3 minutes. If the patient is allowed to cycle the IPPB machine at fast rates or if rest periods are not provided, alveolar hyperventilation and respiratory alkalosis may occur. The clinical signs of hyperventilation include dizziness, fainting, nervousness, numbness and tingling of the extremities, cramps and tremors of the muscles of the hand.

A sharp pain in the chest occurring during IPPB therapy, especially if associated with coughing, should alert the practitioner to terminate the treatment and evaluate the patient for signs of a pneumothorax. The hazard of gastric insufflation is greatest when IPPB is delivered by mask and at cycling pressures greater than 25 cm H_2O in the neurologically obtunded. The patient receiving IPPB by mask should be carefully observed to assure that part of the tidal volume is not entering the stomach. High peak airway pressure may exceed the opening pressure of the esophagus, with variable volumes entering the stomach. The greatest danger of gastric insufflation is rupture of the stomach or vomiting and aspiration of gastric material with low pH into the lungs.

(Q) Which of the following actions should be taken if blood is seen in the sputum during an IPPB treatment?

a. Inspect the sputum and continue the treatment. 324 c
b. Terminate the IPPB treatment and notify the physician. 325 D
c. Continue the IPPB treatment and notify the physician. 325 b

318A (from pages 310–311, frame 175)
Careful. Lyophilized heparin is used to lubricate the syringe and eliminate air that would otherwise fill the dead space in the needle and syringe. The liquid anticoagulant can have a dilutional effect, particularly on CO_2 tensions, and all the excess solution should be expelled. Dilutional effect of heparin can be distinguished from air by the fact that heparin causes little if any change in pH. Please return to pages 310–311, frame 175, and try again.

318B (from pages 312–313, frame 176)
Wrong. The HCO_3^- concentration is below the normal range of 22 to 26 mEq/L, indicating either metabolic acidosis or metabolic compensation of respiratory alkalosis. Review the $Paco_2$ and pH to decide. The Pao_2 would need to be lower than 40 mm Hg to be considered severe hypoxemia. Return to pages 312–313, frame 176, review Table 11-1, and select another answer.

318C (from page 314, frame 177)
Wrong. If the oxyhemoglobin curve is in its normal position, an Sao_2 of 70% would result in a Pao_2 of 40 torr and the patient would be severely hypoxemic. Return to page 314, frame 177, and select another answer.

318D (from page 316, frame 179)
Wrong. The peak pressure represents work done against both elastic and nonelastic forces. Static compliance measurements indicate only changes in elastic forces. Return to page 316, frame 179, and select another answer.

318a (from page 316, frame 179)
Correct. Dividing the tidal volume by the difference between plateau and PEEP will estimate the static compliance. Please continue on page 317, frame 180.

318b (from page 315, frame 178)
Correct. Using the minimal leak technique and tracheal tubes with low-pressure (high volume) cuffs should allow the intracuff pressure to be maintained at less than 20 torr. This will prevent ischemia of the tracheal wall and reduce the chance of tracheal stenosis developing. Please continue on page 316, frame 179.

318c (from pages 310–311, frame 175)
Correct. Only enough lyophilized heparin is used to lubricate the syringe and eliminate air that would otherwise fill the dead space in the needle and syringe. The liquid anticoagulant can have a dilutional effect, particularly on CO_2 tensions, and all the excess solution should be expelled. Dilutional effect of heparin can be distinguished from air by the fact that heparin causes little if any change in pH. Please continue on pages 312–313, frame 176.

318d (from pages 312–313, frame 176)
Wrong. The pH indicates an acidotic state exists. The HCO_3^- concentration is below normal, indicating that a primary disturbance to the metabolic system may exist. Return to pages 312–313, frame 176, review Table 11-1, and select another answer.

319A (from pages 312–313, frame 176)
Correct. The primary disturbance is to the metabolic system and partial respiratory compensation has occurred as alveolar hyperventilation has lowered $Paco_2$ to 32 torr and moved the pH higher toward the normal range. A Pao_2 of 50 torr indicates moderate hypoxemia. Please continue on page 314, frame 177.

319B (from pages 310–311, frame 175)
Careful. Lyophilized heparin is used to lubricate the syringe and eliminate air that would otherwise fill the dead space in the needle and syringe. The liquid anticoagulant can have a dilutional effect, particularly on CO_2 tensions, and all the excess solution should be expelled. Dilutional effect of heparin can be distinguished from air by the fact that heparin causes little if any change in pH. Please return to pages 310–311, frame 175, and try again.

319C (from page 316, frame 179)
Wrong. The PEEP must be subtracted from the plateau pressure not the peak pressure which works against both elastic and nonelastic forces. Static compliance measurements indicate changes in only elastic forces. Return to page 316, frame 179, and select another answer.

319D (from page 315, frame 178)
Wrong. While it is important to record cuff volume every 8 hours to check for overdistention, there is another variable more directly related to tracheal stenosis. Return to page 315, frame 178, and select another answer.

319a (from page 314, frame 177)
Wrong. If the oxyhemoglobin dissociation curve is in its normal position, an Sao_2 of 80% would result in a Pao_2 of 50 torr and the patient would be moderately hypoxemic. Any further drop in arterial oxygen tension will result in a large drop in saturation because the curve is very steep in this portion. Return to page 314, frame 177, and try again.

319b (from page 315, frame 178)
Wrong. Trauma during intubation is not recognized as a major cause of tracheal stenosis. After the tube is in the trachea, weight or tension on the tracheal tube may cause increased pressure on the stoma in addition to the irritation to the tracheal mucosa caused by the cuff. Return to page 315, frame 178, and select another answer.

319c (from page 314, frame 177)
Correct. Maintaining a patient's Sao_2 at 90% or higher will protect the patient from large drops in saturation if the Pao_2 drops, since this part of the oxyhemoglobin dissociation curve is flat. A Sao_2 of 90% normally correlates to a Pao_2 of 60 torr. Please continue on page 315, frame 178.

FRAME 181. AEROSOL THERAPY

Assessment of aerosol therapy relates to the type of drug being delivered and the therapeutic goal. The goal of administering a beta-2 sympathomimetic drug is to reverse constriction of bronchial smooth muscle. Three tests that can be done at the bedside to measure response to inhaled bronchodilators are: forced vital capacity (FVC), forced expiratory volume after 1 second (FEV_1), and forced expiratory flow during the middle half of the FVC (FEF_{25-75}). The amount of improvement needed varies for each test: (1) FVC $\geq$ 10%, (2) $FEV_1 \geq$ 200 mL or 15% of baseline, and (3) $FEF_{25-75} \geq$ 20%. Also, inspection of respiratory pattern and rate, chest auscultation, and questioning the patient about his breathing help to determine if airway obstruction has been reversed. Many bronchodilators have beta-1 side effects that include tachycardia, palpitation, nervousness, muscular tremors, and flushing of the skin. An increase in blood pressure may occur with a limited number of aerosol drugs such as racemic epinephrine that stimulate alpha receptors and cause strong systemic vasoconstriction. Practitioners should monitor vital signs (before, during, and after the treatment) for the potential side effects of inhaled bronchodilators.

Bronchospasm is a hazard whenever aerosol particles are delivered to the airways. Increased airway resistance is likely when 20% acetylcysteine, antibiotics, dry powered cromolyn sodium, water, or hypertonic aerosols are delivered to the lungs. Bronchospasm is also a significant hazard with ultrasonic nebulizers because of the high density of aerosol particles. The practitioner should remain in attendance during ultrasonic therapy with patients who have hyperactive airways, auscultating frequently to check for bronchospasm. Another problem that should be assessed during ultrasonic therapy is the swelling of dried, retained secretions. A 50% decrease in airway caliber will result in a 1600% increase in airway resistance and may result in acute small airway obstruction. Thus, a patient receiving ultrasonic therapy to loosen retained secretions should be monitored for acute dyspnea and respiratory distress that may occur shortly after starting aerosol therapy. Ultrasonic therapy should be given together with chest physiotherapy so that secretions can be moved to the upper airways.

(Q) Which of the following is the most important to monitor before, during, and after administration of an adrenergic bronchodilator?

a. pulse 324 A

b. blood pressure 324 d

c. breath sounds 325 A

FRAME 182. BRONCHIAL HYGIENE THERAPY

The goals of bronchial hygiene therapy are directed at mobilizing retained secretions, reinflation of atelectatic areas, and decreasing the extent and longevity of infection. Four modalities of bronchial hygiene therapy are often combined to accomplish the goals of bronchial hygiene therapy: (1) aerosol therapy, (2) IPPB, (3) chest physical therapy, and (4) incentive spirometry. The following observations are often used to evaluate the effectiveness of the combined treatment plan: sputum, auscultation, work of breathing, blood-gas analysis, pulmonary function studies, and chest x-rays.

Sputum should be evaluated for the quantity produced during each treatment and the total collected over 24 hours. The color, viscosity, and odor of the sputum produced will provide clues regarding the disease state, etiology of the bronchial hygiene problem, and the success of the therapy administered. The normal viscosity of sputum is like water; however, dehydration results in thick, tenacious mucus that tends to stick in the airways. The normal color of sputum is white and translucent. Yellow or green sputum is commonly seen when retained secretions are first raised and may result from a response to an allergic or infectious process. Yellow usually indicates pus, which is a liquid product of inflammation composed of a thin albuminous fluid and dead yellow-tinged leukocytes. Sputum that has been retained long enough to allow enzymes to break mucopolysaccharides into simpler substances looks green. Respiratory infections with *Pseudomonas aeruginosa* typically produce sputum that is thick and green and has a foul, musty odor. Hemoptysis should be evaluated to determine if the blood is fresh (bright red), the result of pulmonary edema (pink and frothy), old (brown), or from the upper airways (bright red, streaked, and not well mixed).

Auscultation of the chest reveals whether the goals of bronchial hygiene therapy are being accomplished. For example, presence of breath sounds where none were apparent may alert the practitioner that previously atelectatic areas are now being ventilated. The sudden absence of breath sounds after therapy has begun may warn of pneumothorax or complete airway obstruction caused by swollen secretions.

Arterial blood-gas measurements may provide objective evidence that collapsed lung segments are now being aerated and that alveolar ventilation and oxygenation have improved. The patient's ventilatory rate and pattern should be monitored to assess use of accessory muscles and the time sequences of inspiration and expiration. The patient's ability to cough effectively and raise retained secretions should be evaluated during each treatment. Measurement of vital and inspiratory capacities will allow the practitioner to determine whether IPPB or sustained maximal inspiration (incentive spirometry) should be used to treat atelectasis or facilitate a productive cough.

(Q) A patient with chronic obstructive airway disease is receiving aerosol therapy via an ultrasonic nebulizer and after 5 minutes suddenly becomes dyspneic; which of the following actions should be taken?

a. Terminate the treatment and chart the adverse reaction. 324 B
b. Combine chest physical therapy (CPT) with the aerosol therapy. 325 B
c. Terminate the treatment and administer a bronchodilator. 325 d

FRAME 183. CPAP/PEEP

Optimal PEEP or CPAP (continuous positive-airway pressure) is the level of end-expiratory pressure that increases functional residual capacity and opens collapsed alveoli and small bronchioles without adversely affecting cardiac output. The amount of PEEP needed will vary according to the extent of pulmonary and cardiovascular dysfunction. Optimal PEEP results in a lower intrapulmonary shunt fraction and substantial improvement in arterial oxygenation with only a small decrease in cardiac output. When PEEP or CPAP is first initiated or increased, the cardiac output may decrease. The blood pressure (BP), urinary output, and oxygen transport should be monitored to assure that the increased intrathoracic pressure does not result in a large decrease in cardiac output. If the cardiac output falls, the difference between arterial and venous oxygen content will increase as the blood flows more slowly through systemic capillaries. If BP drops, blood flow to the kidneys will decrease and urinary output will drop. Also, the mixed venous-oxygen tension will drop below the normal range of 38 to 42 torr. BP and urinary output are the best indicators of low cardiac output, since mixed venous blood samples are required to determine $P\bar{v}O_2$ and a-v O_2 content difference.

Calculating static compliance with different amounts of PEEP or CPAP will also allow the optimal level of end-expiratory pressure to be determined. The optimum PEEP is determined by the level that achieves the highest static compliance (Fig. 11-2). The static compliance will decrease at both low lung volumes and very high lung volumes. Clinically it correlates with lung disorders that produce changes in functional residual capacity (FRC) either by diminishing the FRC, or by overinflating the lung. Adding PEEP will increase peak pressure and plateau pressure and must be taken into account when calculating static compliance.

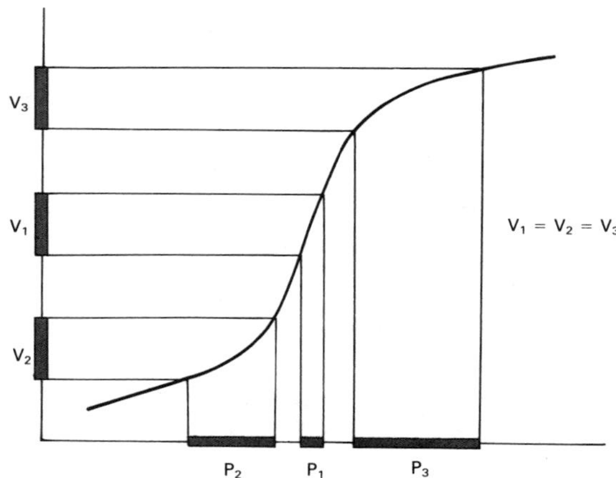

Figure 11-2 Volume-pressure curve illustrates how compliance changes with lung volume.

(Q) After reviewing the volume-pressure curve (Fig. 11-2), select the portion of the curve that correlates with the highest compliance.

a. $C = V_1/P_1$ 325 C
b. $C = V_2/P_2$ 325 a
c. $C = V_3/P_3$ 325 c

FRAME 184. MECHANICAL VENTILATION

Monitoring patient response to mechanical ventilation involves assessing gas exchange, pulmonary mechanics, breath sounds, and the cardiovascular system. Arterial blood gases are always evaluated with respect to the level of ventilatory and oxygenation support a patient is receiving. Changes in arterial CO_2 tension will reflect alveolar ventilation. Alterations in arterial oxygenation are normally a direct result of a change in physiologic shunt or the ventilation-to-perfusion ratio. Noninvasive methods of monitoring gas exchange are available using capnography to monitor end-tidal CO_2, pulse oximeters for Sao_2, and transcutaneous electrodes with infants (and occasionally with adults) to monitor Pao_2 and $Paco_2$. Noninvasive monitoring of blood gases provides real-time indications of blood-gas changes that are particularly useful during initial application of mechanical ventilation. They are also useful during weaning and may reduce the frequency of blood-gas analysis. End-tidal CO_2 monitoring is frequently used in the operating room to assure that intubation of the esophagus has not occurred.

The pulmonary mechanics to monitor during mechanical ventilation include (1) spontaneous tidal volume and rate, (2) vital capacity, (3) maximum inspiratory pressure, (4) static compliance, and (5) airway resistance. Whenever peak airway or plateau pressure increases, the practitioner needs to evaluate the cause and adjust the ventilation parameters accordingly. If the increase in airway pressure is sudden and continuous, a tension pneumothorax, endobronchial intubation, or complete airway obstruction should be suspected. The patient may need to be manually ventilated, suctioned, have the endotracheal tube repositioned or replaced, or have a chest tube inserted. Often the first warning that airway pressure has suddenly increased is the high-pressure alarm, which should be set 10 cm H_2O above the peak inspiratory pressure. Other alarm systems and their thresholds are (1) low pressure, 5 to 10 cm H_2O below average peak airway pressure; (2) loss of PEEP, 3 cm H_2O below PEEP level; (3) oxygen analyzer, 0.05 above and below FIO_2; and (4) exhaled volume, 10% above and below the set V_T.

Breath sounds should be assessed every time a patient ventilator system is evaluated. Absent breath sounds on the left side may be noted with right endobronchial intubation, left-sided pneumothorax, or large left-sided pleural effusions. Breath sounds with right-sided pneumothorax usually are diminished on the right, and normal or decreased on the left. Auscultation of the trachea is also important when the minimal leak technique is used to inflate tracheal tube cuffs.

Increased intrathoracic pressure created during mechanical ventilation may adversely affect the cardiovascular system, which should be evaluated when the ventilator system is checked or when the level of ventilatory support is changed. Heart rate, rhythm, and blood pressure are the most important variables to monitor. If heart rate changes substantially, reconsider the methods used for ventilation. Hypoxemia may cause cardiac arrhythmias and if ventricular arrhythmias develop, steps previously taken to improve tissue oxygenation should be evaluated. Cyanosis, loss of skin turgur, cool skin, and a decrease in urinary output indicate decreased peripheral perfusion and cardiac output.

(Q) Reduced cardiac output seen with mechanical ventilation is a result of

a. increased right ventricular preload. 324 C
b. decreased intra-alveolar pressure. 324 a
c. increased intrathoracic pressure. 324 b

324A (from page 320, frame 181)
Correct. The pulse is the most important clinical sign to monitor when an adrenergic bronchodilator is delivered by aerosol therapy. A bronchodilator such as epinephrine that has both alpha and beta effects may increase systemic resistance and cause the blood pressure to increase. Thus, blood pressure should be monitored when an alpha response is expected. Breath sounds should also be monitored but the pulse is the most important since several bronchodilators have some degree of beta-1 effect (increase in rate and force of cardiac contraction). Please continue on page 321, frame 182.

324B (from page 321, frame 182)
Wrong. The ultrasonic nebulizer is unsuccessful because dry secretions have swollen and caused small airway obstruction. The retained secretion problem still exists and should be treated with one of the other modalities of bronchial hygiene therapy. Return to page 321, frame 182, and select another answer.

324C (from page 323, frame 184)
Wrong. Increased right ventricular preload is not responsible for reduction in cardiac output. Return to page 323, frame 184, and try again.

324a (from page 323, frame 184)
Wrong. Intra-alveolar pressure would be increased during mechanical ventilation. Return to page 323, frame 184, and select another answer.

324b (from page 323, frame 184)
Correct. Increased intrathoracic pressure may restrict venous return to the heart and cause a reduction of cardiac output. Please continue on page 326 and complete the chapter exercises.

324c (from page 317, frame 180)
Wrong. Whenever hemoptysis is seen during IPPB therapy, the physician must be notified. Return to page 317, frame 180, and select another answer.

324d (from page 320, frame 181)
Wrong. A bronchodilator such as epinephrine that has both alpha and beta effects may increase systemic resistance and cause the blood pressure to increase. Thus, blood pressure should be monitored when an alpha response is expected. However, another vital sign is more important to monitor. Return to page 320, frame 181, and select another answer.

325A (from page 320, frame 181)
Wrong. Breath sounds should be monitored but another vital sign is more important. Return to page 320, frame 181, and select another answer.

325B (from page 321, frame 182)
Correct. Chest physiotherapy will help loosen retained secretions as they are hydrated and swell. Combining CPT and aerosol therapy should help to prevent the respiratory distress caused by obstructed airways. Please continue on page 322, frame 183.

325C (from page 322, frame 183)
Correct. This portion of the curve has the highest compliance and correlates with a FRC that is neither diminished or overinflated. Calculating static compliance allows the optimal PEEP level to be determined by finding the level that results in the highest compliance. Please continue on page 323, frame 184.

325D (from page 317, frame 180)
Correct. Whenever hemoptysis is seen during IPPB therapy, the treatment must be terminated immediately and the physician notified. The bleeding may be caused by coughing and usually is bronchial venous bleeding which readily stops. However, the blood may be secondary to left-sided heart failure or tumor, and should be discussed with the patient's physician. Please continue on page 320, frame 181.

325a (from page 322, frame 183)
Wrong. This portion of the curve has a decreased compliance because of low lung volume. Return to page 322, frame 183, and select another answer.

325b (from page 317, frame 180)
Wrong. The physician should be notified but other actions are required. Return to page 317, frame 180, and select another answer.

325c (from page 322, frame 183)
Wrong. This portion of the curve has the lowest compliance of the three segments illustrated. The compliance is low because the lung is overinflated and lung expansion is occurring on the high, flat end of the volume-pressure curve. Return to page 322, frame 183, and try again.

325d (from page 321, frame 182)
Wrong. The problem is not bronchospasm but comes from the swelling of dry secretions. However, high-density bland aerosol therapy can trigger bronchospasm and a bronchodilator is often administered first to patients who have hyperactive airways. Return to page 321, frame 182, and select another answer that will solve the retained secretion problem.

EXERCISES

1. List the items required to obtain blood from the radial artery.
2. Calculate the expected drop in Pa_{CO_2} with compensated metabolic acidosis (assume a $[HCO_3^-]$ of 16 mEq/L).
3. List five applications for the use of pulse oximetry.
4. Measure cuff pressure using the minimal leak technique and two tracheal tubes with low-pressure cuffs. Select the tubes so that one is the right size and the other one smaller than needed. Collect your pressure readings using a thick Tygon tube as a simulated trachea, a test lung, and mechanical ventilator.
5. Calculate the expected plateau pressure of a patient ventilator system given V_T 1.0 L, PEEP 10 cm H_2O, C 0.025 L/cm H_2O.
6. List the clinical signs of a tension pneumothorax and describe the actions that should be taken if one develops during IPPB.
7. List six beta-1 side effects that may be seen when administering aerosolized sympathomimetics.
8. Identify at least one cause for each of the following colors seen in sputum: bright red, pink, brown, black, yellow, green, and white.
9. Draw a pulmonary pressure-volume curve and label the segment that represents normal compliance.
10. List the alarm thresholds for the following alarm systems: F_{IO_2}, high pressure, low pressure, PEEP, and exhaled tidal volume.

POSTTEST

This test is designed to evaluate what you have learned from completing Chapter 11. Check your answers on page 329 and review the topics where your answer is incorrect.

1. The Allen test is negative when the ulnar artery is released and the hand does *not* flush pink within
   A. 3 seconds.
   B. 5 seconds.
   C. 15 seconds.
   D. 30 seconds.
   E. 60 seconds.

2. What size needle should be used to collect a radial artery sample?
   A. 10- to 12-gauge
   B. 12- to 15-gauge
   C. 15- to 17-gauge
   D. 17- to 20-gauge
   E. 23- to 25-gauge

3. What is the acid-base balance and oxygenation of a 55-year-old patient with the following blood-gas data: F_{IO_2} 0.21, pH 7.38, Pa_{CO_2} 60 torr, HCO_3^- 36 mEq/L, Pa_{O_2} 50 torr?
   A. partially compensated respiratory acidosis, moderate hypoxemia
   B. compensated metabolic acidosis, mild hypoxemia
   C. respiratory and metabolic acidosis, moderate hypoxemia
   D. compensated respiratory acidosis, moderate hypoxemia
   E. compensated metabolic alkalosis, mild hypoxemia

4. What is the acid-base balance and oxygenation of a 24-year-old patient with the following blood-gas data: F_{IO_2} 0.21, pH 7.55, Pa_{CO_2} 30 torr, HCO_3^- 28 mEq/L, Pa_{O_2} 110 torr?
   A. compensated metabolic alkalosis, normal oxygenation
   B. compensated respiratory alkalosis, overly corrected hypoxemia
   C. partially compensated respiratory alkalosis, normal oxygenation
   D. partially compensated metabolic alkalosis, normal oxygenation
   E. respiratory and metabolic alkalosis, normal oxygenation

5. When Sa_{O_2} values are above 80%, pulse oximeters used in critical care usually have a precision of
   A. ± 2%.
   B. ± 5%.
   C. ± 10%.
   D. ± 15%.
   E. ± 20%.

6. If the P_{50} is 27 mm Hg, a pulse oximeter reading of 90% will correlate with an arterial oxygen tension of
   A. 40 torr.
   B. 50 torr.
   C. 60 torr.
   D. 70 torr.
   E. 80 torr.

7. If the tracheal tube is the right size and the cuff is of the low-pressure (floppy) type, the intracuff pressure necessary for no-leak ventilation should be less than
   A. 10 torr.
   B. 15 torr.
   C. 18 torr.
   D. 25 torr.
   E. 30 torr.

8. Intracuff pressure will completely stop venous flow and cause tracheal wall congestion when it exceeds
   A. 10 torr.
   B. 15 torr.
   C. 18 torr.
   D. 25 torr.
   E. 30 torr.

9. What is the static compliance of the patient ventilator system given V_T 0.750 L, peak pressure 40 cm H_2O, plateau pressure 35 cm H_2O, PEEP 10 cm H_2O?
   A. 0.010 L/cm H_2O
   B. 0.015 L/cm H_2O
   C. 0.020 L/cm H_2O
   D. 0.025 L/cm H_2O
   E. 0.030 L/cm H_2O

10. What is the resistance of the patient ventilator system for a constant flow generator given peak flow 30 L/min, peak pressure 40 cm H_2O, plateau pressure 35 cm H_2O, PEEP 10 cm H_2O, V_T 1.0 L?
    A. 5 cm H_2O/L/s
    B. 10 cm H_2O/L/s
    C. 20 cm H_2O/L/s
    D. 25 cm H_2O/L/s
    E. 50 cm H_2O/L/s

11. When a mask is used to deliver tidal volume during IPPB, all of the following are complications of gastric insufflation *except*
    A. vomiting and aspiration.
    B. restriction of diaphragm.
    C. mediastinal shift.
    D. gastric discomfort.
    E. epigastric pain.

12. All of the following actions should be used to reduce the hazard of hyperventilation during IPPB *except*
    A. rest periods.
    B. limiting rate to 6 to 8/min.
    C. limiting tidal volume to 10 mL/kg.
    D. providing adequate patient instruction.
    E. 2 to 3 second breath hold with each tidal volume.

13. Which of the following adrenergic receptors when strongly stimulated may cause blood pressure to increase?
    I. alpha
    II. beta-1
    III. beta-2
    A. I only
    B. II only
    C. III only
    D. I and II only
    E. none of the above

14. Which of the following actions may reduce the bronchospasm seen with bland solutions delivered by ultrasonic nebulizer?
    A. Add acetylcysteine to nebulized solution.
    B. Administer a bronchodilator before ultrasonic therapy.
    C. Use a 5% NaCl solution.
    D. Use sterile H_2O.
    E. Discourage coughing until the aerosol has been delivered.

15. Bright red, blood-streaked sputum that is not well mixed may indicate
   A. pulmonary edema.
   B. old blood.
   C. bronchial venous bleeding.
   D. bleeding from the upper airways.
   E. an infectious process.

16. To determine whether IPPB or incentive spirometry should be used to facilitate a strong cough, which of the following should be measured?
   A. vital capacity
   B. FEV_1
   C. FEF_{25-75}
   D. MVV (maximum voluntary ventilation)
   E. peak flow

17. What is the optimal PEEP level in this series of measurements (assume VT 1.0 L)?

	PEEP (cm H_2O)	Plateau Pressure (cm H_2O)	Peak Pressure (cm H_2O)
A.	5	35	38
B.	10	38	41
C.	15	42	45
D.	20	48	51
E.	25	55	58

18. At what time did the resistance of the patient ventilator system increase (assume VT 1.0 L, constant flow of 30 L/min, PEEP 10 cm H_2O)?

	Time	Plateau Pressure (cm H_2O)	Peak Pressure (cm H_2O)
A.	7 A.M.	35	38
B.	9 A.M.	38	44
C.	11 A.M.	38	41
D.	1 P.M.	41	44
E.	3 P.M.	45	48

19. Which of the following end-tidal CO_2 readings indicates that intubation of the esophagus has occurred?
   A. 0%
   B. 3%
   C. 6%
   D. 9%
   E. 12%

20. Which of the following alarm systems may be the first to signal endobronchial intubation?
   A. exhaled tidal volume
   B. inspired tidal volume
   C. high pressure
   D. low pressure
   E. PEEP pressure

ANSWERS TO POSTTEST

1. C (F175)
2. E (F175)
3. D (F176)
4. E (F176)
5. A (F177)
6. C (F177)
7. C (F178)
8. C (F178)
9. E (F179)
10. B (F179)
11. C (F180)
12. C (F180)
13. D (F181)
14. B (F181)
15. D (F182)
16. A (F182)
17. C (F183)
18. B (F183)
19. A (F184)
20. C (F184)

BIBLIOGRAPHY

Barnes, TA: Respiratory Care Practice. Year Book Medical Publishers, Chicago, 1988.

Burton, GG and Hodgkin, JE: Respiratory Care: A Guide to Clinical Practice, ed 2. JB Lippincott, Philadelphia, 1984.

Eubanks, DH and Bone, RC: Comprehensive Respiratory Care, ed 2. CV Mosby, St. Louis, 1990.

Kacmarek, RM and Stoller, JK: Current Respiratory Care. BC Decker, Philadelphia, 1989.

Kirby, RR, Smith, RA, and Desautels, DA: Mechanical Ventilation. Churchill-Livingstone, New York, 1985.

Pilbeam, SP and Youtsey, JW: Mechanical Ventilation. CV Mosby, St. Louis, 1986.

Rau, JL and Pearce, DJ: Understanding Chest Radiographs. Multi-Media Publishing, Denver, 1984.

Riggs, JH: Respiratory Facts. FA Davis, Philadelphia, 1989.

Scanlon, CL, Spearman, CB, Sheldon, RL, and Egan, DF: Egan's Fundamentals of Respiratory Therapy, ed 5. CV Mosby, St. Louis, 1990.

Shapiro, BA, Harrison, RA, Kacmarek, RM, and Cane, RD: Clinical Application of Respiratory Care, ed 3. Year Book Medical Publishers, Chicago, 1985.

Shapiro, BA, Harrison, RA, Templin, RK, and Walton, JR: Clinical Application of Blood Gases, ed 4. Year Book Medical Publishers, Chicago, 1988.

Wilkins, RL, Sheldon, RL, and Krider, SJ: Clinical Assessment in Respiratory Care, ed 2. CV Mosby, St. Louis, 1990.

12

Pulmonary Rehabilitation and Home Care

PRETEST

This pretest is designed to measure what you already know about pulmonary rehabilitation and respiratory home care. Check your answers on page 334 and then continue on page 335, frame 185.

1. Which of the following long-term oxygen therapy systems would be best for a patient living on the second floor of a walk-up apartment building who requires continuous low-flow oxygen therapy?
   A. three H-cylinders of medical oxygen
   B. several E-cylinders of medical oxygen
   C. portable liquid oxygen therapy system with a reservoir
   D. oxygen concentrator
   E. portable liquid oxygen system without a reservoir
2. The member of the respiratory home care team best able to evaluate a patient's residence for equipment service requirements is a
   A. visiting nurse.
   B. hospital-based respiratory therapist.
   C. pulmonologist.
   D. home care respiratory therapist.
   E. the home care equipment driver who makes regular deliveries.
3. The patient and family should have goals for pulmonary rehabilitation that include all of the following *except*
   A. improved level of daily activity.
   B. improved exercise tolerance.
   C. improved pulmonary function.
   D. holding disease progression at current level of dysfunction.
   E. energy conservation.
4. The patient and family should be instructed on all of the following aspects of respiratory home care equipment *except*
   A. transfilling E-cylinders from H-cylinders.
   B. use of oxygen analyzers.
   C. cleaning and disinfecting equipment.
   D. changing cylinder regulators.
   E. maintenance of oxygen concentrators.
5. Work simplification rules include all of the following *except*
   A. use of frequent rest periods.
   B. alternating light and heavy tasks.
   C. completing daily tasks by lunch time.
   D. use of labor-saving devices.
   E. reducing hyperextension.
6. On days with smog alerts which of the following may reduce bronchospasm, shortness of breath, and coughing?
   A. exercising with oxygen
   B. increasing oxygen flow by 50%
   C. increasing use of adrenergic bronchodilators
   D. staying inside in an air-conditioned environment
   E. traveling by car to the country
7. In order to keep bronchial secretions hydrated, COPD patients without cardiac compensation should have a daily fluid replacement plan that totals
   A. 500 to 1000 mL.
   B. 1000 to 1500 mL.
   C. 1500 to 2500 mL.
   D. 3000 to 4000 mL.
   E. 4000 to 5000 mL.

8. The clinical effects of malnutrition include all of the following *except*
   A. weight loss.
   B. skin breakdown.
   C. increased hypoxic response.
   D. decreased macrophage mobilization.
   E. increased irritability.

9. Evidence of not enough oxygen includes all of the following *except*
   A. morning headache.
   B. pulmonary hypotension.
   C. restlessness during sleep.
   D. P wave greater than 3 mm in leads II, III, or AVF.
   E. hematocrit greater than 56%.

10. Oxygen concentrators separate oxygen from air by
    I. absorbing nitrogen with granular zeolite crystals.
    II. using a plastic membrane selectively permeable to oxygen and water vapor.
    III. pressurizing air in sieve beds.
    IV. periodically purging sieve beds of nitrogen.
    A. I only
    B. II only
    C. I and II only
    D. III and IV only
    E. I, III, and IV only

11. What is the duration of a small portable aluminum oxygen cylinder (E size) at 2 L/min?
    A. 2.0 hours
    B. 3.4 hours
    C. 5.7 hours
    D. 13 hours
    E. 20 hours

12. What is the duration of a 14-lb portable liquid oxygen system at 2 L/min?
    A. 2.0 hours
    B. 3.4 hours
    C. 5.7 hours
    D. 13 hours
    E. 20 hours

13. Which of the following would be best to monitor exercise tolerance?
    A. the patient's subjective feelings
    B. serial arterial blood gases
    C. capnography
    D. pulse oximetry
    E. continuous spirometry

14. Exercise sessions for COPD patients should be designed to bring them to what level of their achievable maximal heart rate?
    A. 50%
    B. 70%
    C. 85%
    D. 90%
    E. 100%

15. How long does respiratory home care equipment need to stay submerged in acetic acid (vinegar) to be disinfected?
    A. 5 minutes
    B. 10 minutes
    C. 20 minutes
    D. 1 hour
    E. 12 hours
16. How long can a vinegar solution be used to clean respiratory home care equipment before it is discarded?
    A. 1 day
    B. 2 days
    C. 4 days
    D. 1 week
    E. 2 weeks
17. The accelerated clearance of retained secretions produced with hypertonic saline administered with an ultrasonic nebulizer is most likely the result of
    A. the irritant effect of aerosols.
    B. the hydration of retained secretions.
    C. increased bronchodilation.
    D. breaking of disulfide bonds.
    E. decreased viscosity of secretions.
18. Alpha, beta-1, and beta-2 action occur with which of the following adrenergic bronchodilators?
    I. epinephrine
    II. isoproterenol
    III. isoetharine
    IV. albuterol
    V. racemic epinephrine
    A. I and V only
    B. II and V only
    C. I and III only
    D. I, II, and IV only
    E. II, III, and IV only
19. What is the best pulmonary function test to monitor changes in the degree of airway obstruction in respiratory home-care patients?
    A. vital capacity
    B. FEV_{25-75}
    C. peak expiratory flow
    D. arterial blood-gas study
    E. capnography
20. A dull percussion note will signal a consolidated area with a *minimum* size of
    A. 100 mL.
    B. 200 mL.
    C. 500 mL.
    D. 1000 mL.
    E. 2000 mL.

ANSWERS TO PRETEST

1. D (F185)	6. D (F187)	11. C (F190)	16. C (F192)
2. D (F185)	7. D (F188)	12. D (F189)	17. A (F193)
3. C (F186)	8. C (F188)	13. D (F191)	18. A (F193)
4. A (F186)	9. B (F189)	14. B (F191)	19. C (F194)
5. C (F187)	10. E (F190)	15. C (F192)	20. C (F194)

FRAME 185. DISCHARGE PLANNING

The traditional discharge planning staff, which comprises registered nurses and social workers, will be concerned with the patient as a whole. They will direct their attention to the nursing, emotional, social, and financial aspects of the discharge plan. The respiratory therapist should be actively involved in the respiratory care plan for the homebound patient. The responsibility for determining oxygen and related respiratory care needs requires the education and experience held by the respiratory therapist and supervising pulmonologist. The home care therapist should be actively involved since contact with the patient may last for several months or years. The role of the home care therapist is usually not to provide hands-on medical care in the home. However, the patient, physician, family, and caregivers will look to the therapist for assessment and education and to facilitate the respiratory care being provided.

After the long-term respiratory care orders have been reviewed and the equipment needs identified, the long-term care facility or patient's home must be evaluated for service requirements. Examples of services needed include adequate electrical outlets for an oxygen concentrator and delivery access for oxygen cylinders or a liquid oxygen reservoir. The evaluation of the home or long-term care facility should include the ease with which the tasks of daily living can be accomplished. Exertional dyspnea or oxygen therapy equipment may limit stair climbing, preparing meals, eating, dressing, and bathing. Smoking and air pollution may affect the patient with chronic pulmonary disease. When indoors, patients should avoid all aerosol sprays, dust, and chemical fumes. Adequate air conditioning, with temperature control and filtration, must be provided.

An important part of discharge planning is education, not only for the patient but also for the family and care providers. Communication to the patient and family should be in nontechnical language and cover anatomy and physiology, tobacco abuse, disease pathology, medications, cardiopulmonary resuscitation, a review of equipment operation and adjustment, plan for pulmonary rehabilitation, self-care guidelines, cleaning of equipment, and nutrition.

(Q) Who should be provided with instruction regarding the operation and maintenance of respiratory care equipment for long-term home care?

a. family 340 A
b. family and care providers 341 D
c. family, care providers, and the patient 340 c

FRAME 186. PATIENT AND FAMILY INSTRUCTION

Patient and family instruction should be directed at making the entire family (including the patient) aware of the rehabilitation program. The educational program should emphasize the therapeutic and conditioning goals. Enough basic information should be provided so that the family can understand the disease and the related problems. Goals should be aimed at holding the disease at its current level, improvement in ability to perform certain daily activities, and improved exercise tolerance.

The instruction should include a discussion of how to handle emergencies such as running out of oxygen, power failures, and basic CPR. Prevention and contingency plans are crucial to the well-being of the patient and must be well understood by the family. For example, a manual resuscitator and pneumatically powered ventilator should be ready for use if a power failure or malfunction makes an electrically powered ventilator nonfunctional.

The operation, troubleshooting, and maintenance of respiratory care equipment in use or on standby should be included in the instructional plan. The benefits and dangers involved with oxygen therapy, including information regarding appropriate flow rates and oxygen-induced hypoventilation, should be covered. The patient should be taught how to verify flow from oxygen concentrators and other devices. The cleaning and decontamination of equipment, safety rules, and basics such as attaching cylinder regulators should be taught to the family. If the patient needs to travel with oxygen, instruction on liquid oxygen systems and safety rules for transporting oxygen cylinders must be provided. Some patients may need to be aware of how altitude affects alveolar oxygen tension.

Instruction on task simplification and advice on how to accomplish daily living activities should allow the patient to conserve energy and accomplish more. Exercise is important to keep the patient from becoming depressed and frustrated. Goals for exercise should be set even if they involve less taxing activities.

(Q) Patient instruction on oxygen therapy equipment should include which of the following?

I. safety rules for oxygen administration equipment
II. troubleshooting equipment malfunctions
III. information on how to transfill E-cylinders from larger H-cylinders

a. I only 340 B
b. I and II only 341 A
c. I, II, and III 341 b

FRAME 187. SELF-CARE GUIDELINES

Patients with chronic lung disease often become frustrated and depressed when they become short of breath during routine tasks. Unfortunately, if a patient becomes less active, the ability to complete daily self-care tasks will become even more limited. The principles of work simplification allow the patient to remain active by completing tasks using less energy. Examples include (1) spreading activities evenly throughout the day, (2) alternating light and heavy tasks, (3) working sitting down, (4) grouping supplies within reach of a work station, (5) using a cart to move supplies, (6) frequent rest periods, (7) minimizing hyperextension by working at waist level when standing, (8) performing activities slowly with smooth movements, (9) sliding an object across the floor instead of lifting and carrying, (10) using labor-saving devices, such as an electric can opener.

Being able to dress, wash, and eat are important daily activities taken for granted by most people. Patients with chronic lung disease, even with oxygen, often are not able to accomplish the basics. However, patients can be taught certain guidelines that may allow them to provide their own self-care. For example, eating several small meals is less taxing than two large meals, and sitting while dressing and bathing saves energy.

Patients and their families should be instructed to control the environment to prevent bronchospasm, shortness of breath, and coughing spells. Air pollution, smoking, second-hand smoke, cold air, aerosol sprays, toxic fumes, and dust can irritate the airways. Often dry air during the winter in northern climates promotes nose and throat dryness and humidifiers should be used to maintain relative humidity between 30% and 50%. Humidifiers must be kept clean to avoid contamination with molds or bacteria. Allergic patients should avoid pollens and molds during peak months, and house dust should be kept to a minimum. Air-conditioner and forced-air heating system filters should be changed frequently. On days when there are extremes of temperature or smog alerts, the patient should stay indoors in an air-conditioned environment. It often takes several weeks for patients with chronic lung disease to recover from respiratory tract infections. Thus, people with upper respiratory tract infections should not visit and the patient should avoid large gatherings.

(Q) Patients with chronic obstructive pulmonary disease who cannot sleep at night should

I. receive sleeping pills or tranquilizers.
II. be placed in a supine position.
III. perform bronchial hygiene therapy at bedtime.

a. I only 340 C
b. III only 340 d
c. II and III only 341 B

FRAME 188. NUTRITION

Inadequate nutrition and hydration are common problems seen with patients who have chronic obstructive pulmonary disease (COPD). Patients with COPD may suffer from malnutrition as a result of dyspnea, air swallowing, and nausea. The nausea may be the result of lactic acidosis caused by chronic hypoxemia. Dyspnea triggered by attempts to eat may discourage patients from consuming enough calories. Weight loss is an early sign of malnutrition, although the extent of weight loss may be easily misjudged because some patients have fluid retention. The clinical effects of malnutrition include weight loss, progressive weakness, fat utilization, skin breakdown, apathy, irritability, impaired wound healing, electrolyte and fluid imbalance, decreased hypoxic response, decreased immune response, impaired phagocytosis, and decreased macrophage mobilization. Loss of appetite is a frequent complaint of COPD patients and the cause may be the result of a combination of the following factors: pain, fatigue, stress, depression, nausea, and dyspnea. Six small meals are better tolerated than three large meals by patients with respiratory problems, and oxygen therapy may reduce dyspnea during meals.

Fluid requirements for COPD patients should be carefully monitored. Daily losses of water normally include the following: feces, 100 to 200 mL; urine, 1000 to 1500 mL; lungs, 250 to 400 mL; insensible perspiration, 400 to 600 mL; and visible perspiration, 0 to 10,000 mL. Any condition that increases the minute volume will increase the amount of water lost from the lungs. Under ideal conditions, the minimum adult daily requirement is about 1.5 L of water. COPD patients need a minimum of 3000 to 4000 mL daily to keep bronchial secretions well hydrated. Failure to adequately meet the fluid replacement needs of COPD patients will lead to thick secretions, partial or complete small-airway obstructions, and increased airway resistance.

Nutritional assessment is an important part of rehabilitation of COPD patients. Providing adequate nutrition and fluid requirements becomes more difficult when COPD is accompanied by one or more of the following: cardiac disease and cor pulmonale, diabetes mellitus, allergies, nausea, vomiting, fever, hiatal hernia, and lack of appetite.

(Q) Which of the following is likely to improve the appetite of COPD patients?

I. one or two large meals per day
II. increased levels of daily activity
III. fluid levels held to 2500 mL daily

a. I only 340 b
b. II only 341 C
c. I and III only 341 c

FRAME 189. PORTABLE OXYGEN SYSTEMS

The COPD patient should be encouraged to be as active as possible, and often this means making arrangements for a portable oxygen system. The logical place to begin is by making sure the patient can move around easily at home. Providing the patient a 20- to 50-ft extension tube is an inexpensive way to allow travel around the house. Portable aluminum medical oxygen cylinders can provide 2 to 5.7 hours with flow of 2 L/min, and they weigh approximately one half that of portable steel cylinders. The disadvantages of cylinders include the risk of being dropped and the need to attach a regulator each time a new cylinder is used. There is a danger of grease or oil contaminating the valve if the family or patient changes the regulator. The National Fire Protection Association's recommendations specifically prohibit transfilling small cylinders from larger ones at home because of the danger of fire or explosion. Patients who travel out of town will need to understand cylinder duration, identify home care dealers who can fill cylinders, and make arrangements for billing.

The use of portable liquid oxygen systems may provide advantages over cylinders. One advantage of liquid oxygen is the light weight (5 to 14 lb when full). The duration is 13 hours, which is twice that of an E-cylinder at 2 L/min. Transfilling portable liquid systems is safer and easier for the patient to handle than cylinders. The newest liquid oxygen vessels have optional flow-control valves that provide a wide range of flows from 1/8 to 15 L/min. Some precautions to take when transfilling liquid units from a reservoir include (1) providing an extra supply of oxygen for the patient during the time needed to fill the portable unit, (2) locating a well-ventilated area away from open flames or combustible materials, (3) using protective eyeglasses or goggles to guard against the splashing or spraying of liquid oxygen and insulated gloves to protect the skin from burns caused by the low temperature of fittings, (4) assuring that the connectors of both units are dry and clean (moisture may cause connectors to freeze together), (5) making sure that the flow controller is turned off, (6) connecting the portable unit to the reservoir following manufacturer's instructions, (7) opening the portable unit vent and allowing the unit to fill until the vent valve begins to pass liquid oxygen instead of gas, at which time the valve should be closed, and (8) taking care not to handle with ungloved hands the cold fittings when disengaging the portable unit. The major disadvantage to liquid oxygen systems is the waste and additional expense incurred as a result of evaporative loss if the portable unit is not used on a continuous basis. Regular deliveries are required to fill the reservoir from which the portable unit is transfilled. Finally, injury may occur from handling of extremely cold transfilling fittings (see Figs. 12–1 and 12–2 on p. 343).

(Q) Ice or frost is likely to form on portable or reservoir liquid oxygen systems at which of the following locations?

a. flow-control valve during filling 340 D
b. warming coils at flow rates greater than 3 L/min 340 a
c. vent valve at flow rates of 2 L/min 341 a

340A (from page 335, frame 185)
Wrong. The family certainly should receive instruction about the operation and maintenance of equipment, but what happens when equipment fails and they are not at home with the patient? Return to page 335, frame 185, and select another answer.

340B (from page 336, frame 186)
Wrong. Certainly the safety rules for oxygen cylinders should be taught to patients, but more instruction about oxygen therapy equipment is required. Return to page 336, frame 186, and select another answer.

340C (from page 337, frame 187)
Wrong. Tranquilizers or sleeping pills may depress respirations and coughs. Return to page 337, frame 187, and select another answer.

340D (from page 339, frame 189)
Wrong. The flow-control valve should be closed when the unit is filled with liquid oxygen. It is located after the warming coils. Thus, it is unlikely that frost or ice will accumulate on the valve. Return to page 339, frame 189, and select another answer.

340a (from page 339, frame 189)
Correct. The warming coils may become quite cold at gas flow rates greater than 3 L/min and water may condense and freeze, forming frost or ice. Please continue on page 342, frame 190.

340b (from page 338, frame 188)
Wrong. Several small meals are easier for COPD patients. They need to eat slowly and often need supplemental oxygen. They do not have the energy to prepare or eat large multicourse meals. Return to page 338, frame 188, and select another answer.

340c (from page 335, frame 185)
Correct. The patient, family, and other care providers should all receive instruction about the operation and maintenance of equipment. Please continue on page 336, frame 186.

340d (from page 337, frame 187)
Correct. Performing bronchial hygiene before bedtime will open partially obstructed airways and allow the patient to rest more comfortably. Please continue on page 338, frame 188.

341A (from page 336, frame 186)
Correct. Both the safety rules for oxygen cylinders and the basics of troubleshooting equipment malfunction should be taught to patients receiving oxygen therapy at home. Transfilling oxygen cylinders can be dangerous if done improperly and patients should not be taught to fill their own cylinders. Please continue on page 337, frame 187.

341B (from page 337, frame 187)
Wrong. Placing the patient in the supine position may encumber the patient's breathing, most (COPD) patients are more relaxed when pillows support the head and arms, and some can sleep only in a semi-Fowler's position. Return to page 337, frame 187, and select another answer.

341C (from page 338, frame 188)
Correct. Increasing a patient's daily activity will, if properly planned, increase the appetite of the patient. The patient should have a minimum fluid intake of 3000 to 4000 mL daily. Please continue on page 339, frame 189.

341D (from page 335, frame 185)
Wrong. Care providers and family should receive instruction about the operation and maintenance of equipment, but what about problems when the patient is alone? Return to page 335, frame 185, and try again.

341a (from page 339, frame 189)
Wrong. The liquid oxygen system should not be venting when oxygen is flowing from the system continuously. It is unlikely that frost or ice would form. Also, the vents are either after the warming coils or connected to the upper gas-filled section of the vessel. Return to page 339, frame 189, and select another answer.

341b (from page 336, frame 186)
Wrong. Transfilling oxygen cylinders can be dangerous and patients should not be taught to fill their own cylinders. Return to page 336, frame 186, and select another answer.

341c (from page 338, frame 188)
Wrong. Several small meals are easier for COPD patients. They need to eat slowly and often need supplemental oxygen therapy. They do not have the energy to prepare or eat large multicourse meals. The patient should have a minimum fluid intake of 3000 to 4000 mL daily. Return to page 338, frame 188, and select another answer.

FRAME 190. LONG-TERM OXYGEN THERAPY

The Medicare criteria for low-flow continuous long-term oxygen therapy are an arterial oxygen tension less than or equal to 55 torr (mm Hg) or a saturation equal to or less than 85%. Alternate Medicare criteria that may qualify the patient include a Pa_{O_2} of 56 to 59 torr or an Sa_{O_2} of 86% to 89% plus signs of damage to organs that use oxygen. Evidence of insufficient oxygen include morning headache, impaired cognition, restlessness during sleep, pulmonary hypertension, a hematocrit of greater than 56%, dependent edema, and a P wave greater than 3 mm in leads II, III, or aVF. Oxygen therapy at night may be indicated if criteria for oxygen are reached only during sleep when measured with oximetry and if secondary effects of hypoxemia are seen. Low-flow oxygen therapy may allow a higher level of physical activity and a higher degree of general physical conditioning. Exercise testing with and without oxygen will determine whether oxygen should be prescribed to support a higher level of exercise tolerance.

The four systems commonly used to administer oxygen in the home are oxygen concentrators, membrane-oxygen enrichers, high-pressure cylinders, and liquid oxygen systems. Respiratory care practitioners have an extensive knowledge in handling, storage, transportation, and use of cylinders. This information must be communicated to the patient and family, and should include instruction in (1) use of cylinder carts; (2) danger of oil, grease, and other combustible substances coming in contact with cylinders, valves, hoses, regulators, gauges, and fittings; (3) valve protection caps and safe storage; (4) cracking cylinders before attaching regulators; and (5) fundamentals of safe use of medical gases including a review of the safety systems used to ensure that oxygen regulators are used only with medical oxygen. Patients should not transfill cylinders because of the danger involved and their lack of technical knowledge.

Oxygen concentrators have been widely accepted for long-term low-flow oxygen therapy for the following reasons: (1) especially equipped delivery vehicles are not necessary, (2) the units can be used for several years, since almost every part of the oxygen concentrator is replaceable, (3) no regular deliveries of oxygen are needed, (4) continuous use is possible, (5) they can be easily manipulated by the blind and/or handicapped user, (6) they can be moved around the home easily or placed in a car to be moved to another location, and (7) a low-pressure alarm warns of loss of oxygen supply associated with power failure. Oxygen concentrators separate oxygen from air by absorbing nitrogen in sieve beds. The number of sieve beds will vary from one design to another, and some units have only one sieve bed. The molecular sieve material is a granular zeolite crystal, which has an affinity for nitrogen, water, carbon dioxide, carbon monoxide, and all hydrocarbons. The sieve material allows oxygen and small quantities of argon to pass through. The sieve bed must be purged of nitrogen by special purge reservoirs or by diverting some of the oxygen from the pressurized sieve bed to a second sieve bed, which is simultaneously depressurized with nitrogen being vented. When oxygen is used to purge nitrogen from the sieve bed, the amount of oxygen reaching the storage tank will be the difference between that produced by the pressurized sieve bed and that used to purge the nitrogen-saturated sieve. These cycles typically occur every 10 to 30 seconds and create about 40 to 50 dB of noise.

The oxygen in the storage tank is held at a pressure of 3 to 10 pounds per square inch and flows through a bacteria filter to a flowmeter that is usually pressure compensated. Concentrators produce approximately 93% ± 3% oxygen at flows of 1 to 3 L/min, with most producing 95% at 2 L/min.

Another source of oxygen for long-term use is the oxygen enricher, which uses a plastic membrane selectively permeable to oxygen and water vapor. A pressure gradient is established across a membrane by a vacuum pump that allows the unit to deliver 40% oxygen with three times the ambient humidity without any bacteria, viruses, or airborne particles. The flow rate must be increased by a factor of three to deliver an F_{IO_2} similar to 100% oxygen. Another model of the membrane oxygen enricher allows adjustable levels of absolute humidity up to 38 mg/L.

(Q) When a nasal cannula is used to deliver low-flow oxygen therapy to a COPD patient, it should be connected to

a. an oxygen concentrator at 4 L/min. 350 D

b. a membrane oxygen enricher at 2 L/min. 350 a

c. a membrane oxygen enricher at 6 L/min. 351 c

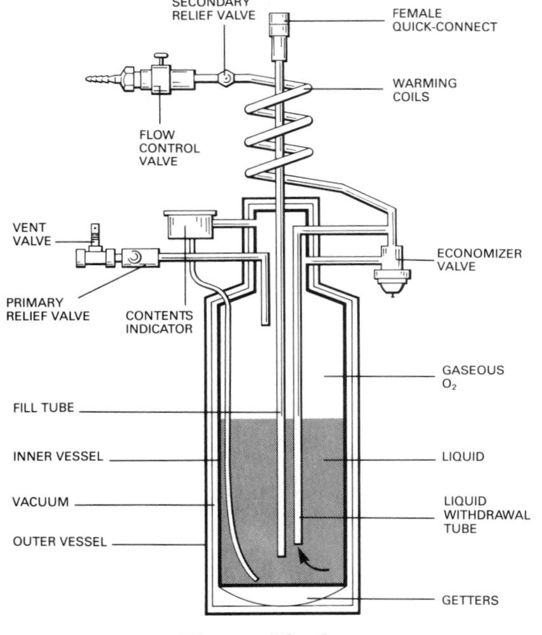

Figure 12–1

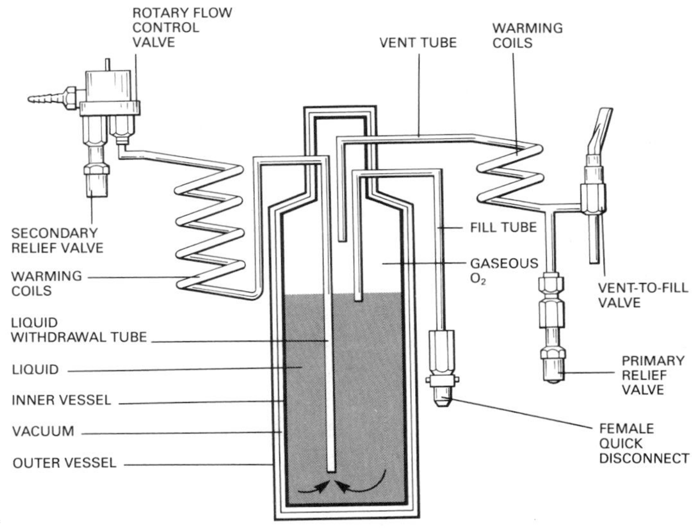

Figure 12–2

Figure 12–1 Liquid oxygen reservoir.

Figure 12–2 Liquid oxygen portable unit.

FRAME 191. PULMONARY REHABILITATION

Patients with COPD are generally inactive and have low exercise endurance. Their sedentary life-style is directly related to the discomfort, dyspnea, and fatigue that results from attempts at physical activity. If exercise tolerance is not improved, a cycle of deconditioning will occur. A schedule of regular exercise should allow the patient to improve exercise endurance, appetite, and overall physical condition. Oxygen therapy administered while exercising may improve the level of activity that is possible. The use of pulse oximetry to monitor oxygen saturation and heart rate is a noninvasive way to evaluate hypoxemia during exercise. Oxygen therapy during exercise should be directed at maintaining arterial oxygen saturation at a minimum of 90%. Exercise sessions should last at least 20 to 30 minutes and occur at least three to four times a week. Exercise should be designed to bring the heart rate to 70% of the achievable maximum. If this level of intensity is not possible at first, exercise should be started at a lower level and gradually increased. A sign that improved conditioning has occurred is when walking distance increases by at least 15%.

Physical therapy exercise programs with appropriate oxygen support may include (1) general conditioning exercise, (2) posture correction, (3) energy conservation and life pacing, (4) chest mobilization and strengthening, (5) breathing exercises (diaphragmatic, segmental, costal, pursed-lip, incentive spirometry, sustained maximal inspiration, and paced breathing), and (6) chest percussion and postural drainage (usually reserved for patients who chronically expectorate 30 mL of sputum daily).

Patient education should always be a major part of the total rehabilitation plan so that the patient and family will understand the disease, its limitations, and the goals of the program. Short- and long-term goals should be discussed with the patient. Long-term plans usually call for improving daily living activities and reducing hospitalizations, and short-term goals address the control of acute symptoms.

(Q) A patient who does not fulfill the criteria for continuous low-flow oxygen therapy may need oxygen when exercising if

a. pulse increases to 70% of maximum during exercise. 350 A
b. arterial oxygen tension falls to 70 torr during exercise. 350 d
c. arterial oxygen saturation falls below 85% during exercise. 351 A

FRAME 192. CLEANING EQUIPMENT

The home care patient and family members should be instructed by respiratory care practitioners on how to clean and make minor repairs to the equipment. Respiratory care equipment such as ventilator circuits, cannulas, aerosol masks, humidifiers, and medication nebulizers should be supplied in duplicate so that equipment can be cleaned twice a week or more often if necessary. The equipment should be washed and soaked in two buckets specifically dedicated for cleaning. The sink should not be used and equipment being rinsed should not touch the sink. The equipment is disassembled and washed in the first bucket with warm water and a mild detergent. All foreign matter should be scrubbed off with a brush and the equipment soaked in the first bucket for 15 minutes. Next the equipment should be rinsed under warm water and shaken dry. Finally, the second bucket should be used to soak the equipment in vinegar for 20 minutes. All parts should be submerged below the surface of the vinegar and air bubbles removed from small tubing and orifices. After soaking in vinegar, the equipment should be rinsed under running water and air-dried. The vinegar used in the final step should be diluted with an equal amount of boiled water. The vinegar solution should be kept in a covered bucket and discarded after 4 days.

Oxygen concentrators need minimal maintenance by the patient or family members, but the following guidelines should be followed: (1) review the prescription for oxygen and show the patient how to check the oxygen flow, (2) explain panel controls such as on/off switch, circuit breakers, and alarms, (3) identify an area of the room that has adequate electrical service with three-pronged outlets, (4) explain the importance of providing space around the concentrator, since the unit may overheat if pushed against curtains, (5) provide information on cleaning filters weekly, (6) review the importance of no smoking and place several signs in the room, including one in the front window, (7) instruct patients on how to check and use the backup oxygen cylinder and point out that subtle internal malfunctions can dramatically reduce oxygen concentration provided by the concentrator, (8) provide instruction on how to check the oxygen analyzer if available on the concentrator or how to use an optional analyzer if one is available, and (9) review the noise that may occur with the pressure-swing cycle as sieve beds are purged every 10 to 30 seconds.

(Q) Which of the following is the best way to dry respiratory care equipment after it has been soaked in a vinegar solution for 20 minutes?

a. rinse in a sink of clean water and wipe dry 351 B
b. rinse under running water and air-dry on a clean towel 350 B
c. remove from vinegar and air-dry by hanging 351 a

FRAME 193. MEDICATIONS

The most commonly ordered medications for COPD patients are beta-adrenergic bronchodilators. Table 12–1 on page 347 should be reviewed and checked for generic and brand names, dosage forms, action on alpha and/or beta receptors, pharmacologic action, and side effects. Patients with chronic sputum production of 30 mL or more daily may benefit from aerosol therapy with mucokinetic agents and bronchial hygiene therapy. Nebulization of bland aerosols has traditionally been used to aid in secretion clearance by liquefaction and hydration of secretions. However, a short 10- to 15-minute bland aerosol treatment with low-output nebulizers probably delivers less than 1 mL of solution to the airways. The accelerated clearance of retained secretions with hypertonic saline administered with an ultrasonic nebulizer is more likely the result of the irritant effect of the aerosol. Thus, high-density, hypertonic solutions behave primarily as an expectorant. The osmotic attraction of water and the alkalinity of nebulized sodium bicarbonate (2% to 7.5% in water) make sputum less adherent, but hypertonic solutions have the disadvantage of breaking down adrenergic bronchodilators. Although it is expensive, the best and most powerful mucokinetic aerosol medication is acetylcysteine (Mucomyst), which works by breaking disulfide bonds in mucus. A normal dose of acetylcysteine would be 10% in normal saline, but the bronchospasm that commonly occurs with its administration may require a bronchodilator to be given first. The foul smell and taste of Mucomyst requires that the patient be instructed to rinse out his or her mouth and nebulizer following each treatment.

Corticosteroids are anti-inflammatory drugs that are frequently given to home care patients to decrease airway caliber that is reduced by inflammation and resultant hyperemia. Steroids delivered by aerosol decrease the incidence of systemic side effects. Beclomethasone (Vanceril), dexamethasone (Decadron), triamcinolone (Azmacort), and flunisolide (AeroBid) are examples of steroids given by a metered-dose inhaler (MDI) for their anti-inflammatory action.

(Q) Which of the following adrenergic bronchodilators has the least rapid onset of beta-2 action?

a. metaproterenol (Alupent) 350 C
b. terbutaline (Brethine, Bricanyl) 350 c
c. albuterol (Proventil, Ventolin) 351 C

TABLE 12–1
ADRENERGIC BRONCHODILATORS

Drug	Dosage Forms	Action	Advantages	Disadvantages
Epinephrine (Adrenalin)	1:1000 for subcutaneous injection; aqueous solution (Susphrine) for IM 1% for aerosol (0.25–0.5 mL)	Alpha, beta-1, beta-2	Potent bronchodilator and reduction of mucosal edema	Tachycardia, hypertension
Racemic epinephrine (Vaponefrin, microNEFRIN)	2.25% for aerosol (0.25–0.5 mL)	Alpha, beta-1, beta-2	Most useful for mucosal congestion	Tachycardia, hypertension
Isoproterenol (Isuprel)	0.5% for aerosol (0.25–0.5 mL); also available in 1:100 for inhalation	Beta-1, beta-2	Potent bronchodilator; rapid onset	Tachycardia, short acting, tachyphylaxis to pulmonary effects but not to cardiac effects
Isoetharine (Bronkosol, Dilabron)	1% for aerosol (0.25–0.5 mL) by MDI, 2 puffs (0.34–0.68 mg)	Beta-1, beta-2	Less beta-1 stimulation and longer duration than isoproterenol	Slower onset
Metaproterenol (Metaprel, Alupent)	5% for aerosol (0.2–0.3 mL) by MDI, 2 puffs (1.3–1.95 mg)	Beta-1, beta-2	Minimal beta-1; long duration; prompt onset	Nervousness and tremors
Terbutaline (Brethine, Bricanyl)	Oral, by MDI 2 puffs (0.40 mg)	Beta-1, beta-2	Minimal beta-1; long duration	Nervousness and tremors
Albuterol (Proventil, Ventolin)	1% for aerosol (0.25 mL) by MDI, 2 puffs (0.18 mg)	Beta-1, beta-2	Minimal beta-1; long duration; prompt onset	Nervousness and tremors

Source: Modified from Bell, CW, Blodgett, D, Goike, CA, Green, M, Kieffer, J, and Smith, MA: Home Care and Rehabilitation in Respiratory Medicine. JB Lippincott, Philadelphia, 1984, p 71. Used with permission.

FRAME 194. PATIENT EVALUATION

Respiratory home care patients need to have an ongoing evaluation that starts with a complete assessment at discharge from the hospital or at the time of the first home care visit. This is necessary to provide a baseline or reference point against which any changes can be measured. The assessment should include historical background on past illness, general state of health, operations, injuries, allergies, current medications, diet, sleep patterns, habits (including exercise, use of coffee, alcohol, other drugs, and tobacco). A brief family and psychosocial history that captures the important and relevant information about the patient as a person should also be collected. A symptom history that includes the chief respiratory complaint should be taken. Typically the major respiratory complaints are dyspnea and cough. Chest pain or discomfort, sputum production, weight loss, hemoptysis, and peripheral edema are other symptoms that occur in a much smaller proportion of the patients. Periodic assessment should include an interval history that attempts to record changes in symptoms and signs over a period of days, weeks, or months.

After a history is obtained, a physical examination that will be primarily directed to the heart and lungs should be done. A first impression or gross inspection will progress to close visual inspection, percussion, palpitation, and auscultation. Commonly seen signs that help to make the first impression include posture when dyspneic, skin color, audible signs of breathing, and equipment in the room. Close inspection of the patient should progress from the patient's head and neck to the chest, abdomen, and finally the extremities. The adult thorax is normally symmetrical when viewed from any aspect. Asymmetry may be caused by unilateral atelectasis or pneumothorax, or by deformities such as kyphoscoliosis, pectus deformities, or rib injuries. Reduced or lack of movement on one side of the chest may reflect pain from fractured ribs or disease of the pleura. Assessment of the work of breathing should include close inspection of the accessory muscles of respiration.

Diagnostic chest percussion is useful in determining the extent of diaphragmatic motion. Hyperresonance is noted over the thorax in conditions with air trapping. Flatness or dullness to percussion may be noted over areas of pleural thickening or pleural effusion or over any consolidated area. Flatness or dullness will be heard only when the effusion or lesion is greater than 500 mL. The chest should be palpated to identify any areas of soreness so that they can be avoided when chest percussion is given. Also, the degree of symmetry and excursion of the chest can be assessed by palpation as well as the position of the trachea. Parenchymal consolidation can be diagnosed by feeling for vibrations with the ulnar surface of the hand as the patient speaks.

The stethoscope can be used both for quantitative and qualitative assessment of breath sounds. One complete respiratory cycle should be listened to at each location. Note the following: (1) the presence or absence of breaths; (2) the intensity and duration of each phase of respiration; (3) the presence, timing, and quality of both normal and abnormal (adventitious) breath sounds. Adventitious (added) sounds are usually in one of three categories: crackles, rhonchi, or wheezes.

Patients should be taught to keep track of their sputum so that any change from normal can be evaluated. Variations in quantity, color, odor, and viscosity may indicate a need for a change in hydration or bronchial hygiene therapy. Microscopic evaluation of the sputum may be necessary if common signs such as fever, changes in color and viscosity of sputum, increasing dyspnea, or changes in breath sounds and percussion notes are present.

Changes in the degree of airway obstruction is normally assessed by measuring timed expiratory volumes such as forced expiratory volume in 1 second (FEV_1) or forced vital capacity (FVC). However, it is usually not practical to perform basic spirometry in the home. A simple test that can be done in the home daily by the patient is the measurement of peak flow as an indicator of changes in degree of airway obstruction.

The goals of bronchial hygiene therapy, if it is prescribed, should be clearly defined and evaluated each time the patient is seen in the home or outpatient clinic. Also, goals established for exercise programs should be regularly reviewed and evaluated based on the patient's progress. Changes in daily living activity should be monitored with a view toward increasing endurance.

(Q) Which of the following measurements is the best for daily monitoring of airway obstruction?

a. peak expiratory flow 351 D
b. sputum production 350 b
c. use of accessory muscles 351 b

350A (from page 344, frame 191)
Wrong. It is normal for the heart rate to rise to this level. This level of exercise is necessary to achieve general physical conditioning. Return to page 344, frame 191, and select another answer.

350B (from page 345, frame 192)
Correct. Home care equipment should be rinsed dry of the vinegar under running water and air-dried by placing equipment on top of a clean towel. Please continue on page 347, frame 193.

350C (from pages 346–347, frame 193)
Wrong. Metaproterenol has a prompt onset and long duration of action with minimal cardiac effects. Return to pages 346–347, frame 193, and try again.

350D (from pages 342–343, frame 190)
Wrong. Oxygen concentrators produce approximately 90% oxygen at a flow of 4L/min. The FIO_2 would be in the range of 30% to 36%, which may induce hypoventilation. Return to pages 342–343, frame 190, and select another answer.

350a (from pages 342–343, frame 190)
Wrong. Membrane oxygen enrichers produce only 40% oxygen and need a flow three times higher than needed with oxygen concentrators that use molecular sieves to produce 95% oxygen at 2 L/min. Return to pages 342–343, frame 190, and select another answer.

350b (from pages 348–349, frame 194)
Wrong. Monitoring sputum production is a useful evaluation device, but is not sensitive enough to assess airway obstruction. Return to pages 348–349, frame 194, and select another answer.

350c (from pages 346–347, frame 193)
Correct. If terbutaline is taken orally, it does not have a rapid onset of bronchial smooth-muscle relaxation. However, it does have the advantages of long duration and minimal cardiac effects. It is also available in metered-dose inhalers, which bring about a more rapid onset of bronchodilation. Please continue on pages 348–349, frame 194.

350d (from page 344, frame 191)
Wrong. The criteria established by Medicare reimbursement for low-flow oxygen therapy during exercise calls for a PaO_2 less than or equal to 55 torr. Alternate criteria state a PaO_2 of 56 to 59 torr, or saturation of 86% to 89%, plus signs of dysfunction from the cardiovascular or central nervous system as a result of hypoxemia. Return to page 344, frame 191, and select another answer.

351A (from page 344, frame 191)
Correct. An arterial oxygen saturation equal to or below 85% during exercise indicates a need for low-flow oxygen therapy to increase exercise tolerance. The arterial oxygen tension would need to drop to 55 torr unless there were signs of dysfunction from other end-user organs before oxygen would be needed. Usually a saturation of 90% corresponds to a Pa_{O_2} of 60 torr. Please continue on page 345, frame 192.

351B (from page 345, frame 192)
Wrong. Home care equipment should not be wiped dry, since the equipment may be reinfected. Return to page 345, frame 192, and select another answer.

351C (from pages 346–347, frame 193)
Wrong. Albuterol has a rapid onset of beta-2 action and brings about relaxation of bronchial smooth muscle with minimal cardiac effects. Return to pages 346–347, frame 193, and select another answer.

351D (from pages 348–349, frame 194)
Correct. It is not practical to do routine spirometry in a patient's home, especially on a daily basis. A peak flow test is the best way to monitor changes in airway obstruction. Please continue on page 352 and complete the chapter exercises.

351a (from page 345, frame 192)
Wrong. The vinegar solution must be rinsed off the equipment. Return to page 345, frame 192, and select another answer.

351b (from pages 348–349, frame 194)
Wrong. Active use of accessory muscles often implies increased airway obstruction but usually is not seen with mild airway obstruction. Return to pages 348–349, frame 194, and select another answer.

351c (from pages 342–343, frame 190)
Correct. Membrane oxygen enrichers produce only 40% oxygen and need a flow three times higher than oxygen concentrators that use molecular sieves to produce 95% oxygen at 2 L/min. Please continue on page 344, frame 191.

EXERCISES

1. Accompany a respiratory therapist to a patient's home to assess the environment and service needs for respiratory equipment.
2. List 10 or more topics that should be included in the instruction provided to a recently discharged ventilator-dependent patient and the patient's family.
3. Prepare a floor plan for an apartment of a COPD patient receiving long-term low-flow oxygen therapy. Include the type and location of the source of oxygen, special adaptations for energy conservation, and environmental control devices.
4. Plan a daily meal and fluid replacement plan for an uncomplicated COPD patient. Include types and quantities of food and fluid to be taken at specific meal times.
5. Locate and read the operation and maintenance manuals for both an oxygen concentrator and a portable liquid oxygen system.
6. Compare the duration time at 1 L/min of a portable aluminum oxygen cylinder and a portable liquid oxygen unit. Select units that have the same weight.
7. Identify two circumstances in which patients who do not meet Medicare criteria for continuous oxygen may qualify for limited oxygen use.
8. Outline in language that a home care patient can easily understand a protocol for cleaning and disinfecting respiratory equipment.
9. Review the charts of five COPD patients who will be discharged and identify orders for bronchoactive adrenergic bronchodilators and mucokinetic agents, noting the means of administration and the dosage.
10. Prepare a guideline for a respiratory home care patient to use for recording daily sputum production.

POSTTEST

This test is designed to evaluate what you have learned from completing Chapter 12. Check your answers on page 355 and review the topics where your answer is incorrect.

1. When evaluating a respiratory home care patient's residence for use of an oxygen concentrator, which of the following is the most important factor?
   A. access to entrance
   B. width of entrance door
   C. location of bedroom
   D. electrical service
   E. heating system
2. Discharge planning for a respiratory home care patient should include instruction in all of the following *except*
   A. anatomy and physiology.
   B. medications.
   C. cleaning of equipment.
   D. replacing the purge pump on an oxygen concentrator.
   E. gas safety and fire prevention rules.
3. All of the following instructions will help a ventilator home care patient and his or her family deal with an electrical power failure *except*
   A. cardiopulmonary resuscitation.
   B. use of a pneumatically powered ventilator.
   C. use of compressed gas cylinders.
   D. use of a manual resuscitator.
   E. use of a battery-powered ventilator.
4. A respiratory home care patient receiving long-term low-flow oxygen therapy should receive instruction in all of the following *except*
   A. maximum oxygen flow allowed.
   B. oxygen-induced hyperventilation.
   C. oxygen-induced hypoventilation.
   D. how to check for oxygen flow from a cannula.
   E. how to check oxygen concentration of gas from a concentrator.
5. Bronchospasm, dyspnea, and coughing may all be caused by the following problems located in a COPD patient's home *except*
   A. secondhand smoke.
   B. hair spray.
   C. heating system filters.
   D. relative humidity of 30% to 50%.
   E. mold formation in humidifiers.
6. Which of the following recommendations regarding daily living activities should be given to a respiratory home care patient?
   A. Eat several small meals.
   B. Eat only twice a day.
   C. Do stretching exercises while dressing.
   D. Take showers rather than using the tub.
   E. Try not to use oxygen when eating.
7. All of the following factors may increase the daily fluid loss of COPD patients *except*
   A. fever.
   B. hypoventilation.
   C. diaphoresis.
   D. hyperventilation.
   E. vomiting.

8. Control of adequate fluid intake for a COPD patient becomes more difficult with all of the following *except*
   A. atelectasis.
   B. cor pulmonale.
   C. chronic heart disease.
   D. diabetes mellitus.
   E. chronic renal failure.

9. The least expensive way to give a respiratory home care patient receiving oxygen more mobility around the home is to teach the patient to
   A. use oxygen only when sleeping.
   B. use oxygen only when exercising.
   C. place oxygen cylinders in each room.
   D. use a 20- to 50-ft extension to oxygen supply tubing.
   E. use a portable liquid oxygen system.

10. What is the range of oxygen flow available on portable liquid oxygen systems?
    A. 1 to 3 L/min
    B. 1 to 4 L/min
    C. 1 to 6 L/min
    D. ½ to 10 L/min
    E. ⅛ to 15 L/min

11. Without signs of end-use damage to other organs, the Medicare "absolute" criteria for long-term continuous low-flow oxygen therapy is a Pa_{O_2} equal to or less than
    A. 50 torr.
    B. 55 torr.
    C. 60 torr.
    D. 65 torr.
    E. 70 torr.

12. Without signs of end-use damage to other organs, the Medicare criteria for long-term continuous low-flow oxygen therapy is an Sa_{O_2} equal to or less than
    A. 60%.
    B. 70%.
    C. 85%.
    D. 90%.
    E. 97%.

13. Criteria for evaluating the effectiveness of pulmonary rehabilitation programs include which of the following?
    I. number of days of hospitalization
    II. level of daily activity
    III. walking distance
    IV. posture evaluation
    V. improvement in vital capacity
    A. I and III only
    B. II, III, and IV only
    C. I, III, and V only
    D. I, II, III, and IV only
    E. II, III, IV, and V only

14. Exercise sessions for COPD patients should be held on which of the following schedules?
    A. 5 to 10 minutes twice a week
    B. 5 to 10 minutes four times a week
    C. 10 to 20 minutes twice a week
    D. 20 to 30 minutes twice a week
    E. 20 to 30 minutes four times a week

15. How often should respiratory home care equipment be cleaned and disinfected?
   A. once a day
   B. every 2 days
   C. twice a week
   D. once a week
   E. every 2 weeks
16. The procedure for cleaning and disinfecting respiratory home care equipment includes all of the following *except*
   A. diluting vinegar with equal parts of boiled water.
   B. soaking equipment in the sink in a detergent solution for 15 minutes.
   C. keeping the vinegar solution in a covered container.
   D. rinsing off vinegar under running water and air-drying equipment.
   E. soaking equipment in a vinegar solution for 20 minutes.
17. Which of the following bronchoactive drugs increases airway caliber by reducing inflammation and hyperemia?
   A. dexamethasone
   B. terbutaline
   C. albuterol
   D. isoproterenol
   E. metaproterenol
18. The shortest duration of action occurs with which of the following adrenergic bronchodilators?
   A. isoetharine
   B. metaproterenol
   C. terbutaline
   D. isoproterenol
   E. albuterol
19. Asymmetry seen during inspection of the thorax may be a sign of which of the following?
   I. rib fracture
   II. bilateral atelectasis
   III. kyphoscoliosis
   IV. use of accessory muscles
   V. cor pulmonale
   A. I and III only
   B. II and IV only
   C. I, II, and III only
   D. II, III, and IV only
   E. II, IV, and V only
20. Which of the following may be suspected by feeling for vibrations with the ulnar surface of the hand as the patient speaks?
   A. pneumothorax
   B. hemothorax
   C. parenchymal consolidation
   D. rib fractures
   E. mediastinal deviation

ANSWERS TO POSTTEST

1. D (F185)
2. D (F185)
3. A (F186)
4. B (F186)
5. D (F187)
6. A (F187)
7. B (F188)
8. A (F188)
9. D (F189)
10. E (F189)
11. B (F190)
12. C (F190)
13. D (F191)
14. E (F191)
15. C (F192)
16. B (F192)
17. A (F193)
18. D (F193)
19. A (F194)
20. C (F194)

BIBLIOGRAPHY

Barnes, TA: Respiratory Care Practice. Year Book Medical Publishers, Chicago, 1988.

Bates, BA: A Guide to Physical Examination and History Taking, ed 4. JB Lippincott, Philadelphia, 1987.

Bell, CW et al: Home Care and Rehabilitation in Respiratory Medicine. JB Lippincott, Philadelphia, 1984.

Burton, GG and Hodgkin, JE: Respiratory Care: A Guide to Clinical Practice, ed 2. JB Lippincott, Philadelphia, 1984.

Eubanks, DH and Bone, RC: Comprehensive Respiratory Care, ed 2. CV Mosby, St. Louis, 1990.

Kacmarek, RM and Stoller, JK: Current Respiratory Care. BC Decker, Philadelphia, 1989.

Lucas, J, Golish, JA, Sleeper, G, and O'Ryan, JA: Home Respiratory Care. Appleton & Lange, Norwalk, CT, 1988.

McPherson, SP: Respiratory Home Care Equipment. Daedalus Enterprises, Dallas, 1988.

McPherson, SP: Respiratory Therapy Equipment, ed 4. CV Mosby, St. Louis, 1990.

Wilkins, RL, Sheldon, RL, Krider, SJ: Clinical Assessment in Respiratory Care, ed 2. CV Mosby, St. Louis, 1990.

13

Oxygen Therapy Equipment

195. Cylinder size and duration
196. Regulators
197. Flowmeters
198. Air/oxygen blenders
199. Simple masks
200. Nasal cannulas
201. Partial rebreathing masks
202. Non-rebreathing masks
203. Air-entrainment nebulizers
204. Air-entrainment masks
205. Oxyhoods
206. Incubators
207. Oxygen tents
208. CPAP devices
209. Manual resuscitators
210. IPPB machines
211. Pulse oximeters
212. Oxygen analyzers

PRETEST

This pretest is designed to measure what you already know about oxygen therapy equipment. Check your answers on page 360 and then continue on page 361, frame 195.

1. What is the cylinder duration of a full E-cylinder set at a gas flow of 15 L/min?
   A. 23 minutes
   B. 41 minutes
   C. 57 minutes
   D. 2 hours, 12 minutes
   E. 7 hours, 40 minutes
2. Which of the following should always be done before a regulator is attached to a cylinder?
   A. The Thorpe tube should be calibrated.
   B. The cylinder should be cracked.
   C. A new label should be placed on the cylinder.
   D. The cylinder valve should be wiped clean.
   E. Teflon tape should be applied to cylinder outlet threads.
3. Which of the following is characteristic of a pressure-compensated Thorpe tube flowmeter?
   I. The flow valve is before the Thorpe tube.
   II. The flow valve is after the Thorpe tube.
   III. The flow can be read when Thorpe tube is in a horizontal position.
   IV. The flowmeter is usually calibrated at 50 pounds per square inch.
   A. I only
   B. II and IV only
   C. III and IV only
   D. I, III, and IV only
   E. II, III, and IV only
4. How will blender performance be affected if the oxygen pressure is significantly higher than air on one side of the dual-inlet mixing valve?
   A. higher FIO_2 than set
   B. lower FIO_2 than set
   C. no change in FIO_2
   D. depends if alarm is sounding
   E. depends on flow rate
5. What is the range of FIO_2 with a simple mask when the oxygen flow is 6 to 10 L/min? 6 to 10 L/min?
   A. 0.24 to 0.28
   B. 0.24 to 0.40
   C. 0.30 to 0.50
   D. 0.30 to 0.60
   E. 0.40 to 0.70
6. What is the highest oxygen flow that should be used with a nasal cannula?
   A. 2 L/min
   B. 4 L/min
   C. 6 L/min
   D. 8 L/min
   E. 10 L/min
7. What is the highest FIO_2 that can usually be achieved with a disposable partial rebreathing mask with oxygen flow of 10 L/min?
   A. 0.28
   B. 0.40
   C. 0.50
   D. 0.60
   E. 0.70

8. What is the range of F_{IO_2} usually obtained with a disposable non-rebreathing mask with oxygen flow of 6 to 10 L/min?
   A. 0.28 to 0.36
   B. 0.30 to 0.40
   C. 0.35 to 0.50
   D. 0.40 to 0.60
   E. 0.55 to 0.70

9. What is the total flow from an air-entrainment mask that delivers an F_{IO_2} of 0.28 with an oxygen flow of 6 L/min?
   A. 12 L/min
   B. 33 L/min
   C. 54 L/min
   D. 68 L/min
   E. 97 L/min

10. What would be the effect of lowering the oxygen flow to an air-entrainment nebulizer from 10 to 6 L/min?
    I. less aerosol produced
    II. lower gas temperture
    III. lower oxygen concentration
    IV. lower total gas flow
    A. I and IV only
    B. II and III only
    C. II and IV only
    D. I, III, and IV only
    E. I, II, III, and IV

11. The gas flow to an oxyhood should *exceed*
    A. 4 L/min.
    B. 7 L/min.
    C. 10 L/min.
    D. 12 L/min.
    E. 15 L/min.

12. When the red paddle on an incubator is elevated to allow oxygen to enter at higher flow rates, F_{IO_2} can range from
    A. 0.24 to 0.35.
    B. 0.30 to 0.40.
    C. 0.40 to 0.50.
    D. 0.60 to 0.70.
    E. 0.80 to 1.00.

13. What is the range of F_{IO_2} obtained in an Air-Shields Corupette model D when supplied with oxygen at 8 to 10 L/min?
    A. 0.24 to 0.35
    B. 0.35 to 0.45
    C. 0.45 to 0.55
    D. 0.50 to 0.60
    E. 0.60 to 0.70

14. Which of the following can be complications of mask continuous positive-airway pressure (CPAP)?
    I. vomiting and aspiration
    II. decrease in ventricular filling pressure
    III. skin ulceration
    IV. eye trauma
    A. I and III only
    B. II and IV only
    C. II and III only
    D. I, II, and IV only
    E. I, II, III, and IV

15. What is the peak inspiratory flow rate that can be obtained with the Bird Mark 7 set to deliver 100% oxygen?
    A. 30 L/min
    B. 40 L/min
    C. 60 L/min
    D. 80 L/min
    E. 100 L/min
16. What is the range of F_{IO_2} delivered by the Bird Mark 7 when set for air entrainment?
    A. 0.35 to 0.45
    B. 0.40 to 0.50
    C. 0.40 to 0.60
    D. 0.60 to 0.90
    E. 0.70 to 1.00
17. The American Society for Testing and Materials standard for the F_{DO_2} delivered by a manual resuscitator with an oxygen reservoir attached and oxygen flowing at 15 L/min is a minimum of
    A. 0.40.
    B. 0.60.
    C. 0.85.
    D. 0.90.
    E. 1.00.
18. Which of the following is likely to increase the F_{IO_2} delivered by a manual resuscitator?
    A. increase bag refill time
    B. increase cycle rate
    C. increase tidal volume
    D. increase bag size
    E. decrease valve dead space
19. Which of these oxygen analyzers could not be safely used with flammable gases?
    A. polarographic
    B. galvanic cell
    C. paramagnetic
    D. volumetric
    E. thermoconductivity
20. The pulse oximeter measures the percent of oxygen saturation of hemoglobin by comparing the amount of infrared light absorbed by oxyhemoglobin with the amount of red light absorbed by
    A. sulfhemoglobin.
    B. deoxyhemoglobin.
    C. carboxyhemoglobin.
    D. methemoglobin.
    E. plasma.

ANSWERS TO PRETEST

1. B (F195)
2. B (F196)
3. B (F197)
4. A (F198)
5. C (F199)
6. C (F200)
7. D (F201)
8. E (F202)
9. D (F204)
10. A (F203)
11. B (F205)
12. D (F206)
13. C (F207)
14. E (F208)
15. B (F210)
16. D (F210)
17. C (F209)
18. A (F209)
19. E (F212)
20. B (F211)

FRAME 195. CYLINDER SIZE AND DURATION

Respiratory care practitioners frequently use oxygen cylinders in transport and CPR situations and must be able to calculate the duration with varying flow rates and cylinder sizes. The volume of gas in the cylinder and the flow needed will determine how long the cylinder will last. Cylinder duration factors can be calculated for each cylinder size by using the following formula:

$$\text{Cylinder duration factor} = \frac{(\text{cubic feet in full cylinder})(28.3\text{ L})}{\text{psig of full cylinder}}$$

Example: Duration factor for an H-cylinder

$$\text{Cylinder duration factor} = \frac{(244)(28.3\text{ L})}{2200\text{ psig}} = 3.14\text{ L/psig}$$

The volume of oxygen is determined by multiplying the cubic feet in a full cylinder by the number of liters in 1 cubic foot (28.3 L). Dividing the total number of liters by the pressure of a full cylinder results in a duration factor for a specific size cylinder. The factor can be used to determine the number of liters of oxygen in the cylinder when the pressure is known. The duration can be calculated by dividing the number of liters available by the oxygen flow per minute. The most commonly used cylinder sizes are D, E, and H, which have duration factors (L/psig) of 0.16, 0.28, and 3.14 respectively. The following formula can be used to calculate cylinder duration:

$$\text{Cylinder duration in minutes} = \frac{(\text{actual gauge pressure})(\text{factor})}{\text{Flow}}$$

Example: D-cylinder with 1000 pounds per square inch and O_2 flow of 10 L/min

$$\text{Cylinder duration in minutes} = \frac{(1000)(0.16)}{10} = 16\text{ minutes}$$

(Q) What is the cylinder duration for a E-cylinder with 1400 psig at 15 L/min?

a. 26 minutes 366 A
b. 41 minutes 366 b
c. 4 hours, 53 minutes 367 B

FRAME 196. REGULATORS

Regulators are used to reduce cylinder gas to a specific working pressure such as 50 psig. If a flowmeter were attached directly to a cylinder without a regulator, the flow would need to be adjusted frequently as the pressure dropped. Most cylinder regulators work by establishing an equilibrium between a spring-loaded diaphragm and gas in the reduction chamber. Flow into the reduction chamber increases pressure on the diaphragm until it is displaced and the inlet valve closes. The amount of pressure reduction is determined by the ratio of the surface area of the diaphragm to the valve inlet. An adjustable diaphragm spring allows the working pressure to be varied further (see Fig. 13–1). Some regulators have two or three reduction chamnbers to minimize the variation in working pressure by stepping down the pressure in stages. Regulators have pressure relief valves (sometimes called spuds), which vent high pressure in the reduction chamber if it reaches a range of 140 to 200 psig. Usually each stage of the regulator has a pressure-relief valve. The most common cause of high pressure in the reduction chamber is a small piece of dirt that holds the inlet valve open. Thus, a cylinder should always be opened (cracked) for 1 second before attaching the regulator to blow away dust from the valve outlet.

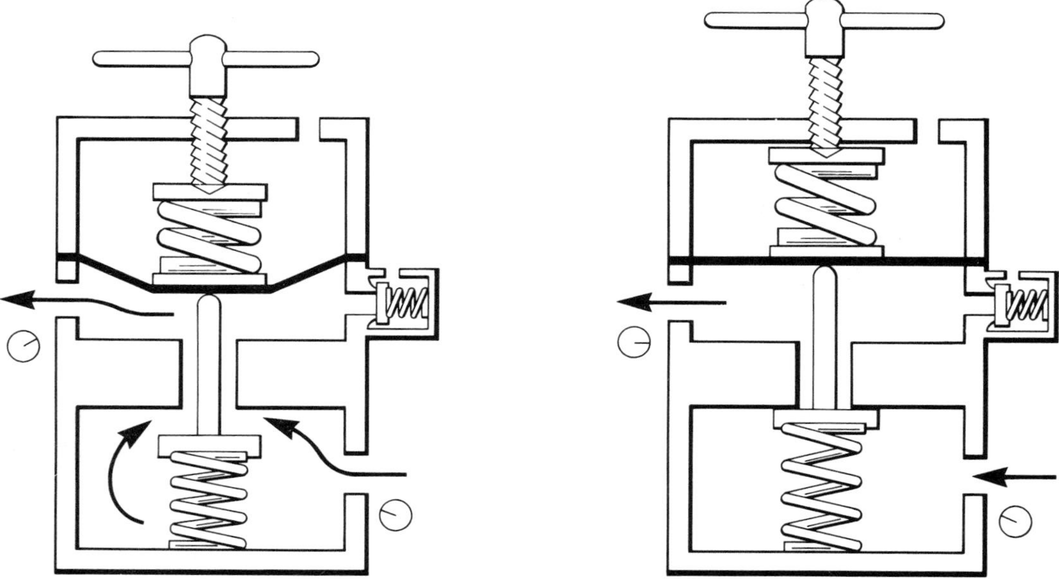

Figure 13–1 Contemporary direct regulator.

(Q) What is the best way to determine if a pressure-relief valve on a regulator is venting gas?

a. Listen for a hissing sound. 366 B
b. Spray regulator spuds with a petroleum-based lubricant. 367 C
c. Cover regulator spuds with soapy water. 366 d

FRAME 197. FLOWMETERS

Flowmeters are used to control the volume of gas per unit of time (L/min) leaving a gas cylinder or piped gas system. The three types of flowmeters in common use are the Bourdon gauge, Thorpe tube, and fixed-orifice flow restrictor. The Bourdon gauge flowmeter has a fixed orifice placed distal to an adjustable pressure regulator. The pressure gauge is calibrated to reflect the flow that occurs as a result of pressure changes before the orifice (Fig. 13–2). Equipment attached downstream to the fixed orifice of the Bourdon flowmeter will reduce the flow without changing the reading on the gauge. If accurate flow is needed, downstream impedance should be held to a minimum. Bourdon gauges are not gravity dependent and can be used on small cylinders placed on their sides during transport.

The pressure-compensated Thorpe tube has a variable orifice and is pressurized at 50 psig. A needle valve allows adjustment of flow through a hollow tube where a float indicates the volume of gas passing through per minute. The placement of the needle valve on the outlet side of the Thorpe tube is critical for accurate flow readings (Fig. 13–3). Downstream impedance has the effect of reducing the caliber of the needle valve and hence the flow through the Thorpe tube, but the flowmeter will accurately indicate the reduced flow. Thorpe tube flowmeters are gravity dependent and must be kept in a vertical position to be read accurately.

A flow restrictor has a fixed orifice and requires a constant inlet pressure. The flow restrictor has no gauge or Thorpe tube and is not adjustable. They are used for applications where there is no need to adjust flow such as with manual resuscitators or oxygen concentrators.

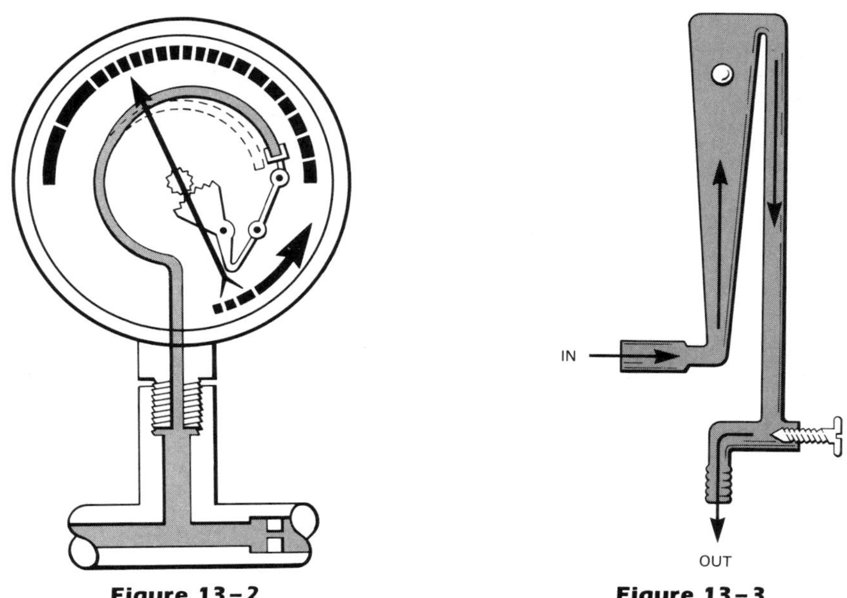

Figure 13–2   **Figure 13–3**

Figure 13–2 Bourdon gauge flowmeter.

Figure 13–3 Compensated Thorpe tube flowmeter.

(Q) Which of the following flowmeters is best for use with a jet nebulizer?

a. flow restrictor 366 c

b. Thorpe tube 367 D

c. Bourdon gauge 367 c

FRAME 198. AIR/OXYGEN BLENDERS

Air/oxygen blenders are used to accurately control oxygen concentration. They mix oxygen and air for use by mechanical ventilators, continuous-flow CPAP systems, add-on intermittent mandatory ventilation (IMV) systems, and control F_{IO_2} for oxygen therapy with oxyhoods. Blenders should receive air and oxygen at pressures as near as possible to 50 psig. Most blenders have an internal pressure-balancing system to accommodate variable inlet gas pressures. Gas flows through spool-shaped valves separated by a flexible diaphragm. Small differences in air or oxygen pressure will move the diaphragm and spool valves to ensure that gases enter the mixing valve at the same pressure. Equal pressure for oxygen and air is important because a dual orifice needle valve controls the proportion of each gas flowing out of the orifices. If the pressure gradient across the orifices is different, an inaccurate oxygen concentration will occur. When inlet pressures of either gas fall below a certain threshold, a reed alarm will sound as gas escapes through a spring-loaded valve. (See Fig. 13–4.)

Other problems encountered with air/oxygen blenders include contamination of one gas supply because of backward flow from the other gas source. This can occur when check valves fail and the higher-pressure gas flows into the opposing gas line. Contaminants from gas lines, such as water, can restrict flow or prevent check valves from sealing.

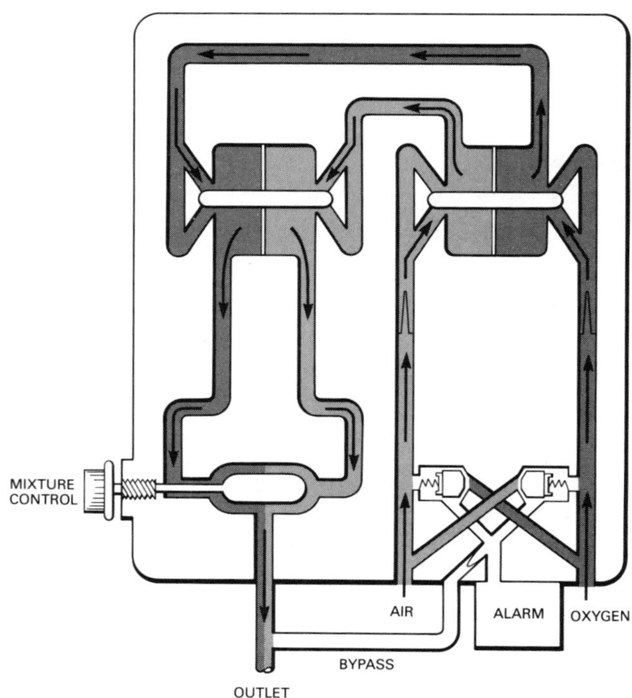

Figure 13–4 Schematic of a typical air/oxygen blender.

(Q) What will the result be of a higher pressure on the air side of a dual orifice needle valve of an air/oxygen blender?

a. higher F_{IO_2} — 366 C
b. lower F_{IO_2} — 367 b
c. no change in F_{IO_2} — 366 D

FRAME 199. SIMPLE MASKS

Simple oxygen masks without reservoir bags supply oxygen concentrations estimated to be in the range of 30% to 50% with oxygen flow of 6 to 10 L/min. The higher end of the range will usually be achieved in patients with slow rates and small tidal volumes. They are easy to apply and offer higher oxygen concentrations than a nasal cannula. They offer better humidification than cannulas, and high flows are possible without mucosal irritation or drying. Simple masks are best used for short periods such as emergency medical transport of a trauma victim, initial oxygen therapy in the emergency room, or in the postoperative recovery room.

Simple masks are uncomfortable for long periods. They are hot and may make the patient feel claustrophobic. They are not good for patients who are severely hypoxemic and breathing at high rates. It is difficult to maintain constant F_{IO_2} because of leaks around the mask especially with variable inspiratory flow patterns. Adequate oxygen flow must be delivered to the mask to wash out exhaled CO_2 from the mask dead space. The mask should not be strapped to the face of a severely hypoxic patient who may vomit while the mask is in place; instead the mask should be held in place or simply set on the face. (See Fig. 13–5.)

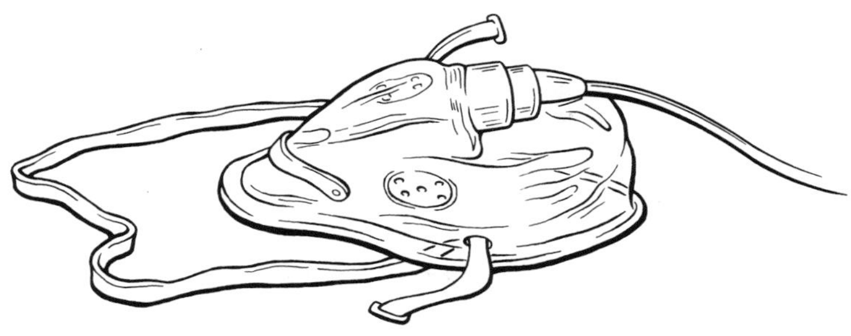

Figure 13–5

(Q) To titrate oxygen flow to a simple mask for a moderately hypoxic patient, which of the following would be best?

a. Set oxygen flow to a maximum of 10 L/min. 367 A
b. Set oxygen flow using a pulse oximeter. 367 a
c. Set oxygen flow using gas-blood measurements. 366 a

366A (from page 361, frame 195)
Correct. Multiplying the duration factor of 0.28 L/psig by 1400 psig and then dividing by 15 L/min results in a cylinder duration of 26 minutes. Please continue on page 362, frame 196.

366B (from page 362, frame 196)
Wrong. Many leaks are too small to be heard, although a missing washer on the valve outlet of a smaller cylinder outlet (size D or E) usually can be heard. Audible leaks on large cylinder (size G or H) outlets usually can be corrected by wrapping them with Teflon tape. Small inaudible leaks from regulator pressure-relief valves (spuds) are more difficult to detect. Return to page 362, frame 196, and select another answer.

366C (from page 364, frame 198)
Wrong. The higher pressure on the air side will fool the dual-orifice needle valve by mixing more air than when the pressure across both apertures was equal. Return to page 364, frame 198, and select another answer.

366D (from page 364, frame 198)
Wrong. The higher pressure on the air side will fool the dual-orifice needle valve by mixing more air than occurred when the pressure across both sides was equal. Return to page 364, frame 198, and select another answer.

366a (from page 365, frame 199)
Wrong. Blood-gas measurements will not take into account variable breathing patterns that will affect the inspired oxygen concentration. Return to page 365, frame 199, and select another answer.

366b (from page 361, frame 195)
Wrong. The cylinder is not full with a pressure of 2200 psig, but has only 1400 psig remaining. Return to page 361, frame 195, and try again.

366c (from page 363, frame 197)
Wrong. A flow restrictor has no gauge or indicator of the flow rate, and it is not pressure compensated. Return to page 363, frame 197, and try again.

366d (from page 362, frame 196)
Correct. Soapy water placed on pressure-relief valves will form bubbles if oxygen is being vented. Petroleum-based lubricants are *never* used on regulators or cylinders due to the fire hazard when oxygen is used. Audible leaks may be caused by a missing washer on smaller cylinders (size D or E), and Teflon tape wrapped around the threads of the valve outlet of larger cylinders (size G or H) may stop leaks. Please continue on page 363, frame 197.

367A (from page 365, frame 199)
Wrong. Variable breathing patterns frequently occur with severely hypoxic patients, and delivered oxygen concentrations will be difficult to estimate with air drawn in around the mask. Return to page 365, frame 199, and select another answer.

367B (from page 361, frame 195)
Wrong. You used the duration factor for an H-cylinder instead of the one for an E-cylinder. Return to page 361, frame 195, and try again.

367C (from page 362, frame 196)
Wrong. Petroleum-based lubricants are *never* used on oxygen regulators or cylinders due to the fire hazard. Return to page 362, frame 196, and select another answer.

367D (from page 363, frame 197)
Correct. If located between the pressure source and the outlet valve, a Thorpe tube will be pressure compensated and accurately indicate the flow. This is important, since the jet nebulizer will cause downstream impedance and cause the flow to decrease. Please continue on page 364, frame 198.

367a (from page 365, frame 199)
Correct. Delivered oxygen concentrations will be hard to predict with the variable breathing pattern commonly seen with severely hypoxic patients. Pulse oximetry will provide continuous monitoring of the effectiveness of oxygen therapy. A blood-gas measurement should be done and compared to the saturation of the oximeter. Please continue on page 368, frame 200.

367b (from page 364, frame 198)
Correct. The higher pressure on the air side will fool the dual-orifice needle valve by mixing more air than occurred when the pressure across both apertures was equal. Please continue on page 365, frame 199.

367c (from page 363, frame 197)
Wrong. A Bourdon gauge is not pressure compensated and will not accurately indicate the flow with the increase in downstream impedance caused by the jet nebulizer. Return to page 363, frame 197, and select another answer.

FRAME 200. NASAL CANNULAS

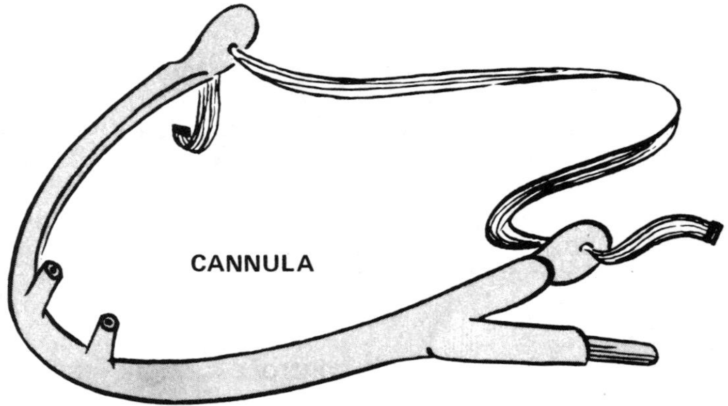

Figure 13–6

Nasal cannulas (Fig. 13–6) are commonly used for oxygen therapy because of the ease with which they can be applied. Compliance is improved since cannulas are relatively unobtrusive, comfortable, and allow the patient to eat and talk while receiving oxygen. The oxygen concentration achieved (FIO_2) will vary greatly with changes in tidal volume, respiratory rate, and pattern of ventilation. Larger tidal volumes and faster rates will decrease FIO_2, and smaller tidal volumes and decreased respiratory rates will increase FIO_2. An ideal patient, with a tidal volume of 500 mL, a respiratory rate of 12/min, and an I:E ratio of 1:2, will have an increase of 0.04 in FIO_2 for every liter per minute change in oxygen flow to the cannula in the range of 1 to 6 L/min. For example, the ideal patient would receive an FIO_2 of 0.24 at 1 L/min and 0.44 at 6 L/min.

The major disadvantage of the nasal cannula is the variable FIO_2 with different breathing patterns. Other problems include drying and irritation of the nasal mucosa at high flow rates (greater than 6 L/min), low to moderate FIO_2 levels, pressure sores on the nose or face, and the possibility of blocked oxygen flow caused by kinking or water in the connecting tubing.

Oxygen flow from the prongs of a nasal cannula should be confirmed by feeling for gas flow or submerging the prongs in water and looking for bubbling. The usual reasons for absent or low flow include (1) flowmeter inaccuracy, (2) a twisted or kinked cannula, or (3) a leaking humidifier. Some humidifiers have audible relief valves that pop off at preset pressure limits to warn of an obstruction to gas flow.

(Q) What would be the FIO_2 delivered by a nasal cannula at 2 L/min to a 70-kg 22-year-old patient with a minute volume of 4 L and a normal respiratory rate?

a. 0.28 374 C
b. 0.36 374 A
c. 0.24 375 A

FRAME 201. PARTIAL REBREATHING MASKS

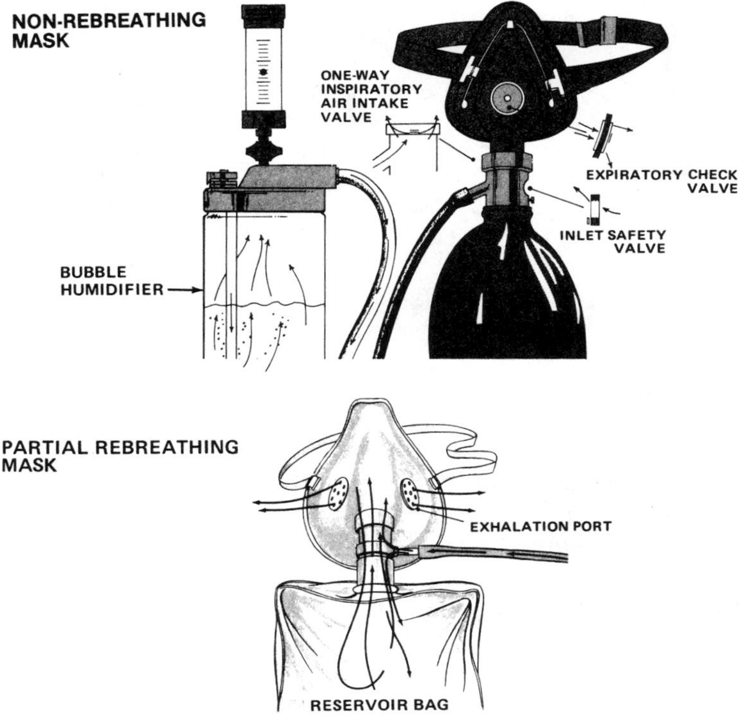

Figure 13–7

Partial rebreathing masks incorporate a reservoir (Fig. 13–7) that increases the amount of oxygen available beyond that in the mask or from the flowmeter. The oxygen concentration delivered will vary with the patient's inspiratory flow rate and ventilatory pattern. The mask does provide moderate to high oxygen concentrations in the range of 35% to 60% when oxygen flow is in the range of 6 to 10 L/min. Since there are no valves, some exhaled gas travels into the reservoir bag; however, the first portion of this gas comes from the anatomical dead space, which is filled with gas from the previous inspiration. The oxygen flow to the mask should be high enough to keep the reservoir bag from collapsing during inspiration.

The advantages of the partial rebreathing mask are (1) it supplies relatively high FIO_2, (2) it is inexpensive, disposable, and easily applied, and (3) high flow is possible. The disadvantages are (1) it is relatively uncomfortable when used for long periods, (2) a good seal is difficult to obtain and air dilution usually occurs, (3) FIO_2 will vary with the ventilation pattern and peak inspiratory flow, and is difficult to predict, and (4) similar to other masks there is a greater potential for aspiration.

(Q) What oxygen flow should be delivered to a partial rebreathing mask for a patient with a normal ventilatory pattern who needs an FIO_2 of 0.60?

a. 6 L/min — 374 B
b. 12 L/min — 375 B
c. enough to keep the bag inflated during inspiration — 374 a

FRAME 202. NON-REBREATHING MASKS

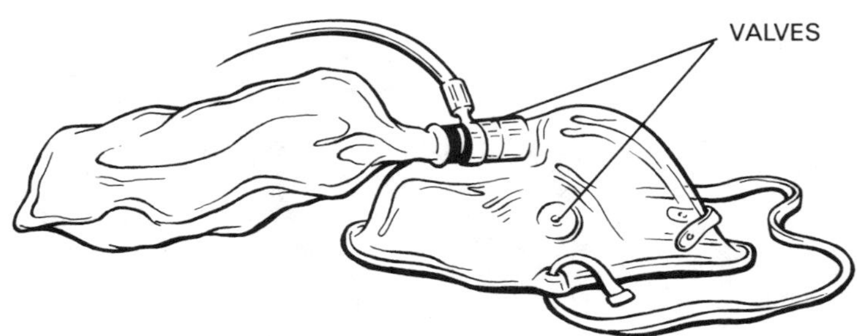

Figure 13–8

The non-rebreathing mask has a valve that prevents exhaled gas from entering the reservoir bag and another set of valves that cover two exhalation ports (Fig. 13–8). The mask can produce oxygen concentrations of 55% to 70% with oxygen flow of 6 to 10 L/min with normal ventilation patterns. The F_{IO_2} is only slightly higher than the partial rebreathing mask unless an anesthesia bag-mask-valve system with a larger reservoir bag and better fitting mask are used. Disposable masks have valves made from thin rubber flaps that may not function as intended, especially when wet. Also, valves may be removed accidentally when the mask has been in use for long periods. The advantages and disadvantages are similar to those observed with partial rebreathing masks.

Non-rebreathing masks are usually used with patients who have moderate to severe hypoxemia and are breathing spontaneously. Examples of clinical problems treated with this mask include carbon monoxide poisoning and congestive heart failure. The key to obtaining high oxygen concentrations is to maintain enough flow to keep the bag from collapsing during inspiration and securing the mask so that it forms a tight seal with the face.

(Q) Which of the following oxygen masks is most likely to deliver an F_{IO_2} of 1.00 to a spontaneously breathing patient with severe hypoxemia?

a. partial rebreathing mask 374 C
b. anesthesia bag-valve-mask system 375 C
c. non-rebreathing mask 375 b

FRAME 203. AIR-ENTRAINMENT NEBULIZERS

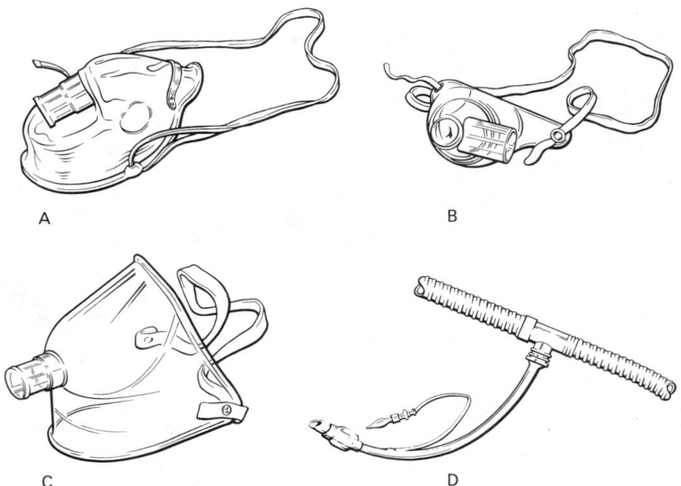

Figure 13–9 Various masks for use with aerosol or high-flow gas delivery systems: (*A*) aerosol face mask; (*B*) tracheostomy collar; (*C*) face tent; (*D*) Briggs adapter or *T*-piece.

All-purpose air-entrainment nebulizers are used to provide humidified oxygen to a variety of masks and adapters for tracheal tubes (Fig. 13–9). The F_{IO_2} is usually controlled by changing the size of the air-entrainment port to deliver oxygen concentrations of 0.40, 0.60, 0.70, and 1.00 or by continuously adjusting port size to achieve an F_{IO_2} that ranges from 0.30 to 1.00. The small size of the jet in the nebulizer limits the source gas to < 15 L/min and total flow may be inadequate to meet a severely dyspneic patient's inspiratory flow needs at high F_{IO_2} settings. The use of two air-entrainment nebulizers with their output connected together will double the available flow when high F_{IO_2} settings limit air entrainment. A T-tube extension may be added to reduce the amount of air dilution that occurs when peak inspiratory flow exceeds total flow delivered to a tracheal tube. If aerosol particles can be seen leaving the extension tube throughout inspiration, air dilution of the F_{IO_2} is not occurring. Air dilution is more difficult to control with other types of attachments such as tracheostomy collars, face tents, and aerosol masks. When the air-entrainment nebulizer is used with tracheal tubes, the gas must be humidified at 100% body humidity (100% relative humidity at 37°C). Thus, many of these nebulizers have provisions for heating the inspired gas, and water commonly collects in the wide-bore delivery tubing as the gas cools on the way to the patient. The water that collects in the tubing impedes gas flow and causes the pressure proximal to the entrainment port to increase, which causes less air to mix with oxygen. The results of this downstream impedance are that F_{IO_2} increases and total gas flow decreases.

(Q) What is the total flow that occurs when an air-entrainment nebulizer is set at an F_{IO_2} of 0.60 and an oxygen flow of 15 L/min?

a. 15 L/min 374 b
b. 25 L/min 375 a
c. 30 L/min 375 c

FRAME 204. AIR-ENTRAINMENT MASKS

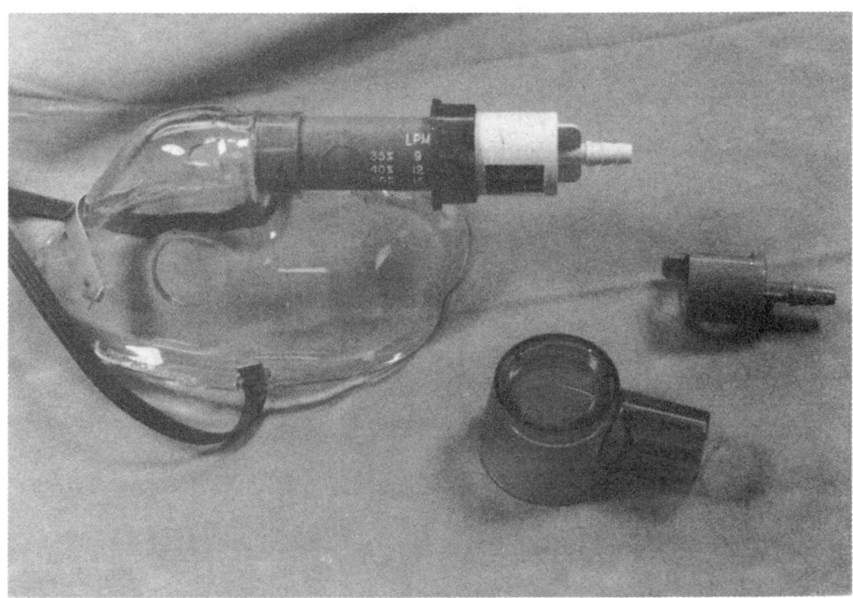

Figure 13–10 Variable FIO_2 air-entrainment mask. (Source: Barnes, TA: Respiratory Care Practice. Year Book Medical Publishers, Chicago, 1988. Used with permission.)

Air-entrainment masks are used when high flow rates are needed to meet the inspiratory demands of patients with fast respiratory rates and large tidal volumes. A consistent FIO_2 can be delivered to patients who frequently change their breathing pattern. These masks can deliver an FIO_2 with a range of 0.24 to 0.50 with total gas flow that varies from 33 L/min (0.50) to 97 L/min (0.24). (See Fig. 13–10.) The high total flow to the face and accurate control of low oxygen concentrations make this mask a good choice for patients with chronic obstructive pulmonary disease. These patients may hypoventilate if exposed to moderate-to-high FIO_2 levels.

The principles that allow air-entrainment masks to deliver an accurate FIO_2 are (1) the size of the jet orifice and entrainment port determine the amount of air mixed with oxygen, (2) downstream impedance will raise the pressure proximal to entrainment ports and reduce the amount of air mixed with oxygen, and (3) any condition that reduces air entrainment will lower total flow. The smaller the jet, the lower the pressure that will be generated proximal to the entrainment ports, and more air will be mixed with oxygen to produce a lower FIO_2 and higher total flow. Reducing the size of the entrainment port will limit the amount of air that can be mixed with the oxygen jet stream at any proximal pressure, will increase the FIO_2, and will decrease total flow. A larger jet size may be used with masks that are designed to deliver higher FIO_2, such as 0.50, since the velocity of gas leaving the jet will be lower, proximal pressure will be lower, and less air will be entrained. An alternative design is to make the jet size and velocity constant and to vary the size of the entrainment ports.

Disadvantages of air-entraiment masks are (1) entrainment ports can become occluded and raise FIO_2, (2) a false sense of security may occur if total mask flow does not meet the patient's inspiratory flow demands, (3) a humidity deficit may be created if only a bubble humidifier is used, (4) they are uncomfortable when used for long periods, and (5) downstream impedance may raise FIO_2.

(Q) Which of the following would be the result of increasing the oxygen flow to an air-entrainment mask designed to deliver an FIO_2 of 0.50?
  a. Total flow will increase and FIO_2 will remain the same. 374 D
  b. Total flow will increase and FIO_2 will increase. 375 D
  c. Total flow will decrease and FIO_2 will increase. 374 d

374A (from page 368, frame 200)
Correct. A minute volume of 4 L is lower than normal, and the smaller tidal volume will mix less air with the oxygen that has accumulated in the pharynx. This will result in a higher F_{IO_2}. Please continue on page 369, frame 201.

374B (from page 369, frame 201)
Wrong. A higher flow would be necessary to decrease the amount of air that leaks in around the mask. Return to page 369, frame 201, and select another answer.

374C (from page 370, frame 202)
Wrong. A partial rebreathing mask can deliver an F_{IO_2} of only 0.35 to 0.60 and may deliver much lower oxygen concentrations if air leaks in where the mask contacts the face. This air dilution is most likely to occur when the ventilatory pattern is abnormal, which is often the case with severe hypoxemia. Return to page 370, frame 202, and select another answer.

374D (from pages 372–373, frame 204)
Correct. The mixing ratio of air to oxygen (1.7 : 1) will stay the same and the F_{IO_2} will not change. However, since the source gas is higher, the total flow will increase proportionately. The total increase in flow can be calculated by adding both parts of the ratio together (1.7 + 1 = 2.7) and then multiplying the sum by the increase in oxygen flow. Please continue on pages 376–377, frame 205.

374a (from page 369, frame 201)
Correct. Oxygen flow to a partial rebreathing mask should be set high enough to keep the reservoir bag from deflating during inspiration. An F_{IO_2} of 0.60 is the upper end of the range for this type of mask and a flow of 10 L/min should be the minimum used. A flow higher than 10 L/min should be used if the bag collapses during inspiration. Please continue on page 370, frame 202.

374b (from page 371, frame 203)
Wrong. The air-to-oxygen mixing ratio is 1 : 1 and source gas alone is 15 L/min. Return to page 371, frame 203, and select another answer.

374c (from page 368, frame 200)
Wrong. A minute volume of 4 L is lower than normal and the smaller tidal volume will be composed of less air and more oxygen that has accumulated in the pharynx. Return to page 368, frame 200, and select another answer.

374d (from pages 372–373, frame 204)
Wrong. The mixing ratio of air to oxygen (1.7 : 1) will stay the same and since the source gas is higher, the total flow will increase proportionately. The total increase in flow can be calculated by adding both parts of the ratio together (1.7 + 1 = 2.7) and then multiplying the sum by the increase in oxygen flow. What will be the result on the F_{IO_2} if the mixing ratio stays the same? Return to pages 372–373, frame 204, and try again.

375A (from page 368, frame 200)
Wrong. A minute volume of 4 L is lower than normal and the smaller tidal volume will mix less air with the oxygen that has accumulated in the pharynx. Return to page 368, frame 200, and select another answer.

375B (from page 369, frame 201)
Wrong. An oxygen flow of 12 L/min may be too high when the ventilation pattern and peak inspirtory flow are normal. Return to page 369, frame 201, and select another answer.

375C (from page 370, frame 202)
Correct. The tighter seal possible with an anesthesia mask, the larger oxygen reservoir, and the higher-quality one-way valves may result in an F_{IO_2} of 1.00 provided the peak flow is not too high. Please continue on page 371, frame 203.

375D (from pages 372–373, frame 204)
Wrong. The mixing ratio of air to oxygen (1.7 : 1) will stay the same, and since the source gas is higher the total flow will increase proportionately. The total increase in flow can be calculated by adding both parts of the ratio together ($1.7 + 1 = 2.7$) and then multiplying the sum by the increase in oxygen flow. What will be the result on the F_{IO_2} if the mixing ratio stays the same? Return to pages 372–373, frame 204, and try again.

375a (from page 371, frame 203)
Wrong. The air-to-oxygen ratio is 1 : 1 and the source gas is 15 L/min. Return to page 371, frame 203, and select another answer.

375b (from page 370, frame 202)
Wrong. A non-rebreathing mask can deliver an F_{IO_2} of only 0.55 to 0.70 and may deliver much lower oxygen concentrations if air leaks in where the mask contacts the face. This air dilution is most likely to occur when the ventilatory pattern is abnormal, which is often the case with severe hypoxemia. Return to page 370, frame 202, and select another answer.

375c (from page 371, frame 203)
Correct. The air-to-oxygen entrainment ratio is 1 : 1 and the source gas is 15 L/min. The two parts of the ratio are added together ($1 + 1 = 2$) and multiplied by the source gas flow to calculate the total flow ($2 \times 15 = 30$). Please continue on pages 372–373, frame 204.

FRAME 205. OXYHOODS

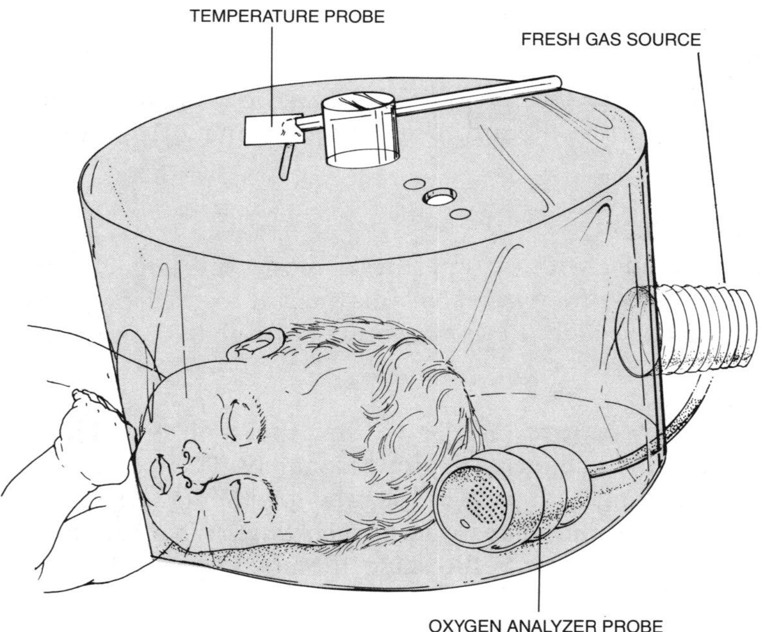

Figure 13–11

Oxyhoods are used with neonates and small infants to administer controlled amounts of oxygen and heated humidification. They cover only the head and allow access to the rest of the body. Oxygen is delivered to the hood by wide-bore tubing from a heated humidifier (cascade, wick, pass-over, or large-volume nebulizer), which must deliver the gas mixture at a temperature that is neither too hot nor too cool. The hood temperature should be monitored continuously and maintained at a thermally neutral temperature. For example, if the oxyhood is used inside an Isolette, the Isolette and hood temperature should be the same. Total gas flow should exceed 7 L/min to wash out carbon dioxide that accumulates under the hood. Since oxygen can layer within the hood with highest concentration found at the base, an oxygen analyzer with high and low alarm settings should be in continuous use with the sensor placed near the infant's face (Fig. 13–11).

Air-entrainment devices should not be used with oxyhoods because the noise they create is close to the danger limit of 65 dB, which may cuase a hearing loss in the infant. A blender can be used to supply source gas to a large nebulizer set on 100% (without air entrainment), cascade, wick, or pass-over humidifier. If a blender is not available and a large mainstream nebulizer must be used, then a bleed-in adapter connected to the nebulizer port can be used to mix oxygen and air with the air-entrainment port closed. The air and oxygen flowmeters should be adjusted not only to deliver the desired F_{IO_2} but must also provide a combined flow greater than 7 L/min. When two flowmeters are used, it will take a few minutes for the oxygen concentration to stabilize. An alternate source of oxygen therapy should be available in case the oxyhood needs to be removed.

The oxyhood is a simple device that, if proper care is taken, should be relatively trouble free. However, besides continuous monitoring of F_{IO_2} and temperature, often a pulse oximeter or transcutaneous oxygen monitor is also used to ensure against hypoxemia or complications of oxygen. The appropriate size hood should be used so that there is enough space for the infant to be comfortable. Disposable hoods are available, and using the right size will avoid necrosis around the infant's neck.

(Q) Which of the following would be the best gas source for an oxyhood?
- a. a heated nebulizer set on 40% with oxygen flow of 10 L/min 384 c
- b. 4 L/min from a blender (F_{IO_2} 0.40) with a cascade humidifier 390 a
- c. a heated nebulizer set on 100%, using air as a source gas and oxygen bleed into the nebulizer to deliver an F_{IO_2} of 0.40 and a total flow to the oxyhood of 10 L/min 384 A

FRAME 206. INCUBATORS

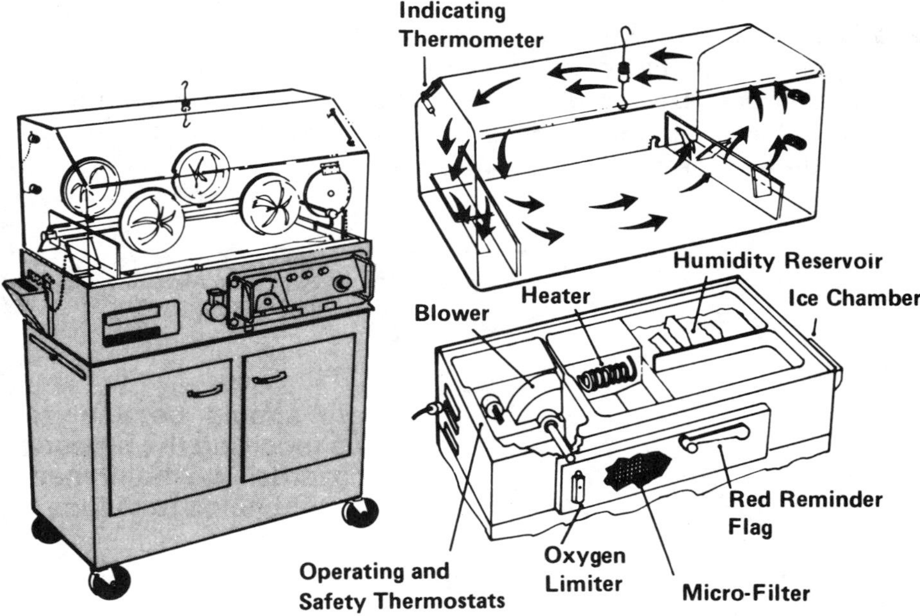

Figure 13–12

Incubators are designed to control temperature, humidity, and oxygen concentration, and to filter incoming gas (Fig. 13–12). They are used primarily with infants born prematurely. Controlling the oxygen concentration inside incubators is difficult because of the relatively large volume and because the opening of the access ports dilutes the accumulated oxygen. Oxygen is added to the incubator via a nipple adapter from a flowmeter. The appropriate F_{IO_2} is a result of a recommended liter flow. Some incubators have systems to limit the flow of oxygen into the chamber and thus limit oxygen concentration to a maximum of 0.40. This was done to reduce the risk of retrolental fibroplasia from a high F_{IO_2}. A red paddle on the back must be elevated to allow oxygen to enter at higher flow rates, which potentially can result in oxygen concentrations that range from 0.60 to 0.70. When an F_{IO_2} greater than 0.30 is needed, the safest method is to use an oxyhood inside the incubator (see frame 205). An Oxygen In Use sign should be prominently displayed on the side of the incubator to encourage the nursing staff to keep the ports closed. Another disadvantage of the incubator, besides difficulty in controlling F_{IO_2}, is the increased risk of bacterial growth inside the incubator because of the moist, warm, oxygen-enriched environment.

(Q) What is the highest F_{IO_2} that can be achieved when the red flag is *not* displayed on an incubator?

a. 0.70 if the ports are closed most of the time 384 B
b. 0.50 if the ports are opened frequently 385 A
c. 0.40 if the ports are closed most of the time 390 b

FRAME 207. OXYGEN TENTS

THE CROUPETTE
(A MINIATURIZED OXYGEN TENT)

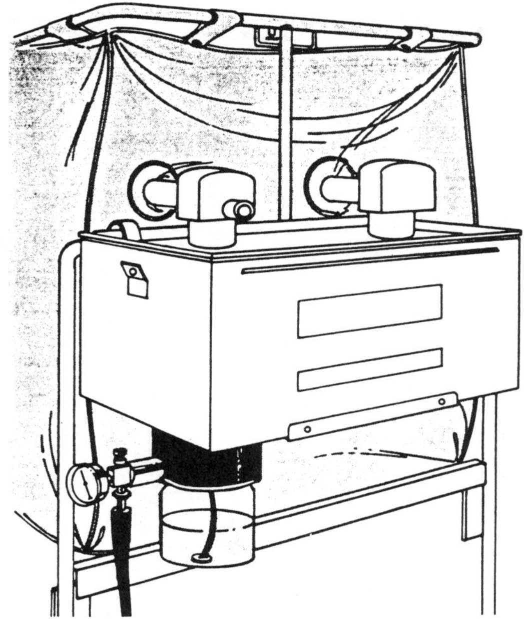

- ICE CHAMBER COOLING
- SELF-CONTAINED ATOMIZER
- PRODUCTION OF HIGH OXYGEN CONCENTRATION, IF NEEDED
- OPERATION BY COMPRESSED GAS SOURCE

Figure 13–13

Oxygen tents were used for both adult and pediatric patients prior to hospital air conditioning. The tents were used to provide the patient with an oxygen-enriched, temperature- and humidity-controlled environment. The oxygen concentration was generally limited to less than 50% because of problems with air leaking under the canopy. An oxygen flow 12 to 15 L/min was needed to wash out exhaled CO_2 and maintain an F_{IO_2} of 0.40 to 0.50.

Today tents are primarily used with pediatric patients who require a short-term high-humidity environment, such as those with croup or cystic fibrosis. Temperature control on some small tents, such as the Croupette (Fig. 13–13), is by ice. Gas is entrained through a duct surrounded by ice and water. Heat is absorbed and the gas is mixed with aerosol from a jet nebulizer and returned to the canopy. The Air-Shields Croupette model D for infants has an aerosol output of 0.8 to 1.3 mL/min and an F_{IO_2} of 0.45 to 0.55 when supplied with oxygen at 8 to 10 L/min. The ice in the chamber will reduce the temperature of the tent environment 7° to 10°F below room temperature. The larger Croupette model for children has an aerosol output of 1.3 ml/min and an F_{IO_2} of 0.45 to 0.55 when supplied with oxygen at 10 to 12 L/min. Use of ice in the chamber of the larger Croupette lowers the canopy temperature by 4° to 5°F below room temperature. Other manufacturers of pediatric and infant tents use a refrigeration cycle to cool the canopy. These tents with direct exposure of tent gas to refrigeration coils have the capability of lowering the canopy environment to 10° to 12°F below room temperature.

Fire is the biggest hazard when oxygen tents are used. The canopy should have three No Smoking signs and one should be readable from the inside. A No Smoking sign should be placed on the door to the patient's room, and visitors and other patients should be advised not to smoke. Static charge sparks, nurse call devices, toys, radios, electric razors, and other electric appliances are all potential fire starters and should be kept out of the canopy. Temperature and CO_2 wash-out problems may occur if young children stick stuffed animal or toys into ducts that circulate gas under the canopy.

(Q) What should be the minimum oxygen flow to a Croupette tent used with children?

a. 5 to 7 L/min 384 C
b. 8 to 10 L/min 385 B
c. 10 to 12 L/min 385 a

FRAME 208. CPAP DEVICES

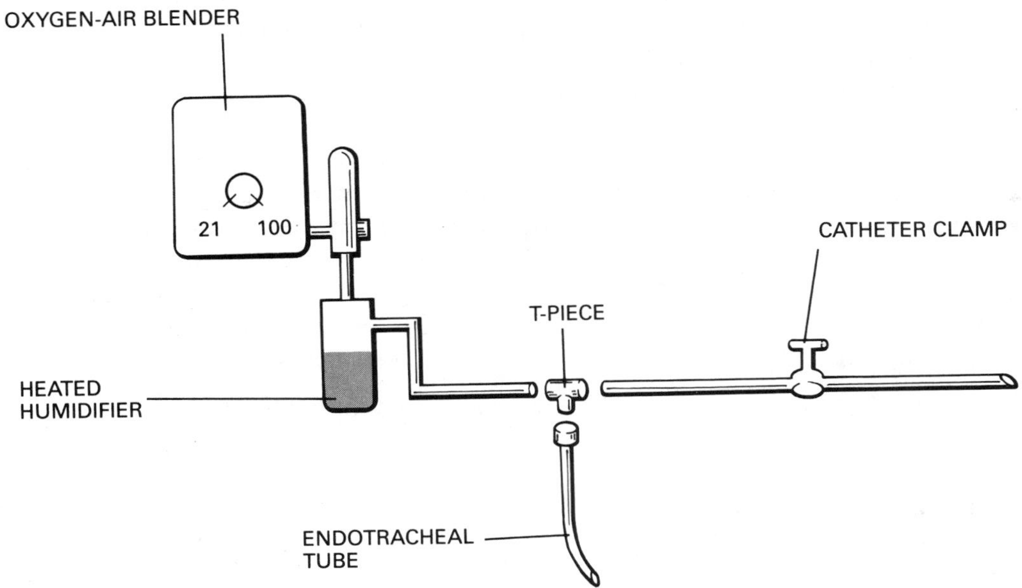

Figure 13–14 Simplified model of continuous positive-airway pressure (CPAP) system that uses a flow resistor.

The components of a representative CPAP system include (1) a blender to control F_{IO_2} and regulate the flow through the breathing circuit, (2) an oxygen monitor with a sensor placed in a dry part of the circuit before the humidifier, (3) a humidifier (heated if the system is used with an intubated patient), (4) a reservoir bag, (5) a one-way valve, (6) a thermometer (needed if humidifier is heated), (7) a pressure manometer, (8) a pressure-release valve, and (9) a threshold resistor. Many of the components may not be necessary for more basic applications, such as a nasal CPAP system used for obstructive sleep apnea, which may comprise only a blower unit, cushioned nasal mask, and spring-loaded positive end-expiratory pressure (PEEP) valve. A more sophisticated system will be required for infants with respiratory distress syndrome, high-permeability pulmonary edema, cardiogenic pulmonary edema, and weaning from mechanical ventilation.

The administration of CPAP by face mask may avoid tracheal intubation, with its potential to increase the risk of nosocomial infection and tracheal injury. CPAP masks should be cushioned and formfitting to create a leak-free seal with the face. If applied properly the mask can be relatively comfortable and safe. Complications include (1) vomiting and aspiration (do not use opaque black rubber anesthesia masks), (2) decreased ventricular filling pressure and increased pulmonary vascular resistance, (3) skin ulceration and facial trauma, and (4) eye trauma if the mask compresses the eye. An alternative to taut head straps is the use of a soft silicone elastomer mask in combination with high flow rates so that the prescribed level of CPAP can be maintained even with small leaks.

CPAP systems use either a threshold resistor or flow resistor. A threshold resistor uses a force such as a calibrated weight, a water column placed against a diaphragm, or one-way valve to prevent the airway pressure from falling below the CPAP level. A flow resistor creates back pressure at the airway by restricting flow through an orifice that is adjusted to the prescribed level of CPAP (Fig. 13–14). A demand valve system uses a threshold resistor because there is not a continuous flow of gas through the circuit. A continuous-flow CPAP system can use either a threshold resistor or flow resistor.

To reduce the work of breathing, positive airway pressure should be held constant during inspiration. A low-resistance system providing a high flow on demand (usually higher than 60 L/min for adults) during spontaneous breathing usually meets this requirement. The flow available is inadequate if the airway pressure, when observed at the patient connection during inspiration, falls by more than a few centimeters H_2O. Continuous-flow CPAP systems should have flow through the circuit equal to or exceeding the patient's peak inspiratory flow.

(Q) A CPAP system that uses a demand valve to supply inspiratory gas flow has what type of PEEP device?

a. flow resistor 384 a
b. threshold resistor 390 d
c. flow or threshold resistor 385 D

FRAME 209. MANUAL RESUSCITATORS

Manual resuscitators are commonly used to provide high oxygen concentrations and ventialtion during CPR, suctioning, and transport, and as a backup to mechanical ventilators. The basic components found with most manual resuscitators include (1) a bag, the compressible unit that is squeezed to deliver the tidal volume, (2) a patient valve, a one-way valve that directs gas to the patient connection and prevents rebreathing of exhaled gas, (3) a bag refill valve, which allows ambient air or oxygen to enter the bag during the expiratory phase, (4) an oxygen reservoir, which attaches to the bag refill valve to supply oxygen instead of air, (5) an auxiliary air intake valve, which allows the bag to refill if the oxygen reservoir is collapsed, (6) reservoir pressure release valve to prevent the oxygen reservoir from filling to the breaking point, and (7) a patient connection pressure release valve, which is used with infant models. An oxygen reservoir should always be used when high oxygen concentrations (≥0.85) are needed, since manual resuscitators with oxygen attached directly to the bag refill valve deliver an FIO_2 of only about 0.40.

When a resuscitator has to be used without a reservoir, slowing the bag refill time will allow less air to mix with oxygen and the FIO_2 delivered will increase up to about 70%. The best technique for slowing bag refill time is to apply hand pressure so that the bag is full only at the instant before the next compression. The oxygen flow to the resuscitator should always be at 15 L/min when ventilating adults, and it should always be higher than the minute volume being delivered. Seldom, if ever, is it necessary to use oxygen flows higher that 20 L/min, because high flow has little or no effect on increasing FIO_2. It is absolutely incorrect to turn an oxygen flowmeter to flush, since the flow can be as high as 50 L/min, which may lock the patient valve and cause high airway pressure.

Respiratory care practitioners should become familiar with the tidal volume that they can deliver with a one-hand squeeze of the bag compared with that of two hands. The average practitioner can deliver only 600 mL with one hand, compared with 800 mL with two hands. When "bagging" a patient using a mask, the volume leaking around the seal between the mask and the face should be considered, especially since only one hand will be available to squeeze the bag. It is important to use infant bags that have a large enough volume (300 to 400 mL) to compensate for the leaks. A pressure-release valve set to limit pressure to 40 cm H_2O and that can be turned off when higher pressures are needed should be used with infant manual resuscitators.

Several manual resuscitators are designed with large low-resistance non-rebreathing valves so that the patient can breathe spontaneously from the bag during transport. If a non-rebreathing mask is not available in emergency situations, allowing the patient to breathe from a resuscitator will provide oxygen therapy with a high FIO_2.

(Q) What is the best way to ensure the highest FIO_2 when using a manual resuscitator without an oxygen reservoir?

a. Turn the oxygen flowmeter to flush. 384 b
b. Retard the refill of the bag. 384 D
c. Turn the oxygen flowmeter to 20 L/min. 385 C

384A (from pages 376–377, frame 205)
Correct. The combined flow of 10 L/min should be enough to wash out exhaled CO_2. Since there is no air-entrainment, noise should not be a problem. Finally running the nebulizer with air and titrating the oxygen allows the FIO_2 to be controlled. Please continue on page 378, frame 206.

384B (from page 378, frame 206)
Wrong. When the red flag is down (not displayed), the oxygen flow through the oxygen nipple is limited. Return to page 378, frame 206, and select another answer.

384C (from pages 379–380, frame 207)
Wrong. The oxygen flow is inadequate to wash out exhaled CO_2. Return to pages 379–380, frame 207, and select another answer.

384D (from page 383, frame 209)
Correct. Slowing the refill time will allow less air to mix with oxygen and the delivered oxygen concentration may rise as high as 70%. Please continue on page 386, frame 210.

384a (from pages 381–382, frame 208)
Wrong. A flow resistor needs a continuous flow through the circuit to create CPAP. A demand valve provides flow through the circuit only during inspiration. Return to pages 381–382, frame 208, and select another answer.

384b (from page 383, frame 209)
Wrong. Setting the oxygen flowmeter to flush may result in flow rates as high as 50 L/min, which could lock the patient valve and expose the airways to high pressure. Return to page 383, frame 209, and try again.

384c (from pages 376–377, frame 205)
Wrong. The noise created by air entrainment would approach the 65 dB danger threshold for hearing loss. The combined flow of 40 L/min would be too high and might cause hypothermia and an increased oxygen consumption. Return to pages 376–377, frame 205, and select another answer.

384d (from pages 388–389, frame 212)
Correct. The polarographic analyzer can be used for continuous monitoring of FIO_2 with high and low alarm settings. Remember to place the sensor in a dry part of circuit before the humidifier and to calibrate the analyzer on 21% and 100% oxygen at regular intervals. Please continue on page 391 and complete the chapter exercises.

385A (from page 378, frame 206)
Wrong. When the red flag is down (not displayed), the oxygen flow through the inlet nipple is limited. Return to page 378, frame 206, and select another answer.

385B (from pages 379–380, frame 207)
Wrong. This is the amount of oxygen flow that you would use on the smaller model D Croupette, designed for use with infants. The model D Croupette tent has a smaller canopy volume than the larger Croupette used with older children. Return to pages 379–380, frame 207, and select another answer.

385C (from page 383, frame 209)
Wrong. Turning the oxygen flow from 15 to 20 L/min will not raise the delivered oxygen concentration by any significant amount unless the minute volume is greater than 15 L. Return to page 383, frame 209, and select another answer.

385D (from pages 381–382, frame 208)
Wrong. A flow resistor needs a continuous flow through the circuit to create CPAP. A demand valve provides flow through the circuit only during inspiration. Return to pages 381–382, frame 208, and select another answer.

385a (from pages 379–380, frame 207)
Correct. This is the amount of oxygen flow that you would use on the larger model Croupette tent designed for use with older children. This model has a larger canopy volume than the smaller model D Croupette used with infants. Accordingly, the larger model requires a higher oxygen flow to wash out exhaled CO_2. Please continue on pages 381–382, frame 208.

385b (from page 386, frame 210)
Wrong. The Bird Mark 7 powered with oxygen and set for air entrainment will deliver oxygen concentrations that can vary form 0.60 to 0.90 depending on the amount of back pressure. A COPD patient with chronic hypercarbia and a hypoxic respiratory drive will have breathing depressed by an F_{IO_2} this high. Return to page 386, frame 210, and select another answer.

385c (from pages 388–389, frame 212)
Wrong. The thermoconductivity analyzer could be used for a spot check, but could not be used for continuous monitoring of F_{IO_2}. Return to pages 388–389, frame 212, and select another answer.

385d (from page 387, frame 211)
Wrong. Although this patient has a low pulse-oximeter reading of 85% and 2 g/dL of dysfunctional sulfhemoglobin, which the pulse oximeter will ignore in calculating saturation, one of the other patients has a lower oxygen content. Return to page 387, frame 211, and try again.

FRAME 210. IPPB MACHINES

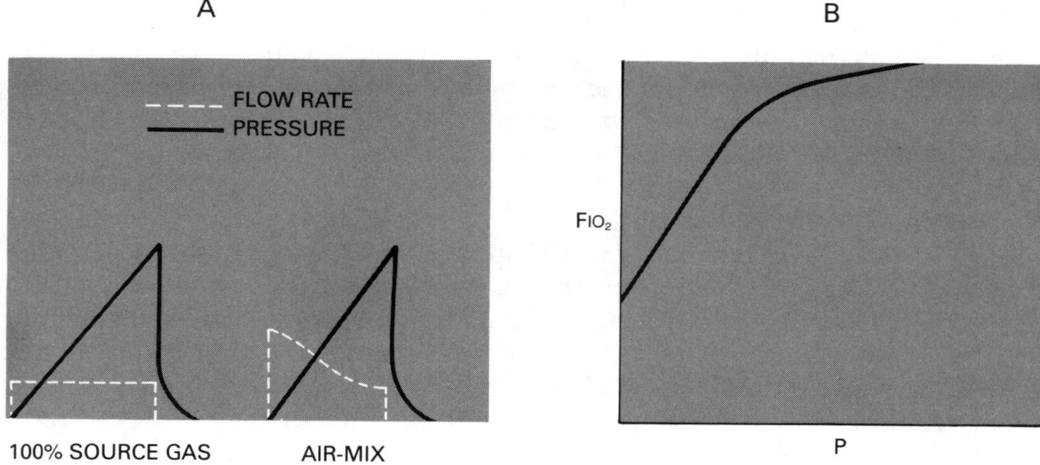

Figure 13–15 *(A)* the effect of the air-mix control on the inspiratory flow waveform of a Bird Mark 7; *(B)* the effect of the back pressure on the FIO_2 of a Bird Mark 7 when set on air dilution.

Intermittent positive-pressure breathing (IPPB) machines control delivered oxygen concentrations with air-entrainment devices that are affected by back pressure created by downstream impedance. For example, the Bird Mark 7 will deliver 100% oxygen when the air-mix control closes the Venturi system. When the Venturi is activated the FIO_2 will vary from 0.60 to 0.90 dependent on how much back pressure is encountered. When controlled oxygen concentrations are needed for chronically hypercarbic patients who breathe on a hypoxic drive, IPPB machines should be powered by compressed air at 50 psig and an oxygen reservoir attached to the air entrainment port. The FIO_2 can be controlled by monitoring the oxygen concentration with an analyzer and varying the amount of oxygen flow to the entrainment port reservoir. Operating the IPPB machine with source gas from a blender with no air entrainment will significantly decrease the peak flow rate. For example, the Bird Mark 7 has a peak flow of 0 to 80 L/min when the Venturi system is used and 0 to 40 L/min with the Venturi is closed (100% O_2 setting). Switching from air mix to 100% oxygen will cause the respiratory rate to decrease as a result of a longer inspiratory time.

The inspiratory flow will be constant and have a square wave flow pattern when the Bird Mark 7 is set to deliver 100% oxygen. When the Venturi is activated, the Mark 7 will deliver an FIO_2 that sharply increases during inspiration as back pressure decreases the amount of air entrained. (See Fig. 13–15.)

(Q) What is the best way to deliver an IPPB treatment to a dyspneic COPD patient using a Bird Mark 7?

a. Set air-mix control for 100% O_2, power Mark 7 with air. 390 A

b. Set air-mix control for entrainment, power Mark 7 with 100% O_2. 385 b

c. Set air-mix control for entrainment, power Mark 7 with air, and bleed oxygen into the entrainment port reservoir. 390 D

FRAME 211. PULSE OXIMETERS

Pulse oximeters use light absorption to continuously measure arterial saturation of hemoglobin with oxygen and pulse rate. Oxygen saturation is determined by comparing the amount of red light absorbed by deoxygenated hemoglobin with the amount of infrared light absorbed by oxygenated hemoglobin. Each heart beat brings a surge of oxygenated blood into the tissues. Pulse rate is determined by the change in saturation between heart beats. The sensor probe is usually placed over a toe or finger and consists of a light source and the receiver. Only functional hemoglobin is considered, which may lead to a false sense of security when other dysfunctional forms of hemoglobin are present, such as carboxyhemoglobin, sulfhemoglobin, and methemoglobin. Clinical situations in which abnormal forms of hemoglobin may be present include cases of smoke inhalation, heavy smoking, and exposure to automobile exhaust like that experienced by toll takers and tunnel policemen.

Two major advantages of pulse oximetry are that the monitoring can be continuous and noninvasive without the discomfort and risk of complications from serial arterial blood-gas studies. Other advantages are real-time saturation data, lack of need for calibration, ease of application, use with patients of all ages, and a reusable sensor. The pulse oximeters can be used to adjust oxygen therapy of home care patients. They can also be used to evaluate oxygen saturation during exercise, sleep, and rehabilitation studies. Application of oximetry include use during bronchoscopy, surgery, and emergency room screening.

The problems and disadvantages of pulse oximeters include a lack of understanding on the user's part about what the measurements represent. For example, the knowledge required to correctly interpret an Sao_2 reading includes an understanding of the shape of the oxyhemoglobin curve and a knowledge of which factors can shift the curve. Practitioners must be able to appreciate the large drop in oxygen tension that can occur with small changes in saturation. The oxygen-carrying capacity of the arterial blood can easily be overestimated if dysfunctional hemoglobin is not taken into account. Other disadvantages include inaccurate measurements when vasoactive drugs are used or when the patient is in shock. Elevated bilirubin concentrations greater than 10 mg/100 mL and bright light sources can also cause erroneous readings.

(Q) All of the following patients have a hemoglobin concentration of 15 g/dL. Which one has the lowest total oxygen content?

a. pulse oximeter 90% and 4 g/dL of carboxyhemoglobin — 390 B
b. pulse oximeter 85% and 2 g/dL of sulfhemoglobin — 385 d
c. pulse oximeter 85% and 2 g/dL deoxygenated hemoglobin — 390 c

FRAME 212. OXYGEN ANALYZERS

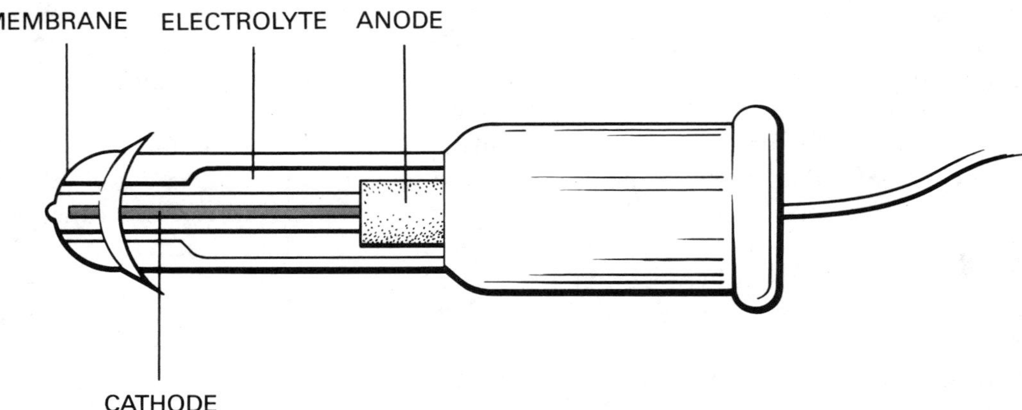

Figure 13–16 Clark electrode used with polarographic oxygen analyzers.

There is no substitute for confirming FIO_2 by monitoring the inspired oxygen concentration, preferably on a continuous basis but at a minimum at regular scheduled intervals. Commonly used analyzers can be grouped based on how they work: (1) paramagnetic principle, (2) thermoconductivity principle, and (3) polarographic and galvanic fuel cell.

Paramagnetic oxygen analyzers operate on the principle that oxygen increases the strength of a magnetic field. Nitrogen and other gases do not exhibit the paramagnetic properties of oxygen. Changes in the amount of oxygen in the sample chamber are measured by the effect of the magnetic field on a glass dumbbell suspended on a quartz wire that has a small mirror attached. The changes in the magnetic field will cause the wire to rotate and a light beam focused on the mirror is reflected to a translucent scale calibrated to read oxygen concentration. The changes in the magnetic field are in response to changes in the partial pressure of oxygen and the analyzer scale can be calibrated to read oxygen tension. If an FIO_2 scale is used, it must be corrected for changes in barometric pressure at higher altitudes such as is found in Denver. Since the gas sample is drawn through a drying tube of silica gel before it enters the analyzer, no correction is necessary for the partial pressure of water vapor. The analyzer can safely be used to measure FIO_2 in flammable gas mixtures. Paramagnetic oxygen analyzers are expensive and easily broken, and they cannot be used for continuous monitoring.

Thermoconductivity analyzers operate on the principle that increased concentrations of oxygen will dissipate more heat from a metallic resistor. The Wheatstone bridge has metallic resistors and the sample gas is exposed to only one of the resistors. Changes in resistance will create an imbalance in the circuit, causing a change in voltage, which can be calibrated to oxygen concentration. This type of oxygen analyzer is not suitable for measuring flammable gases. It is not accurate when the sample has gases other than nitrogen and oxygen.

Polarographic and galvanic oxygen analyzers both work on the principle that increased amounts of oxygen will increase a chemical reaction and cause increased electrical activity. The major advantage of this type of analyzer is that it can be used for continuous monitoring and sampling probes can be placed directly in the circuit. Polarographic oxygen analyzers work by having oxygen molecules diffuse through a semipermeable membrane into a potassium chloride electrolyte solution (Fig. 13–16). Both galvanic and polarographic analyzers produce electrical current flow when oxygen causes a reduction reaction to occur. The reduction reaction takes place at the charged cathode and the more oxygen molecules that migrate to the cathode, the more electrons will be generated. The sensor is made of platinum or gold and the anode of silver-silver chloride. Galvanic cells generate current when oxygen molecules are reduced at a gold cathode and move to a lead anode through a cesium hydroxide electrolyte solution. The precautions that should be taken when using polarographic or galvanic cells include placing sensors in a dry part of the circuit. Most analyzers are calibrated on dry gas; humidified gas will lower the oxygen concentration. Polarographic analyzers must be periodically calibrated on room air and 100% oxygen and are accurate to within ± 2% and a few brands to ± 1%. The most common reasons why they fail to calibrate are (1) torn membranes, (2) not enough electrolyte, or (3) dead or low battery charge. Both galvanic and polarographic analyzers have sensor and battery combinations that have limited life spans and need to be periodically checked and replaced.

(Q) Which of the following types of oxygen analyzers would be best to check the F_{IO_2} of a ventilator?

a. paramagnetic analyzer 390 C
b. thermoconductivity analyzer 385 c
c. polarographic analyzer 384 d

390A (from page 386, frame 210)
Wrong. Powering the Bird Mark 7 on compressed air will prevent high oxygen concentrations from depressing the patient's breathing. However, a patient who is dyspneic will need a higher peak inspiratory flow than the Mark 7 can deliver when set to deliver 100% O_2 (e.g., with no air entrainment). Return to page 386, frame 210, and select another answer.

390B (from page 387, frame 211)
Correct. Although this patient has the highest pulse-oximeter reading, 4 g/dL of dysfunctional carboxyhemoglobin are present, which the pulse oximeter ignores. If the dysfunctional hemoglobin is considered, the saturation drops to approximately 70%, which would leave this patient in severe hypoxemia. Please continue on pages 388–389, frame 212.

390C (from pages 388–389, frame 212)
Wrong. The paramagnetic analyzer can be used for spot checks but is not capable of continuously monitoring F_{IO_2}. Return to pages 388–389, frame 212, and select another answer.

390D (from page 386, frame 210)
Correct. A COPD patient with chronic hypercarbia and a hypoxic respiratory drive may have breathing depressed by a high F_{IO_2}. A dyspneic patient will need a higher peak inspiratory flow than the Mark 7 can deliver when set to deliver 100% O_2 (e.g., with no air entrainment). Please continue on page 387, frame 211.

390a (from pages 376–377, frame 205)
Wrong. The flow to the oxyhood should exceed 7 L/min to wash out exhaled CO_2. A blender can be used to control F_{IO_2}. The cascade does have the advantage of quiet operation and provides 100% body humidity. Return to pages 376–377, frame 205, and select another answer.

390b (from page 378, frame 206)
Correct. When the red flag is down (not displayed), the oxygen flow through the inlet nipple is limited and the F_{IO_2} will be no higher than 0.40. When the red flag is displayed, the oxygen flow through the inlet nipple can be higher and the F_{IO_2} may be as high as 0.60 to 0.70. However, the wide fluctuations in oxygen concentrations observed with incubators is of concern. An oxyhood should be used when an F_{IO_2} greater than 0.30 is needed. Please continue on page 379, frame 207.

390c (from page 387, frame 211)
Wrong. Although this patient has a below-normal oxygen saturation, there is no dysfunctional hemoglobin reported. The patient has a higher oxygen content than the other two patients. Return to page 387, frame 211, and select another answer.

390d (from pages 381–382, frame 208)
Correct. A threshold resistor is needed with demand-valve-type CPAP, since flow through the circuit occurs only during inspiration. A flow resistor needs a continuous flow through the circuit to create CPAP. Continue on page 382, frame 209.

EXERCISES

1. Determine the size and number of oxygen cylinders necessary to transport a patient by ambulance to another hospital 2 hours away if the oxygen flow is 10 L/min.
2. If a full H-cylinder has a single-stage regulator attached with an inlet valve with a cross-sectional area of 1 mm^2 and the surface of the pressure regulator diaphragm is 40 mm^2, calculate the outlet pressure.
3. Identify two situations in which a Bourdon gauge flowmeter would be more appropriate than a Thorpe tube flowmeter.
4. What effect will condensed water in compressed air piping systems have on blenders?
5. List two advantages that a simple oxygen mask has over a nasal cannula.
6. Describe the effect of changes in tidal volume and respiratory rate on the FIO_2 delivered by a nasal cannula.
7. Compare and contrast the differences in design of the partial rebreathing and non-rebreathing masks.
8. Describe how the size of the oxygen jet and air-entrainment port on the Venturi mask can affect FIO_2.
9. Describe two situations in which an air-entrainment nebulizer would deliver a FIO_2 that is higher than expected.
10. List five potential complications that may result from the use of oxyhoods.
11. Describe why oxyhoods are often used inside incubators.
12. List five electrical appliances that children are likely to bring into oxygen tents that may cause a fire.
13. Diagram and label nine components used in a CPAP system.
14. Explain how you would modify a Bird Mark 7 to safely administer IPPB to a COPD patients on low-flow oxygen therapy.
15. Describe the factors that affect the oxygen concentration delivered by a manual resuscitator.
16. List three advantages of oxygen analyzers that work on the polarographic principle versus the paramagnetic or thermoconductivity principle.
17. List three problems that commonly cause polarographic oxygen analyzers to read inaccurately.
18. Describe the problems that may occur as a result of pulse oximeters not measuring the amount of dysfunctional hemoglobin.
19. Explain how pulse oximeters measure heart rate.
20. What conclusion can be made regarding a pulse oximeter that has a pulse rate substantially lower than the radial pulse?

POSTTEST

This test is designed to evaluate what you have learned from Chapter 13. Check your answers on page 394 and review the topics where your answer is incorrect.

1. How long will a full H-cylinder last if the oxygen flow is 1 L/min?
   A. 6 hours
   B. 11 hours
   C. 21 hours
   D. 4 days, 19 hours
   E. 5 days, 12 hours
2. Oxygen regulators have pressure-relief valves that vent gas at pressures exceeding
   A. 20 to 40 psig.
   B. 40 to 60 psig.
   C. 50 to 100 psig.
   D. 140 to 200 psig.
   E. 500 to 1000 psig.
3. Which of the following is true regarding Bourdon gauge flowmeters?
   I. Placement of the flow valve on the outlet side guarantees accurate readings.
   II. Bourdon gauges have a fixed outlet orifice.
   III. Downstream impedance has the effect of reducing the size of the valve and lowering the output.
   IV. Flow will read accurately when downstream impedance is added.
   A. I only
   B. III only
   C. II and III only
   D. II and IV only
   E. I, II, III, and IV
4. Small variation in oxygen and air inlet pressure to a blender results in
   A. accurate F_{IO_2} delivered by the blender.
   B. inaccurate F_{IO_2} delivered by the blender.
   C. the reed alarm sounding continuously.
   D. damage to the blender.
   E. inaccurate flowmeter readings.
5. To achieve an F_{IO_2} that falls in the range of 0.30 to 0.50 with a simple mask, the oxygen flow should be
   A. 1 to 2 L/min.
   B. 2 to 4 L/min
   C. 4 to 6 L/min
   D. 6 to 10 L/min.
   E. 12 to 15 L/min.
6. An ideal patient with a tidal volume of 500 mL, a respiratory rate of 12/min, I:E ratio of 1:2, and receiving oxygen via a nasal cannula with oxygen flow of 4 L/min will receive an F_{IO_2} of
   A. 0.24.
   B. 0.30.
   C. 0.36.
   D. 0.40
   E. 0.46.
7. To achieve an F_{IO_2} in the range of 0.35 to 0.60 with a partial rebreathing mask the oxygen flow needed to keep the oxygen reservoir from collapsing is usually
   A. 2 to 4 L/min.
   B. 4 to 8 L/min.
   C. 6 to 10 L/min.
   D. 12 to 15 L/min.
   E. 15 to 20 L/min.

8. Which of the following is (are) true regarding the advantages of the anesthesia bag-valve-mask system over a disposable non-rebreathing mask?
   I. A higher FIO_2 can be achieved.
   II. The oxygen reservoir is bigger.
   III. The valves are more reliable.
   IV. The mask may make a better seal with the face.
   A. I only
   B. I and II only
   C. II and III only
   D. II, III, and IV only
   E. I, II, III, and IV

9. What is the lowest oxygen concentration usually available from air-entrainment nebulizers that have a continuously adjustable entrainment port?
   A. 0.24
   B. 0.28
   C. 0.30
   D. 0.35
   E. 0.40

10. Which of the following would increase the FIO_2 and decrease the total flow from an air-entrainment mask?
   A. Increase the diameter of the oxygen jet.
   B. Increase the number of air-entrainment ports on the mask.
   C. Increase oxygen flow to the mask.
   D. Attach an aerosol collar proximal to the air-entrainment ports.
   E. Decrease oxygen flow to the mask.

11. Which of the following are disadvantages of using a jet nebulizer with an oxyhood?
   I. It is dangerously noisy if air-entrainment is used.
   II. Aerosol particles act as a carrier for bacteria.
   III. It requires more oxygen flow.
   IV. It requires a blender to lower FIO_2.
   A. I only
   B. I and II only
   C. II and III only
   D. I, III, and IV only
   E. I, II, and III only

12. Which of the following are disadvantages of incubators?
   I. increased risk of bacterial growth inside the incubator
   II. difficult to control oxygen concentration
   III. ambient temperature too cool
   IV. inadequate removal of exhaled CO_2
   A. I only
   B. III only
   C. I and II only
   D. II, III, and IV only
   E. I, II, III, and IV

13. All of the following can start fires in oxygen tents *except*
   A. radios.
   B. electric razors.
   C. static sparks.
   D. books.
   E. toys.

14. Continuous-flow CPAP may use which of the following PEEP devices?
   I. flow resistor
   II. threshold resistor
   III. calibrated orifice
   A. I only
   B. II only
   C. III only
   D. I and II only
   E. I, II, and III

15. Pressure release valves on infant manual resuscitators should limit pressure to
    A. 25 cm H_2O.
    B. 30 cm H_2O.
    C. 35 cm H_2O.
    D. 40 cm H_2O.
    E. 50 cm H_2O.
16. Which of the following would be the best way to deliver an accurate and adjustable F_{IO_2} with a Bird Mark 7?
    A. Use oxygen to drive Mark 7 with air entrainment.
    B. Use blender to drive Mark 7 with no air entrainment.
    C. Use blender to drive Mark 7 with air entrainment.
    D. Use air to drive Mark 7 with gas entrained from an O_2 reservoir.
    E. Use air to drive Mark 7 with no air entrainment.
17. Which of the following pulse-oximeter values normally correlate with an arterial oxygen tension of 60 torr?
    A. 85%
    B. 90%
    C. 95%
    D. 97%
    E. 100%
18. A pulse oximeter measures heart rate by monitoring pulsatile changes in
    A. Sa_{O_2}.
    B. electrical activity.
    C. pulse pressure.
    D. heart sounds.
    E. temperature.
19. Which of the following O_2 analyzers work(s) best with dry sample gas?
    I. paramagnetic
    II. thermoconductivity
    III. polarographic
    IV. galvanic cell
    A. I only
    B. III only
    C. I and II only
    D. III and IV only
    E. I, III, and IV only
20. Which of the following types of oxygen analyzers work(s) by a reduction of oxygen molecules at a platinum or gold cathode?
    I. paramagnetic
    II. thermoconductivity
    III. polarographic
    IV. galvanic cell
    A. I only
    B. III only
    C. I and II only
    D. III and IV only
    E. II, III, and IV only

ANSWERS TO POSTTEST

1. D (F195)	5. D (F199)	9. C (F203)	13. D (F207)	17. B (F211)
2. D (F196)	6. C (F200)	10. A (F204)	14. E (F208)	18. A (F211)
3. C (F197)	7. C (F201)	11. B (F205)	15. D (F209)	19. E (F212)
4. A (F198)	8. E (F202)	12. C (F206)	16. D (F210)	20. D (F212)

BIBLIOGRAPHY

Aloan, CA: Respiratory Care of the Newborn: A Clinical Manual. JB Lippincott, Philadelphia, 1987.

Barnes, TA: Respiratory Care Practice. Year Book Medical Publishers, Chicago, 1988.

Eubanks, DH and Bone, RC: Comprehensive Respiratory Care, ed 2. CV Mosby, St. Louis, 1990.

Kirby, RR, Smith, RA, and Desautels, DA: Mechanical Ventilation. Churchill Livingstone, New York, 1985.

Koff, PB, Eitzman, DV, and Neu, J: Neonatal and Pediatric Respiratory Care. CV Mosby, St Louis, 1988.

Lucas, J, Golish, JA, Sleeper, G, and O'Ryan, JA: Home Respiratory Care. Appleton & Lange, Norwalk, 1988.

McPherson, SP: Respiratory Home Care Equipment. Daedalus Enterprises, Dallas, 1988.

McPherson, SP: Respiratory Therapy Equipment, ed 4. CV Mosby, St. Louis, 1990.

Riggs, JH: Respiratory Facts. FA Davis, Philadelphia, 1989.

Wilkins, RL, Sheldon, RL, and Krider, SJ: Clinical Assessment in Respiratory Care, ed 2. CV Mosby, St. Louis, 1990.

14

Humidity and Aerosol Therapy Equipment

213. Pass-over humidifiers
214. Bubble humidifiers
215. Cascade humidifiers
216. Heated wick humidifiers
217. Small-medication nebulizers
218. Metered-dose inhalers
219. Large mainstream nebulizers
220. Ultrasonic nebulizers
221. Babington nebulizers
222. Heat-moisture exchangers

PRETEST

This pretest is designed to measure what you already know about humidity and aerosol therapy equipment. Check your answers on page 399 and then continue on page 400, frame 213.

1. Humidity is produced by pass-over humidifiers by
   A. evaporation.
   B. Babington principle.
   C. hydronamic principle.
   D. cascade effect.
   E. a jet system.
2. Which of the following may be a limitation of pass-over humidifiers?
   A. volume of water held by reservoir
   B. control of inspired gas temperature
   C. transmission of nosocomial infection
   D. excessive noise level above 65 dB
   E. no provision for heating water in reservoir
3. Bubble humidifiers are normally *not* used unless oxygen flow exceeds
   A. 2 L/min.
   B. 4 L/min.
   C. 6 L/min.
   D. 8 L/min.
   E. 10 L/min.
4. Which of the following is true about jet humidifiers?
   A. The jet is below the surface of the water.
   B. No diffuser is necessary.
   C. Water is pulled up a capillary tube to the jet.
   D. Aerosol particles are created above the water level.
   E. Particles produced by the jet are broken by a baffle.
5. What factor may lower the efficiency of a cascade humidifier?
   A. F_{IO_2}
   B. PEEP/CPAP level
   C. tidal volume
   D. inspiratory flow rate
   E. inspiratory flow-wave pattern
6. How often should a Bennett Cascade I humidifier be checked?
   A. every 2 hours
   B. every 4 hours
   C. every 8 hours
   D. every 12 hours
   E. every 24 hours
7. What is the internal compliance of a Bird wick humidifier?
   A. 0.23 mL/cm H_2O
   B. 0.50 mL/cm H_2O
   C. 1.3 mL/cm H_2O
   D. 2.6 mL/cm H_2O
   E. 4.0 mL/cm H_2O
8. Heated wick humidifiers are capable of producing 100% body humidity with continuous flow up to
   A. 30 L/min.
   B. 40 L/min.
   C. 60 L/min.
   D. 80 L/min.
   E. 100 L/min.

9. What size aerosol particle is produced by disposable sidestream medication nebulizers?
   A. 0.1 to 1.0 μm
   B. 1 to 7 μm
   C. 5 to 10 μm
   D. 7 to 12 μm
   E. 10 to 15 μm

10. Which of the following are likely to affect the particle size produced by a small-medication nebulizer?
    I. mainstream versus sidestream placement
    II. flow rate to jet
    III. missing baffle
    IV. volume of medication used
    V. molecular weight of medication
    A. I only
    B. I and III only
    C. II and IV only
    D. III and V only
    E. I, II, III, IV, and V

11. The ratio of metered-dose inhaler (MDI) dose (2 to 3 puffs) compared with the dose given by inhalant-solution jet nebulizer treatment is
    A. 1:1.
    B. 1:5.
    C. 5:1.
    D. 1:10.
    E. 10:1.

12. Without the use of spacer or reservoir, an MDI will deliver what proportion of the aerosol droplets to the lung periphery?
    A. 10%
    B. 25%
    C. 40%
    D. 80%
    E. 90%

13. Water collecting in the delivery tubing of a large air-entrainment nebulizer will have which of the following effects?
    I. decrease F_{IO_2}
    II. decrease total flow
    III. decrease oxygen flow
    IV. decrease inspired-gas temperature
    V. decrease aerosol density
    A. I only
    B. II only
    C. I, IV, and V only
    D. II, III, and IV only
    E. I, II, III, IV, and V

14. Which of the following are true regarding large air-entrainment nebulizers?
    I. Aerosol particles grow in size after leaving an unheated nebulizer.
    II. Aerosol density will increase when F_{IO_2} is increased.
    III. Heating the nebulizer has no effect on body humidity produced.
    IV. Increased downstream resistance will increase F_{IO_2}.
    V. Increased downstream resistance will increase air entrainment.
    A. I and III only
    B. II and V only
    C. II and IV only
    D. IV and V only
    E. I, II, III, IV, and V

15. The size particle produced by an ultrasonic nebulizer depends on
    A. amplitude of the sound wave generated.
    B. radio frequency applied to the crystal.
    C. size of the nebulization cup.
    D. size of the couplant chamber.
    E. molecular weight of the solution nebulized.

16. Variables that may decrease the aerosol density produced by an ultrasonic nebulizer include which of the following?
    I. baffling and condensation in the tubing
    II. increase in carrier gas flow
    III. increase in viscosity of the solution
    IV. residue from soaps or plastics
    V. decreased fluid in the couplant chamber
    A. I and III only
    B. II and V only
    C. IV and V only
    D. I, III, and IV only
    E. I, II, III, IV, and V

17. Which of the following humidifiers produces aerosol particles with a high-pressure source exiting from a small hole in a glass sphere?
    A. Bird wick humidifier
    B. Babington nebulizer
    C. Ohmeda mainstream nebulizer
    D. Bennett Cascade humidifier
    E. Bird mainstream medication nebulizer

18. What size particle is produced by a hydronamic nebulizer?
    A. 0.1 to 1 μm
    B. 1 to 3 μm
    C. 3 to 5 μm
    D. 5 to 10 μm
    E. 10 to 15 μm

19. What is the maximum absolute humidity produced by a heat-moisture exchanger?
    A. 20 mg/L
    B. 25 mg/L
    C. 30 mg/L
    D. 35 mg/L
    E. 44 mg/L

20. What is the maximum pressure a heat-moisture exchanger should be able to tolerate without leaking when used with a ventilator?
    A. 40 cm H_2O
    B. 50 cm H_2O
    C. 60 cm H_2O
    D. 80 cm H_2O
    E. 100 cm H_2O

ANSWERS TO PRETEST

1. A (F213)
2. B (F213)
3. B (F214)
4. A (F214)
5. D (F215)
6. A (F215)
7. A (F216)
8. C (F216)
9. B (F217)
10. B (F217)
11. D (F218)
12. A (F218)
13. B (F219)
14. C (F219)
15. B (F220)
16. E (F220)
17. B (F221)
18. C (F221)
19. C (F222)
20. E (F222)

FRAME 213. PASS-OVER HUMIDIFIERS

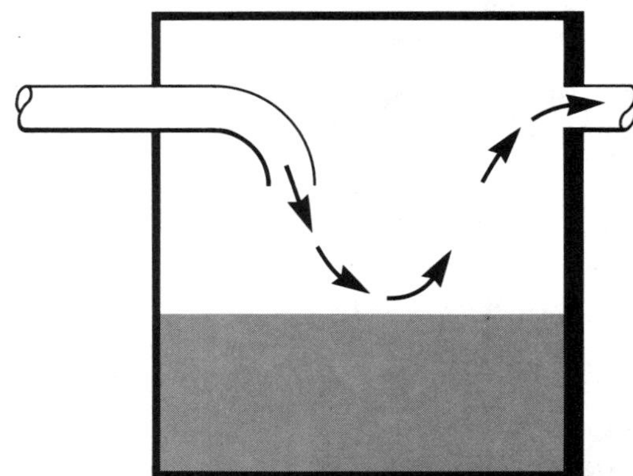

Figure 14–1

Pass-over humidifiers are used with the Emerson ventilator and with some models of incubators. Humidity is added by evaporation as gas travels across the surface of a water reservoir (Fig. 14–1). The humidifier is heated when used with a ventilator to increase the amount of evaporation, since warmer gas will hold more water vapor. The amount of humidity provided by pass-over humidifiers also depends on the surface area of the reservoir. Wick humidifiers, which are discussed in frame 216, enhance humidification by increasing the surface area for evaporation and by heating the gas.

One advantage of pass-over humidifiers is the ability to add water vapor rather than produce aerosol particles. If the reservoir of a nebulizer becomes contaminated with pathogens, the infection may be carried to the patient by airborne particles. A pass-over humidifier, since it does not produce an aerosol, will not transport pathogens from the reservoir to the patient. The quiet operation of pass-over humidifiers is an advantage when using the device with infants who may suffer a hearing loss when the background noise exceeds 65 dB.

Disadvantages of pass-over humidifiers include inadequate humidification for ventilator patients if the inspired gas is not heated to 32° to 34°C. A problem common to all heated humidifiers for ventilators is the collection water in the delivery tubing caused by condensation as the gas cools. One solution to this problem is to install water traps in the inspiratory and expiratory lines with one-way valves and effusion bags. Most often this problem is handled by frequent draining of the water from the delivery tubing into a disposable container. It is absolutely incorrect to drain the water in the tubing back into the reservoir, since this may contaminate the humidifier with pathogens from the tubing. Incubators with pass-over humidifiers must be carefully disinfected at periodic intervals and between patient use because the environment of a warm oxygen-enriched gas facilitates bacterial growth.

(Q) What level of humidity does a heated pass-over humidifier provide?

a. 70% body humidity	406 A
b. 36 mg/L of absolute humidity	406 b
c. 75% relative humidity at 37°C	407 A

FRAME 214. BUBBLE HUMIDIFIERS

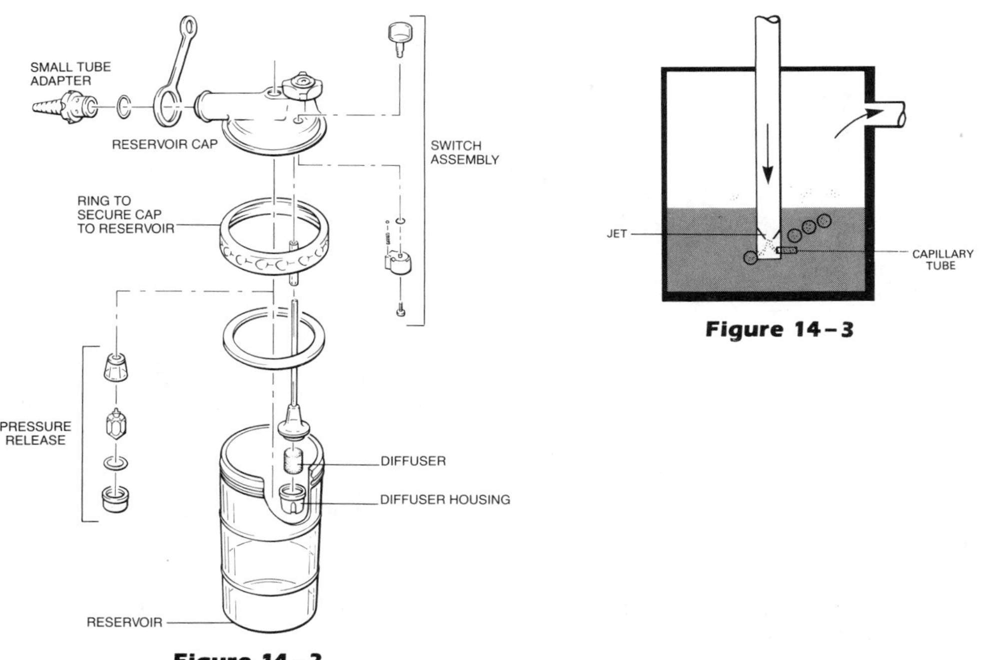

Figure 14–2 Assembly of Bennett Bubble-Jet humidifier.
Figure 14–3 Underwater jet humidifier.

Bubble humidifiers are used for humidification of oxygen delivered by nasal cannula or by mask. Bubble humidifiers are usually not used unless the oxygen flow is more than 4 L/min, since the proportion of dry oxygen to room air inhaled is small at low flow. The relative humidity at 37°C of these devices ranges from 30% to 40% depending on the flow. The typical bubble humidifier (Fig. 14-2) consists of a flowmeter, a small-bore down tube submerged in sterile water with a diffuser at the end, and a pressure-relief valve. The function of the diffuser is to cause the gas to be broken into very small bubbles, increasing the surface area and relative humidity. A high-pressure release valve is incorporated into the top of the humidifier. This valve will whistle and release gas when the pressure exceeds 2 pounds per square inch gauge. Occluding the outlet allows the pressure relief valve to be checked and ensures that gas is not leaking from the humidifier. The relief valve releases pressure and whistles or clicks when there is an obstruction in the tubing or when the oxygen flow is excessive.

Jet humidifiers are devices that mix water with oxygen through a jet system and force the aerosolized water through a diffuser. Gas travels through the down tube to a jet that is below the surface of the water; as gas streams through the jet, it pulls in water through an adjacent capillary tube on the side of the down tube. The aerosolized water is forced though a diffuser, and bubbles containing aerosol particles float to the surface. The gas within the bubbles contain more vapor because of the evaporation that occurs from the aerosol particles (Fig. 14–3).

(Q) The best way to ensure that a pressure relief valve works correctly is
a. to occlude the humidifier outlet. 406 B
b. to turn the oxygen flowmeter to flush. 407 C
c. to loosen the reservoir jar. 407 a

FRAME 215. CASCADE HUMIDIFIERS

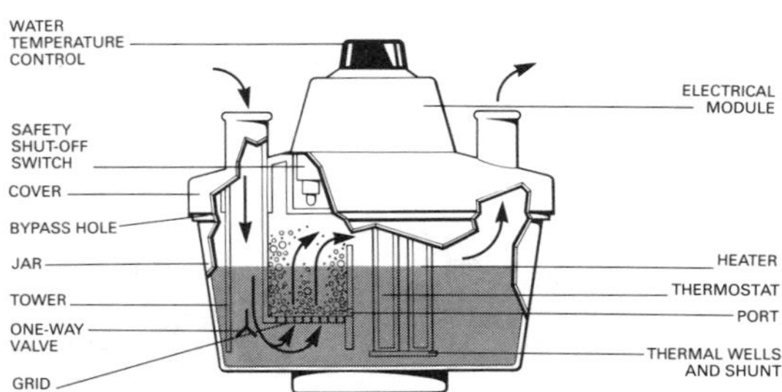

Figure 14–4

The main advantage of servo-controlled cascade-heated humidifiers is their ability to deliver 100% relative humidity at body temperature (37°C). Other considerations include (1) the device operates quietly, making it suitable for use with oxyhoods, (2) pathogens in the humidifier reservoir will not be carried to the patient, since aerosol particles are not generated, (3) the heating element can be servo-controlled to maintain a preset gas temperature (20° to 40°C) by means of a thermistor (sensor) at the proximal airway, (4) a high temperature alarm can be set, and (5) low water level results in an alarm function. A tower in the cascade humidifier channels the gas below the surface of the water and through a one-way valve. Water displaced by this gas flow raises the water level in the reservoir and causes water to enter through a port above the diffusion grid in the tower. Concurrently, gas exiting from the tower's one-way valve flows up through the grid and mixes with water to form a cascade of small bubbles. The cascade effect increases the surface area of the gas and water interface, which produces a relative humidity at body temperature of 80% to 100% at flows of 8 to 14 L/min.

The earlier Bennett Cascade I humidifier (Fig. 14-4) is not servo-controlled and must have its heating element manually adjusted using control numbers and an in-line thermometer proximal to the airway. The heating element must be set high enough so that gas is delivered at 32° to 37°C. Since the Bennett Cascade I does not have a low-water alarm, the reservoir water level needs to be checked at frequent intervals (e.g., ventilator checks every 2 hours). If the humidifier runs dry, super-heated gas may burn the patient's airway and the plastic reservoir jar may melt or burn if a thermoswitch in the heating element fails to shut off the power. If the heating element is adjusted properly, the inspiratory line will need to be frequently emptied of water that condenses as the gas cools.

A bypass hole in the tower of the cascade humidifier allows the patient to trigger an assisted breath. Without the hole in the tower the patient would have to generate an inspiratory effort equal to the depth of the water in the reservoir in addition to the effort required to trigger an assisted breath. A safety shut-off switch built into the heater control shuts off the power when the unit is removed from the heating element well.

(Q) When the reservoir of a Bennett Cascade I humidifier runs dry, which of the following is likely to happen?

a. A low-water alarm will sound. 406 C
b. A high-gas temperature alarm will sound. 406 d
c. A high-gas temperature may be delivered to the airways. 407 B

FRAME 216. HEATED WICK HUMIDIFIERS

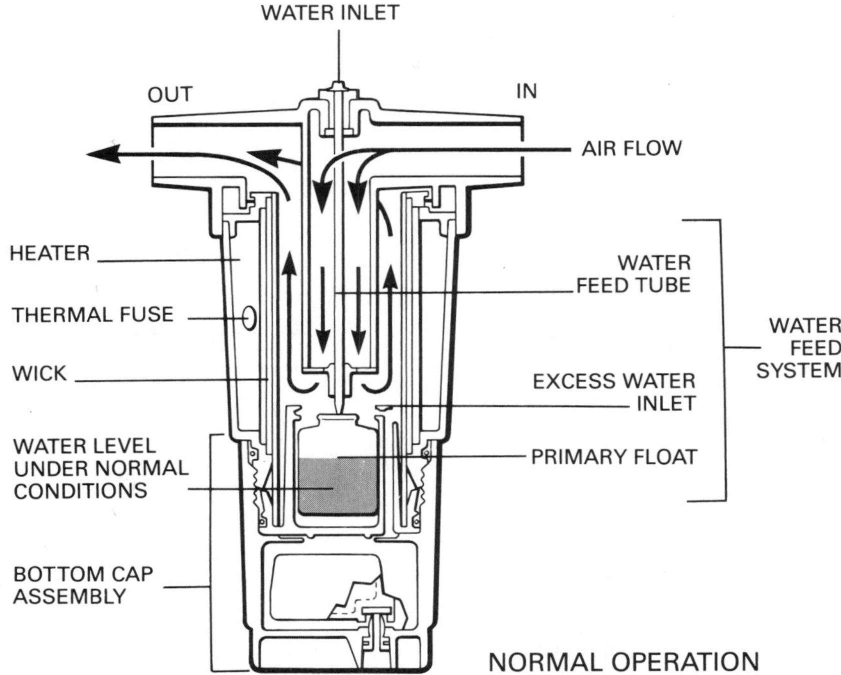

Figure 14–5 Internal components of the Bird humidifier.

The Bird wick humidifier is able to maintain 100% relative humidity at body temperature at continuous flow of up to 60 L/min. The wick absorbs water and is warmed by a cylindrical heating element. The gas flows around the wet cylinder-shaped wick, which provides a large surface area for evaporation. The ability to maintain 100% body humidity at high flow make this unit a good choice for continuous-flow intermittent mandatory ventilation (IMV) or continuous positive-airway pressure (CPAP). The internal volume of the Bird wick humidifier is significantly smaller than the cascade or pass-over devices, and the internal compliance is low. The internal compliance of the Bird wick humidifier (Fig. 14–5) is only 0.23 mL/cm H_2O, and the resistance is 0.3 cm H_2O at 60 L/min. The Bird wick humidifier is servo-controlled by a thermistor close to the airway.

Alarm systems are commonly incorporated into servo-controlled devices and provide an audiovisual warning when the proximal probe detects a high temperature (38° to 40°C). When a high temperature is sensed, the power to the heating element is turned off. Other features of the servo-controlled Bird wick humidifier are alarm modes for low temperature and probe unplug, and a digital temperature display.

(Q) Which of the following advantages does a Bird heated wick humidifier have over the heated Bennett Cascade II humidifier?

a. 100% relative humidity at body temperature at high flow 406 D
b. servo control of the proximal airway temperature 407 D
c. high-temperature alarm is operative 407 c

FRAME 217. SMALL-MEDICATION NEBULIZERS

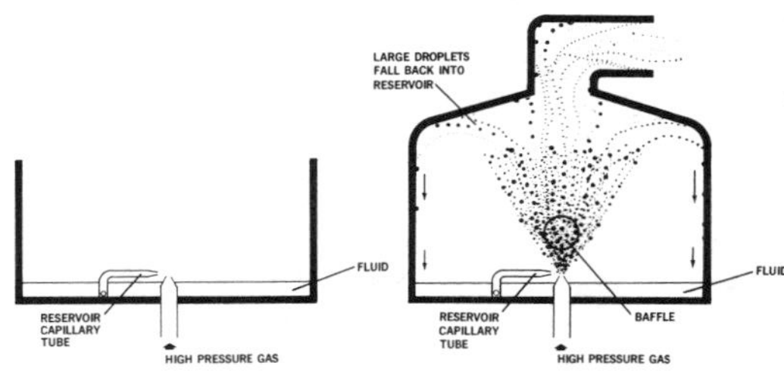

Figure 14–6 Schematic of a jet nebulizer: (*A*) production of a primary spray (e.g., atomizer); (*B*) baffling of droplets (medication nebulizer).

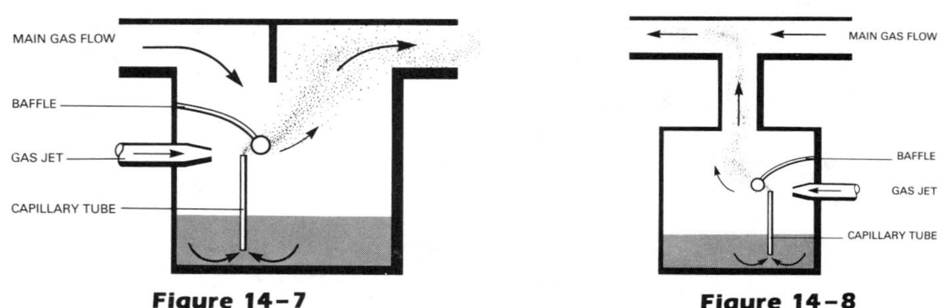

Figure 14–7 Mainstream nebulizers: (*A*) schematic of mainstream nebulizer; (*B*) cutaway of Bird micronebulizer.

Figure 14–8 (*A*) schematic of sidestream nebulizer; (*B*) cutaway of Bennett sidestream nebulizer.

Small-medication nebulizers are frequently used to deliver bronchoactive aerosol medications to the lung periphery. Disposable nebulizers are frequently used to limit the spread of nosocomial infections. The numerous brands of disposable nebulizers all have the following: a jet, capillary tube, baffle, small-volume medication cup of 5 to 30 mL, mouthpiece, and gas delivery tube. Baffles must be incorporated into the design of the nebulizer (Fig. 14–6) to produce particles in the therapeutic range of 1 to 10 μm. Two basic designs for jet medication nebulizers are mainstream (Fig. 14–7) and sidestream (Fig. 14–8).

Troubleshooting problems include ensuring that the capillary tube and jet are not plugged and adjusting the flow to the jet so that an adequate amount of aerosol is produced. Some medication nebulizers must be held in a vertical position to prevent spilling while others are designed with an antispill barrier to prevent loss of solution if the nebulizer is tipped or inverted during therapy. In order for the particle size to be small enough (1 to 5 μm) to reach the lung periphery, the nebulizer baffle must be in place. More evaporation and baffling will occur with sidestream nebulizers and they tend to produce smaller particles than mainstream medication devices. When particles leaving a medication nebulizer feel wet or fail to bounce off a glass surface, they are too large to reach the lung periphery. Disposable nebulizers are designed to nebulize 3 to 5 mL in 5 to 10 minutes when the source gas is 5 to 10 L/min.

(Q) What size aerosol droplets are commonly produced by disposable sidestream medication nebulizers?

a. 1 to 7 μm — 406 a
b. 4 to 10 μm — 407 b
c. 7 to 12 μm — 406 c

FRAME 218. METERED-DOSE INHALERS

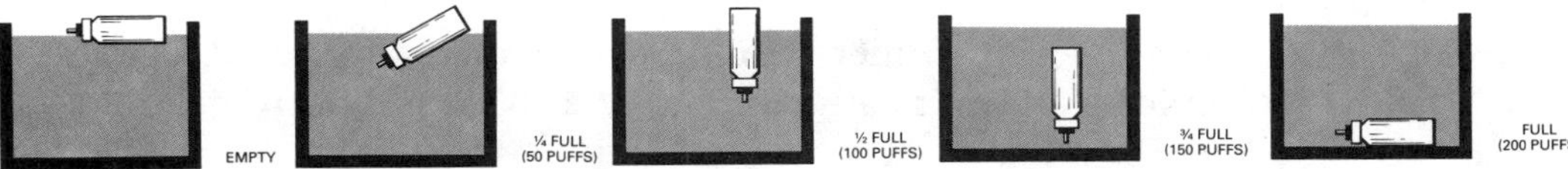

Figure 14–9 The amount of medication left in a metered-dose inhaler can be estimated by the position of the canister when placed in a bowl of water. The prescription should be refilled when the inhaler is one-quarter full.

Metered-dose inhalers (MDIs) are self-contained devices powered by an inert gas. Discharging the pressurized canister will provide a single dose of medication (a puff). A full canister usually contains 200 puffs. The number of puffs remaining in an MDI can be estimated by floating the canister in water (see Fig. 14–9). The inhaler should be shaken before use, held with the metal canister on top, and placed 1½ inches in front of an open mouth. The canister is pressed down with the index finger after a slow, deep inhalation has begun, and a breath-hold period lasting 10 seconds should be followed by exhaling through pursed lips. Disposable sidestream medication nebulizers deliver varying amounts of inhalant solution, e.g., from 0.15 to 0.85 mL/min with a significant amount lost during exhalation. The equivalent MDI dose is ¹⁄₁₀ that given with an inhalation-solution treatment. Table 14–1 shows the corresponding dose for MDI versus delivery with sidestream medication nebulizers.

Holding an MDI 4 cm (1½ in) away from the mouth and starting inhalation before discharging the aerosol reduces the amount of aerosol impacting in the oropharynx. A reservoir chamber or extension tube can be added to the MDI to reduce aerosol impaction in the mouth. These attachments require less coordination than holding the canister 4 cm away, aiming for the mouth, and actuating the canister after inhalation has begun. The extension chambers are available with a soft mask on the end for very young children. Several devices are available for attachment to the MDI that incorporate a reservoir/spacer, and a few have an incentive indicator for a deep breath and a pause. Deposition of aerosols in the periphery will be increased if the MDI is used with a breath hold of 10 seconds.

(Q) How many puffs from an MDI of metaproterenol (Alupent) would be equivalent to the typical dose administered by a disposable hand-held jet nebulizer?

a. 2 to 3 puffs — 412 a
b. 8 to 10 puffs — 412 C
c. 15 to 23 puffs — 413 D

TABLE 14-1 DOSES OF BRONCHODILATORS DELIVERED BY AEROSOLIZATION

Bronchodilators	Dose/Puff of MDI* (mg)	Typical Dose of Inhalant (mL)	Range Solution (mg)
Albuterol	0.09	0.25–0.5	1.2–2.5
Epinephrine	0.16–0.22	0.25	6
Isoetharine	0.34	0.25–0.5	2.5–5
Isoproterenol	0.08–0.13	0.25–0.5	2.5–5
Metaproterenol	0.65	0.20–0.30	10–15
Terbutaline	0.20	1–2	1–2

*The usual dose of a metered-dose inhaler (MDI) is 2 to 3 puffs. The corresponding dose from an inhalation-solution treatment is about 10 times as much for each bronchodilator. For each delivery system, about 10% of the dose is deposited in the lungs.

Source: Zimet, I: Editorial: A prescription for prescription writers. Respir Care 33:841–843, 1988. Used with permission.

406A (from page 400, frame 213)
Wrong. A heated pass-over humidifier should be able to be adjusted to deliver at least 82% body humidity (100% relative humidity at 33°C). Return to page 400, frame 213, and select another answer.

406B (from page 401, frame 214)
Correct. This is the most logical way to create enough pressure (greater than 2 psig) to check to see if the pressure-relief valve releases gas and whistles or clicks. If the pressure does not increase, the reservoir jar could be misthreaded, a gasket could be missing, a crack may have developed in the humidifier assembly or reservoir, or the flowmeter may be loosely connected to the humidifier. Please continue on page 402, frame 215.

406C (from page 402, frame 215)
Wrong. The Bennett Cascade I does not have a low-water alarm. The newer Bennett Cascade II humidifier is servo-controlled and has a low-water alarm system. Return to page 402, frame 215, and try again.

406D (from page 403, frame 216)
Correct. The Bird heated wick humidifier has the capability of delivering 100% relative humidity at body temperature at high flow up to 60 L/min. The Bennett Cascade II humidifier can deliver 100% relative humidity only at 86°F with flows of up to 40 L/min. Please continue on page 404, frame 217.

406a (from page 404, frame 217)
Correct. Aerosol particles in this range are commonly produced by disposable hand-held medication nebulizers. Particles of this size will deposit in the lower airways. Some disposable nebulizers produce droplets with a more limited range of 1.5 to 4 μm, which will deliver more medication to the peripheral airways. Please continue on page 405, frame 218.

406b (from page 400, frame 213)
Correct. If the gas is delivered to the patient at 33°C, a heated pass-over humidifier should be capable of providing absolute humidity of 36 mg/L under ideal conditions. However, variables that decrease water vapor delivery are water-reservoir temperature, ambient temperature, water-reservoir dead space, and high gas flow. Please continue on page 401, frame 214.

406c (from page 404, frame 217)
Wrong. Aerosol particles in this range would deposit only in the upper airways. For example, 75% of all 12-μm droplets will deposit in the mouth, and 80% of all 7-μm particles will be deposited between the mouth and larynx. Return to page 404, frame 217, and try again.

406d (from page 402, frame 215)
Wrong. The Bennett Cascade I does not have a high-gas temperature alarm. The Bennett Cascade II has servo-controlled gas temperature and a high-temperature alarm. Return to page 402, frame 215, and try again.

407A (from page 400, frame 213)
Wrong. If the gas is delivered to the patient at 33°C, a heated pass-over humidifier should be capable of delivering a relative humidity of approximately 82% at 37°C. Return to page 400, frame 213, and try again.

407B (from page 402, frame 215)
Correct. Unless the thermoswitch in the heating element shuts off the power, gas with a high temperature may be delivered to the airways. The Bennett Cascade II humidifier servo-controls proximal gas temperature and has an alarm system for high-temperature and low-reservoir water level. Please continue on page 403, frame 216.

407C (from page 401, frame 214)
Wrong. This is not the most logical way to create enough pressure (greater than 2 psig) to see if the pressure relief valve releases gas and whistles or clicks. Also, it does not duplicate an obstruction in the delivery tubing, which is a common cause of high pressure in the humidifier. Return to page 401, frame 214, and select another answer.

407D (from page 403, frame 216)
Wrong. Both the Bird wick humidifier and the Bennett Cascade II humidifier servo-control the proximal airway temperature using proximal airway probes and display the gas temperature sensed at the airway. Return to page 403, frame 216, and select another answer.

407a (from page 401, frame 214)
Wrong. This will lower the pressure in the humidifier. Return to page 401, frame 214, and select another answer.

407b (from page 404, frame 217)
Wrong. Aerosol particles in this range would have a small proportion of deposit in the peripheral airways. For example, 65% of 10-μm particles would deposit in the mouth, and 99% of the remaining 10-μm particles would deposit in the larynx. Aerosol particles that are 4 μm in size would have 65% deposit in the upper airways and only 24% in the periphery. Return to page 404, frame 217, and select another answer.

407c (from page 403, frame 216)
Wrong. Both the Bird wick humidifier and the Bennett Cascade II humidifier have alarm systems for high proximal temperature. Return to page 403, frame 216, and select another answer.

FRAME 219. LARGE MAINSTREAM NEBULIZERS

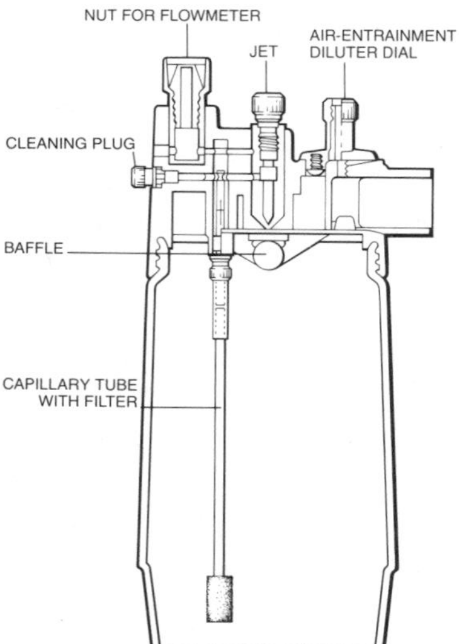

Figure 14–10 Cutaway view of the Ohio Deluxe mainstream nebulizer.

Heated mainstream nebulizers can be used to provide humidity for intubated patients because they have the capability to deliver 100% relative humidity at body temperature. All of these devices have air-entrainment ports that allow the FIO_2 to be adjusted by varying the amount of air that is mixed with oxygen. The FIO_2 will be increased substantially if downstream impedance creates back pressure that results in less air being entrained. Typically this occurs when water accumulates in the delivery tube due to the condensation that occurs as the gas cools on the way to the patient. Devices of this type deliver both water vapor and aerosol particles of water. The particle size of the aerosol produced is small (1 to 10 μm) and the output high enough (1 to 3 mL/min) that a large surface for evaporation from aerosol particles creates 50% to 75% relative humidity at body temperature when the humidifier is unheated. The particle size generated by a heated mainstream nebulizer will grow as the gas cools on the way to the patient and becomes saturated with water vapor; that is, the dew point is reached and water condenses on the particles, making them bigger. When mainstream nebulizers are used unheated, the aerosol particles decrease in size as the gas is warmed to ambient temperature as gas travels through the delivery tube.

Mainstream nebulizers can have both humidity and FIO_2 lowered if the total flow does not meet the patient's peak inspiratory flow. The aerosol mist should continue to flow from the ports of an aerosol mask or a T-tube throughout inspiration. To increase the total flow to an aerosol mask or T-tube, the oxygen flow to the jet on the nebulizer should be increased especially if the nebulizer is already set for air entrainment. When the nebulizer is set to deliver an FIO_2 of 0.40, a flow of 12 L/min through the jet combined with entrained air will provide a total flow that will match most patients' peak inspiratory flow (12 L/min O_2 + 36 L/min air = 48 L/min).

(Q) Which of the following should be the first action taken if aerosol is exiting from the delivery tube of a heated mainstream nebulizer in a series of puffs?

a. Increase the flow to 12 L/min. 412 D

b. Drain the delivery tube. 413 B

c. Add an extension to the T-tube. 413 b

FRAME 220. ULTRASONIC NEBULIZERS

Ultrasonic nebulizers generate aerosol particles by converting electrical energy into mechanical energy. A special ceramic (piezoelectric) crystal has the ability to change shape in resonance with a high-frequency radio-wave generator. The usual frequency applied to the piezoelectric crystal is 1.35 million cycles per second. The radio frequency applied to the crystal determines the size of the aerosol particles generated as sound waves impact the surface of the fluid reservoir. The sound energy is focused on the surface of the solution in the medication cup, where a geyser is formed. Aerosol particles are generated as surface tension and cohesive forces are overcome. The height (amplitude) of the sound wave generated determines the amount of aerosol produced. Changing the amplitude will vary the output from 0 to 6 mL/min depending on the model used. The sound waves created by the vibration of the piezoelectric crystal are transmitted to the solution cup via the couplant chamber, in the base of which is the transducer, which contains the vibrating crystal. The couplant chamber is filled with water that acts as a transfer medium and absorbs heat created by the transducer. A blower is used to provide a carrier gas to move the aerosol to the patient. Usually the fluid level in the solution cup must be kept at a specific level by a continuous feed system for aerosol to be produced. Variables that may decrease the amount of aerosol actually delivered to the patient include (1) baffling and condensation in the tubing, (2) increase in carrier gas flow, (3) the temperature of the liquid in the solution cup, (4) high-viscosity solutions, (5) residue from soaps or plastics entering the solution cup, and (6) decreased fluid in the couplant chamber.

Ultrasonic nebulizers can be used to deliver bland aerosols to hydrate retained secretions. The high-density aerosol output and average 3 μm particle size is optimal for deposition in peripheral airways. Bronchodilators and mucolytics are not suitable for ultrasonic nebulizers, since they may be reconcentrated. Reconcentration occurs because water and saline nebulize faster than other medications due to their molecular weights. The high-density output of ultrasonic nebulizers is a potential hazard because of the large amount water delivered to the lungs during long-term administration. This is especially a problem with small children, where their use may be contraindicated. Since ultrasonic nebulizers produce very large amounts of aerosol, they are unsuitable for use as humidifiers for artificial airways. Other hazards of the high-density aerosol produced by ultrasonic nebulizers include increased airway resistance, bronchospasm, and dyspnea.

(Q) Which of the following is *not* an appropriate use for ultrasonic nebulizers?

a. to deliver sterile water to induce sputum for culture and sensitivity studies 412 A
b. to treat croup in small children 412 b
c. to thin retained thick, dry secretions 413 C

FRAME 221. BABINGTON NEBULIZERS

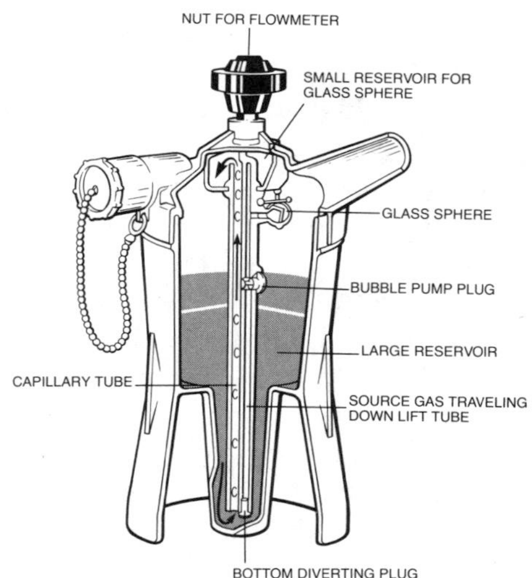

Figure 14–11 The Solo-Sphere nebulizer and its component parts illustrate the Babington principle.

The Babington nebulizer differs from the jet nebulizer by using a hollow glass sphere to generate high-density aerosol particles. Gas from a high-pressure source enters the hollow sphere and exits through a small hole at very high velocity. Gravity causes solution from a small reservoir to drain over the sphere and form a thin liquid layer. Gas emitting from the hole in the sphere tears the thin liquid film into particles that are impacted against a baffle. The aerosol particle size generated by a Babington (hydronamic) nebulizer is 3 to 5 μm (same size as produced by ultrasonic nebulizers). The small reservoir is filled from the larger reservoir below by the source gas forcing small bubbles up a capillary tube. Each bubble lifts a small amount of solution to the reservoir above the sphere. The Solo-Sphere nebulizer (Fig. 14–11) is an example of a larger capacity nebulizer that works on the Babington principle. Particle size is determined by the thickness of the film, velocity of fluid flow, and configuration of the sphere surface. The aerosol density produced is determined by the number of orifices in the sphere and the gas flow through the nebulizer. The high-density aerosol output is inappropriate for small children, infants, and ventilator patients. The particle size is similar to that of an ultrasonic nebulizer and too small for the treatment of croup.

The nebulizer is attached to a flowmeter to control source gas and has an air-entrainment port for controlling F_{IO_2} and total gas flow. The Solo-Sphere has a heater that clips on the base to control the inspired gas temperature. The heater is designed to deliver aerosol at a temperature of 35°C at the maximum heat setting and low flow. The Solo-Sphere has an aerosol output capacity of approximately 2 mL/min.

(Q) Which of the following applications would be appropriate for a nebulizer that works on the Babington principle?

a. delivery of a mucolytic — 412 c
b. humidification for an artificial airway — 413 A
c. delivery of a bronchodilator — 413 c

FRAME 222. HEAT-MOISTURE EXCHANGERS

A device that serves as a heat-moisture exchanger for patients who have their upper airways bypassed is sometimes referred to as the *hygroscopic condenser* humidifier or the *artificial nose*. The devices are placed between the endotracheal tube and the breathing circuit, and during exhalation heat and moisture pass through the core containing the hygroscopic material. During the next breath the heat and moisture retained in the core warm and humidify the inspired gas. Newer heat-moisture exchangers use a hygroscopic material such as a woven fiber coated with lithium salts, which makes them more efficient than heat-moisture exchangers that use a stainless steel core. Endotracheal tubes have been shown to serve as inefficient heat-moisture exchangers, adding 5 to 8 mg/L and 3° to 5°C to inspired gas. A minimal level of humidity of 25 to 30 mg/L (57% to 68% relative humidity at 37°C) and a temperature of close to 32°C at the proximal end of the trachea is necessary to preserve normal mucociliary function. Several hygroscopic condenser humidifiers produce 25 to 30 mg/L of humidity, which when combined with the 5 to 8 mg/L contributed by artificial airways provides enough humidity to condition inhaled gas for short periods of time.

Heat-moisture exchangers are appropraite when intubated patients are being transported to special procedures or surgery. When used in mechanical ventilation circuits, they must have the ability to withstand 100 cm H_2O of internal pressure and there should be little if any gas leakage. Dead space and resistance to airflow should be low. Heat-moisture exchangers are commonly used when heated humidifiers are not practical, since they are inexpensive, disposable, and do not require water or electrical power. However, they should not be used with patients who have retained secretions or impaired mucociliary clearance. If the patient needs frequent suctioning or bronchial lavage, a conventional heated humidifier should be used.

(Q) What is the minimum amount of absolute humidity that a heat-moisture exchanger should provide during transport of a ventilator patient?

a. 15 mg/L 412 B
b. 25 mg/L 412 d
c. 35 mg/L 413 a

412A (from page 409, frame 220)
Wrong. Ultrasonic nebulizers can be used to stimulate a cough to produce sputum for culture and sensitivity studies. Return to page 409, frame 220, and select another answer.

412B (from page 411, frame 222)
Wrong. More humidity is needed to provide adequate humidity so that the mucociliary escalator is not adversely affected. Remember the endotracheal tube alone adds only 5 to 8 mg/L to inspired gas. Return to page 411, frame 222, and select another answer.

412C (from page 405, frame 218)
Wrong. The dose by weight of 8 to 10 puffs from an Alupent MDI would be 5.2 to 6.5 mg, which is considerably less than the typical dose for Alupent inhalant solution given by a hand-held jet nebulizer. Return to page 405, frame 218, and select another answer.

412D (from page 408, frame 219)
Wrong. Increasing the flow to the jet on the nebulizer may reduce the puffing effect, but there is still a problem with the F_{IO_2} reading higher than set on the nebulizer. Return to page 408, frame 219, and try again.

412a (from page 405, frame 218)
Wrong. The dose by weight of 2 to 3 puffs from an Alupent MDI would be 1.30 to 1.95 mg, which is considerably less than the typical dose range for Alupent inhalant solution given by a hand-held jet nebulizer. Return to page 405, frame 218, and select another answer.

412b (from page 409, frame 220)
Correct. Ultrasonic nebulizers produce aerosol particles suitable for deposition in small airways. Since croup is an upper airway disease, the ultrasonic nebulizer is not appropriate and may be contraindicated for small children due to fluid overload. Please continue on page 410, frame 221.

412c (from page 410, frame 221)
Wrong. The Babington-type devices are used in the same manner as the large-capacity jet nebulizer. A small-volume medication nebulizer would be used to administer a mucolytic. Return to page 410, frame 221, and select another answer.

412d (from page 411, frame 222)
Correct. A minimum of 25 to 30 mg/L of humidity is needed to provide adequate humidity so that the mucociliary escalator is not adversely affected. Please continue on page 414 and complete the chapter exercises.

413A (from page 410, frame 221)
Correct. Since a heater can be added to the bottom of Babington-type nebulizers, they have an aerosol output similar to large heated jet nebulizers. Thus the nebulizer can be used to humidify gas delivered to an artificial airway. Please continue on page 410, frame 222.

413B (from page 408, frame 219)
Correct. Condensate water has collected in the delivery tube as the gas cooled. This causes the aerosol to exit in puffs as the water periodically obstructs gas flow. This downstream impedance lowers air entrainment, which increases the F_{IO_2} and decreases the total gas flow to the patient. Please continue on page 409, frame 220.

413C (from page 409, frame 220)
Wrong. Ultrasonic nebulizers can be used to hydrate and thin secretions. Caution should be taken with thick, dry secretions because they may swell as they become hydrated and cause an increase in airway resistance, wheezing, and dyspnea. However, the ultrasonic nebulizer may be indicated when dry retained secretions need to be thinned so that chest physical therapy can be more effective. Return to page 409, frame 220, and select another answer.

413D (from page 405, frame 218)
Correct. The dose by weight of 15 to 23 puffs from an Alupent MDI would be approximately 10 to 15 mg, which is the same dose range of Alupent inhalant solution given by a hand-held jet nebulizer. Caution is warranted when making these types of comparisons since a dose given by MDI may have less medication wasted. Remember that a typical dose of an MDI is only 2 to 3 puffs. The point to consider is that repeat MDI doses may be warranted more often than the 6- to 8-hour intervals recommended for inhalant solutions used with pneumatic jet nebulizers. Please continue on page 408, frame 219.

413a (from page 411, frame 222)
Wrong. A heat and moisture exchanger is not as efficient as a heated humidifier. The best-designed hygroscopic condenser humidifiers produce a maximum of 29 mg/L of absolute humidity. Return to page 410, frame 222, and select another answer.

413b (from page 408, frame 219)
Wrong. Adding an extension tube to the patient's T-tube or to the ports of an aerosol mask will not solve this puffing problem. The F_{IO_2} is also reading higher than set on the nebulizer. Return to page 408, frame 219, and select another answer.

413c (from page 410, frame 221)
Wrong. The Babington-type devices are used in the same way as large-capacity jet nebulizers. A small-volume nebulizer or metered-dose inhaler should be used to administer a bronchodilator. Return to page 410, frame 221, and select another answer.

EXERCISES

1. Identify three clinical applications in which pass-over humidifiers would be better than heated mainstream nebulizers.
2. Connect a bubble humidifier to an oxygen flowmeter and simulate three clinical situations that will make the pressure-relief valve click or whistle.
3. Inspect a Bennet cascade I and Bennett cascade II humidifier and make a list of the components that are similar to both units. Also make a list of the improvements incorporated in the design of the newer model.
4. Calculate circuit compliance for a ventilator circuit with a cascade humidifier attached and then again with a Bird wick humidifier attached. Describe why there is a difference in compliance.
5. Gather six disposable jet medication nebulizers and list the differences in the design of the jet, capillary tube, baffles, and reservoir cup. Determine if they must be held in a vertical position so as to not lose any medication.
6. Locate and inspect three different types of spacers or reservoir systems for metered-dose inhalers. Describe the advantage of each device in terms of how it will improve delivery of the medication.
7. Connect a 6-ft piece of aerosol tubing to the outlet of a large mainstream air-entrainment nebulizer set to deliver an F_{IO_2} of 0.40 and adjust the oxygen flowmeter to 10 L/min. Place a polarographic oxygen analyzer probe and a Wright respirometer at the end of the aerosol tubing. Measure the F_{IO_2} and total flow exiting the tubing. Repeat the measurements after you have created a lazy loop in the aerosol tube and have added 100 mL of water. Repeat the measurements (with and without water in the tubing) with the nebulizer set to deliver an F_{IO_2} of 1.00.
8. Weigh an ultrasonic nebulizer cup before use and after 10 minutes of operation at the lowest setting and calculate the volume nebulized. Repeat the measurements with the nebulizer set at its highest setting. Describe how the output compares with the amount of aerosol produced by large heated jet nebulizers.
9. Obtain a hydronamic (Babington) nebulizer and locate the following components: (1) glass sphere, (2) small reservoir feeding the glass sphere, (3) larger reservoir feeding the small reservoir, (4) baffles adjacent to holes in the sphere, (5) capillary tube between small and large reservoirs, and (6) connection for gas source.
10. List four clinical situations in which heat-moisture exchangers could safely be used to replace a heated mainstream humidifier.

POSTTEST

This test is designed to evaluate what you have learned from completing Chapter 14. Check your answers on page 415 and review the topics where your answer is incorrect.

1. Pass-over humidifiers are not likely to be a source of nosocomial infection because of which of the following factors?
   I. The humidifier is unheated.
   II. Aerosol particles are not produced.
   III. There is no air entrainment.
   IV. The reservoir volume is limited.
   V. Gas passes through a bacterial filter located at the humidifier outlet.
   A. I only
   B. II only
   C. II and III only
   D. III and V only
   E. I, II, III, IV, and V
2. How does a Bird wick humidifier differ from a pass-over humidifier?
   A. The internal gas volume is substantially smaller.
   B. It has air-entrainment capability.
   C. It delivers a higher FIO_2.
   D. It is heated.
   E. It is disposable.
3. What is the relative humidity at 37°C produced by bubble humidifiers?
   A. 20% to 30%
   B. 30% to 40%
   C. 40% to 60%
   D. 60% to 80%
   E. 80% to 100%
4. Jet humidifiers produce more water vapor than bubble humidifiers because of which of the following factors?
   A. high-speed jet
   B. lack of a diffuser
   C. extra baffles
   D. flow is limited to 4 L/min
   E. aerosol particles trapped inside oxygen bubbles
5. What is the purpose of the bypass hole found in the cascade humidifier tower?
   A. to monitor FIO_2
   B. to baffle out very large aerosol particles
   C. to allow triggering of an assisted breath
   D. to measure airway pressure during CPAP
   E. to monitor inspiratory temperature
6. How often does a Bennett Cascade II humidifier need to be checked?
   A. every 2 hours
   B. every 4 hours
   C. every 8 hours
   D. every 12 hours
   E. every 24 hours

7. Which of the following account(s) for the ability of the Bird wick humidifier to deliver 100% body humidity at a flow of 60 L/min?
   I. large surface area for evaporation
   II. wick warmed by a heating element
   III. high internal gas volume
   IV. water level maintained by external reservoir
   A. I only
   B. II only
   C. I and II only
   D. I, II, and IV only
   E. I, II, III, and IV

8. The Bird wick humidifier has alarm systems for all of the following *except*
   A. high temperature.
   B. low temperature.
   C. probe unplugged.
   D. torn wick cartridge.
   E. automatic shutdown of element.

9. Which of the following is a disadvantage of a *mainstream* medication nebulizer when compared to a *sidestream* nebulizer?
   A. less solution nebulized
   B. smaller particle size produced
   C. less baffling of large particles occurs
   D. reconcentration of medication
   E. rebreathing of exhaled gas

10. What size aerosol particles feel wet and impact on a glass surface?
    A. 0.1 to 1 μm
    B. 1 to 3 μm
    C. 3 to 5 μm
    D. 5 to 10 μm
    E. 10 to 15 μm

11. What is the dose/puff from an MDI of metaproterenol (Alupent)?
    A. 0.09 mg
    B. 0.16 mg
    C. 0.20 mg
    D. 0.34 mg
    E. 0.65 mg

12. How far away from an open mouth should an MDI be held?
    A. 1 cm
    B. 2 cm
    C. 4 cm
    D. 8 cm
    E. 10 cm

13. What is the aerosol output of a large unheated mainstream nebulizer?
    A. 0.5 to 1 mL/min
    B. 1 to 3 mL/min
    C. 3 to 6 mL/min
    D. 6 to 10 mL/min
    E. 10 to 15 mL/min

14. The body humidity produced by unheated mainstream nebulizers is
    A. 20% to 30%.
    B. 30% to 40%.
    C. 40% to 50%.
    D. 50% to 75%.
    E. 75% to 100%.

15. What determines the aerosol output of an ultrasonic nebulizer?
   A. amplitude of the sound wave generated
   B. radio frequency applied to the crystal
   C. size of the nebulization cup
   D. size of the couplant chamber
   E. molecular weight of the solution nebulized

16. Which of the following solutions would be most appropriate to nebulize using an ultrasonic nebulizer?
   A. 0.5 normal saline
   B. 10% acetylcysteine (Mucomyst)
   C. 15 mg of metaproterenol (Alupent, Metaprel)
   D. 50% ethyl alcohol
   E. cromolyn sodium (Intal)

17. What is the aerosol output produced by a Solo-Sphere nebulizer?
   A. 1 mL/min
   B. 2 mL/min
   C. 3 mL/min
   D. 6 mL/min
   E. 10 mL/min

18. A Babington nebulizer would be inappropriate for which of the following types of patients and clinical situations?
   I. small children
   II. infants
   III. as humidifiers for ventilator patients
   IV. treatment of croup
   A. I only
   B. II only
   C. I and II only
   D. I, II, and IV only
   E. I, II, III, and IV

19. Heat-moisture exchangers for intubated patients would be indicated in all of the following *except*
   A. after bronchial lavage.
   B. for transport to another hospital.
   C. during surgery.
   D. during helicopter transport.
   E. during short-term mechanical ventilation.

20. What is the *minimum* absolute humidity required to preserve normal mucociliary function?
   A. 20 to 25 mg/L
   B. 25 to 30 mg/L
   C. 30 to 35 mg/L
   D. 35 to 40 mg/L
   E. 40 to 44 mg/L

ANSWERS TO POSTTEST

1. C (F213)
2. A (F213)
3. B (F214)
4. E (F214)
5. C (F215)
6. A (F215)
7. D (F216)
8. D (F216)
9. C (F217)
10. E (F217)
11. E (F218)
12. C (F218)
13. B (F219)
14. D (F219)
15. A (F220)
16. A (F220)
17. B (F221)
18. E (F221)
19. A (F222)
20. B (F222)

BIBLIOGRAPHY

Barnes, TA: Respiratory Care Practice. Year Book Medical Publishers, Chicago, 1988.
Eubanks, DH and Bone, RC: Comprehensive Respiratory Care, ed 2. CV Mosby, St. Louis, 1990.
Kacmarek, RM and Stoller, JK: Current Respiratory Care. BC Decker, Philadelphia, 1988.
McPherson, SP: Respiratory Home Care Equipment. Daedalus Enterprises, Dallas, 1988.
McPherson, SP: Respiratory Therapy Equipment, ed 4. CV Mosby, St. Louis, 1990.
Riggs, JH: Respiratory Facts. FA Davis, Philadelphia, 1989.

15

Airway Care Equipment

223. Pharyngeal airways
224. Esophageal obturator airways
225. Endotracheal tubes
226. Laryngoscopes
227. Suction catheters
228. Vacuum regulators
229. Sputum specimen collectors
230. Tracheostomy tubes and buttons
231. Incentive spirometers
232. Chest percussors

PRETEST

This pretest is designed to measure what you already know about airway care equipment. Check your answers on page 422 and then continue on page 423, frame 223.

1. Which of the following will reduce the trauma to the nasal mucosa caused by a nasal pharyngeal airway?
   A. leaving the tube untaped so it can move as patient's head turns
   B. alternating the tube between nares
   C. lubricating the tube with petroleum gel
   D. inserting the tube without lubricant
   E. using the size tube that creates a tight fit
2. All of the following are advantages of oropharyngeal airways *except*
   A. relieving obstruction caused by the tongue.
   B. providing a pathway for oropharyngeal suctioning.
   C. providing a pathway for orotracheal suctioning.
   D. protecting the tongue from being bitten during seizure.
   E. protecting an endotracheal tube from becoming crimped.
3. Clinical signs of esophageal rupture when using an EOA include which of the following?
   I. subcutaneous emphysema
   II. pneumomediastinum
   III. bleeding
   IV. hypoxemia
   V. chest pain
   A. I and III only
   B. II and V only
   C. I, III, and V only
   D. II, III, IV, and V only
   E. I, II, III, IV, and V
4. All of the following should be done before removing an esophageal obturator airway *except*
   A. turning the patient into a supine position.
   B. ventilating with 100% oxygen.
   C. removing one-way valve from cuff pilot tube.
   D. preparing suction equipment with a large catheter.
   E. intubating the trachea with an endotracheal tube.
5. A tracheostomy tube with a properly inflated Fome cuff will exert a pressure on the airway wall of
   A. 5 mm Hg.
   B. 15 mm Hg.
   C. 20 mm Hg.
   D. 25 mm Hg.
   E. 30 mm Hg.
6. How is the size of endotracheal tubes designated?
   A. outside diameter
   B. inside diameter
   C. length
   D. wall thickness
   E. cross-sectional area
7. Which of the following laryngoscope blades is appropriate to intubate a neonate?
   A. size 0 straight blade (Miller)
   B. size 2 straight blade (Miller)
   C. size 3 straight blade (Miller)
   D. size 0 curved blade (Macintosh)
   E. size 1 curved blade (Macintosh)

8. Which of the following should be on an intubation tray?
   I. needles and syringes
   II. MDI bronchodilator canisters
   III. tonsil sucker (Yankauer)
   IV. Magill forceps
   V. oral and nasal pharyngeal airways
   A. I and III only
   B. II and IV only
   C. III, IV, and V only
   D. I, III, IV, and V only
   E. I, II, III, IV, and V

9. Which of the following suction catheters is least likely to traumatize the airway?
   A. whistle-tip (one side hole)
   B. whistle-tip (two opposing side holes)
   C. straight-tip (without side holes)
   D. straight-tip (two opposing side holes)
   E. straight-tip (four opposing side holes)

10. Which of the following will reduce trauma caused by a suction catheter?
   A. apply suction pressure for only 15 seconds at one time
   B. release suction pressure when moving catheter in the airway
   C. apply and release pressure when catheter is moving in the airway
   D. use a suction catheter that is one size larger than normal
   E. suction the patient only during inspiration

11. What range of tracheal suction pressure should be used with adults?
   A. 60 to 80 mm Hg
   B. 80 to 100 mm Hg
   C. 80 to 120 mm Hg
   D. 100 to 140 mm Hg
   E. 140 to 180 mm Hg

12. Inability to suction secretions from the airway may be the result of
   I. kinked suction tubing.
   II. disconnected suction tubing.
   III. secretions too thin and watery.
   IV. too large a volume of secretions.
   V. full collection reservoir.
   A. I and III only
   B. II and V only
   C. I, II, and V only
   D. III, IV, and V only
   E. I, II, III, IV, and V

13. When collecting a sputum specimen for bacterial and cytologic evaluation the specimen should be
   A. collected at any time (24 hrs/day).
   B. brought dry to the clinical lab.
   C. taken from the hypopharynx.
   D. induced with hypertonic saline.
   E. mixed with sterile water to move it into specimen trap.

14. A sputum specimen collector should be placed between
   A. catheter and suction tubing.
   B. vacuum regulator and suction reservoir.
   C. ultrasonic nebulizer cup and aerosol mask.
   D. tonsil (Yankauer) sucker and suction tubing.
   E. tracheostomy tube and suction tubing.

15. All of the following are early complications of tracheostomy tubes *except*
    A. bleeding.
    B. tracheoesophageal fistula.
    C. subcutaneous emphysema.
    D. pneumothorax.
    E. air embolism.

16. To allow a patient with a fenestrated tracheostomy tube to cough more effectively, which combination of the following could be done?
    I. cork tracheostomy tube
    II. deflate cuff
    III. inflate cuff
    IV. add an Olympic Trach-Talk valve to tracheostomy tube
    V. remove inner cannula
    A. I and III only
    B. I and II only
    C. III and IV only
    D. I and IV only
    E. II, IV, and V only

17. How long should a patient hold the balls at the top of the Triflo II incentive breathing exerciser?
    A. 1 second
    B. 2 seconds
    C. 3 seconds
    D. 6 seconds
    E. 8 seconds

18. How many sustained maximal inspirations should a patient complete when using an incentive spirometer every hour while awake?
    A. 1
    B. 2
    C. 5
    D. 10
    E. 20

19. How long on one location of the chest should a percussor be held?
    A. 1 minute
    B. 2 minutes
    C. 5 minutes
    D. 10 minutes
    E. 20 minutes

20. Which of the following is the best way to determine the force being generated by a chest percussor?
    A. Grasp percussor applicator tightly with one hand.
    B. Place a hand on the chest next to percussor applicator.
    C. Evaluate the amount of vibrations delivered to the arm.
    D. Grasp percussor loosely with two hands.
    E. Direct therapist body weight to applicator.

ANSWERS TO PRETEST

1. B (F223)
2. C (F223)
3. E (F224)
4. A (F224)
5. C (F225)
6. B (F225)
7. A (F226)
8. D (F226)
9. E (F227)
10. B (F227)
11. C (F228)
12. C (F228)
13. B (F229)
14. A (F229)
15. B (F230)
16. E (F230)
17. C (F231)
18. D (F231)
19. A (F232)
20. B (F232)

FRAME 223. PHARYNGEAL AIRWAYS

Oropharyngeal Airways Oropharyngeal airways are used to relieve an obstruction caused by the tongue falling backward against the pharyngeal wall. The obstruction often may be relieved without use of an oral airway by repositioning the head or by forward displacement of the mandible. Oral airways have a hollow tube or open side channels to provide a pathway for breathing and suctioning (Fig. 15–1). A rigid material behind the flange prevents patients from crimping the tube with their teeth. Oral airways can trigger gag and vomit reflexes by touching the pharyngeal wall and should be used only with unconscious patients whose protective reflexes are obtunded. Oral airways can be inserted behind the tongue after it has been moved forward by a wooden tongue blade. Frequently the oral airway is inserted with tip pointing toward the hard palate; then it is advanced and turned 180 degrees so that it slides behind the tongue.

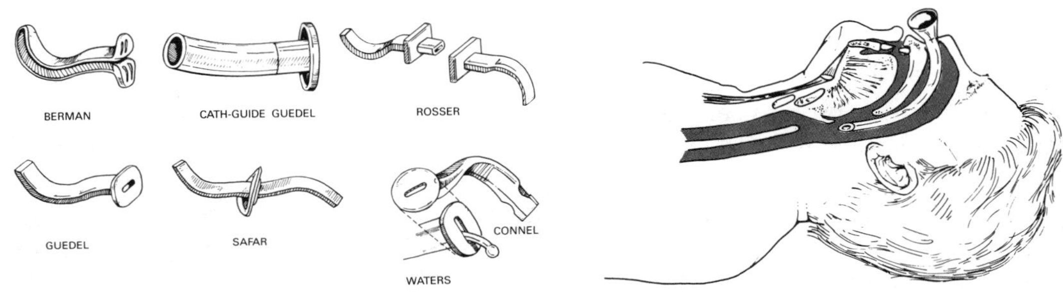

Figure 15–1 **Figure 15–2**

Figure 15–1 Various types of oropharyngeal airways.

Figure 15–2 Nasopharyngeal airway in place.

Nasopharyngeal Airways Nasopharyngeal airways are used with patients who need frequent tracheal suctioning (Fig. 15–2). The airway helps to guide the suction catheter to the trachea and protects the nasal and pharyngeal mucosa. Nasal airways are usually made of soft latex and should have a ring, cone, or pin through the proximal end to prevent the tube from slipping into the esophagus or trachea. The nasal airway should be lubricated with viscous lidocaine or water-soluble gel and gently inserted. If resistance is encountered, the airway should be withdrawn and the other nare or a smaller size airway should be used. The tube should be anchored with tape to keep it from moving. Nasal airways can precipitate laryngospasm, vomiting, nosebleeds, or tissue necrosis. Alternating the tube between the nares may reduce trauma to the nasal mucosa.

(Q) Which of the following would be appropriate for use during a seizure (*before the tonic phase begins*) to prevent the tongue from falling posteriorly and obstructing the airway?

a. nasopharyngeal airway 428 A
b. oropharyngeal airway 428 d
c. endotracheal tube 429 B

FRAME 224. ESOPHAGEAL OBTURATOR AIRWAYS

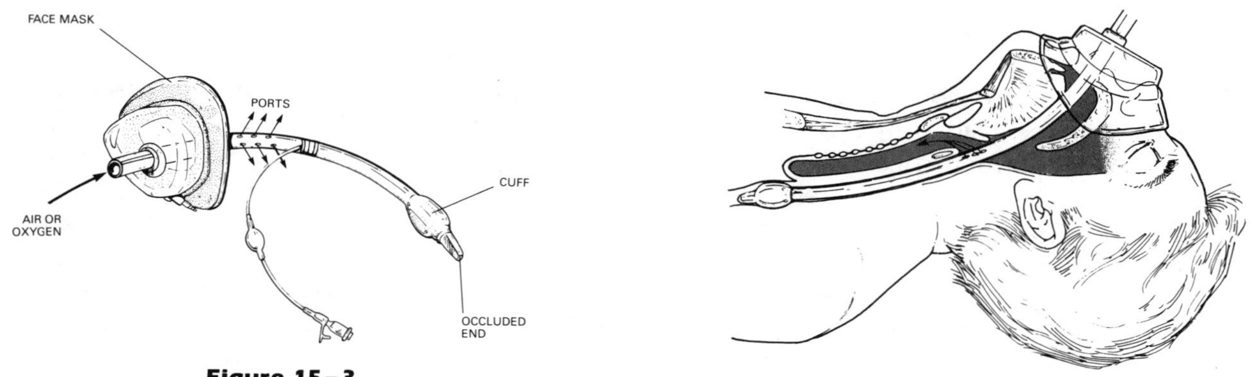

Figure 15–3 Esophageal obturator.

Figure 15–4 Esophageal obturator in place.

An esophageal obturator airway (EOA) may be used outside of hospitals during cardiopulmonary resuscitation of adults by emergency medical technicians who are unskilled in endotracheal intubation (Figs. 15–3 and 15–4). The EOA is used outside of hospitals to establish a patent airway if one or more of the following criteria are met: (1) a laryngoscope and endotracheal tube are not available, (2) circumstances do not allow the use of an endotracheal tube, (3) oral or nasal pharyngeal airways are not appropriate because the possibility of aspiration of gastric contents must be reduced, or (4) attempts at orotracheal intubation have been unsuccessful.

The three major complications of EOAs are tracheal intubation, esophageal rupture, and vomiting with possible aspiration pneumonia during acute retching episodes or as the tube is removed. If the EOA slips into the trachea, the patient will not be able to be ventilated because the end of the tube is occluded (see Fig. 15–3). If chest movement or breath sounds are absent, the EOA should be removed at once because it is obstructing the airway. The clinical signs of esophageal rupture include subcutaneous emphysema, pneumomediastinum, bleeding, and chest pain. Overinflation of EOA cuffs may tear the esophagus, and the inflation volume used should be limited to approximately 35 mL of air. To prevent aspiration an endotracheal tube should be placed before the EOA is removed. If the patient regains consciousness before an endotracheal tube can be substituted for the EOA, the EOA must be removed immediately before the patient gags, vomits, and aspirates. Suction equipment must be ready with a large catheter, since most patients will vomit when the airway is removed. Turn the patient to one side, deflate the cuff by removing the one-way valve, and withdraw the EOA from the esophagus and upper airway.

(Q) The mask on an esophageal obturator is removed for which of the following reasons during CPR in a hospital emergency room?

a. to use a manual resuscitator to ventilate the patient 428 C
b. to intubate the trachea with an endotracheal tube 429 A
c. to pass a nasogastric tube to decompress the stomach 429 c

FRAME 225. ENDOTRACHEAL TUBES

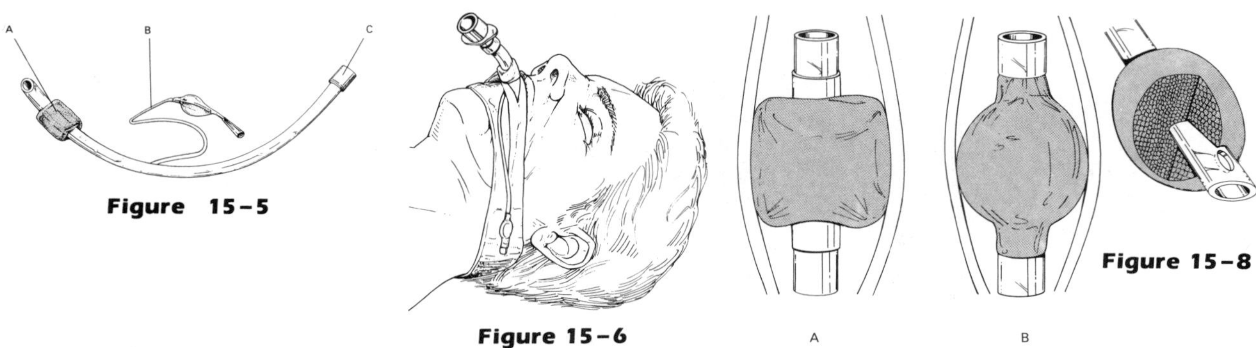

Figure 15-7

Figure 15-5 Oral endotracheal tube: (*A*) cuff; (*B*) pilot tube for inflating cuff; (*C*) 15/22 mm connector.

Figure 15-6 Endotracheal tube secured in place.

Figure 15-7 Comparison of (*A*) high-residual-volume, low-pressure cuff and (*B*) low-residual-volume, high-pressure cuff.

Figure 15-8 **Figure 15-8** Kamen-Wilken- son Fome cuff.

Endotracheal tubes are the airway of choice to protect the lungs from aspiration pneumonia and to provide a pathway for ventilation of the lungs. The Z-79 denotes a standard specified for endotracheal tubes by the American National Standards Institute (ANSI) Z-79 Committee for Anesthesia Equipment. If *IT* is stamped on the side, the material the tube is made from has been tested to ensure that it is nonreactive when implanted in a rabbit muscle. Other markings on the tube (Fig. 15–5) include (1) length markings in centimeters where the tube extends from the mouth, (2) inside diameter in millimeters (ID), and (3) outside diameter in millimeters (OD). Endotracheal tubes are sized according to the inside diameter with a 7.5 to 8.0 being appropriate for the average adult female and 8.0 to 8.5 for the average adult male. One size above and below the estimated size needed should be available before an intubation is attempted. (See placement, Fig. 15–6.)

High-volume cuffs on endotracheal tubes will allow low pressure to create a seal. However, high pressure may be needed if the tube is too small and the area of the cuff making contact with the trachea is reduced (Fig. 15-7). If the appropriate size tube is used with the minimum-leak technique, a high-volume cuff should seal at a pressure of less than 25 mm Hg. The Fome cuff is filled with a soft foam (Fig. 15–8). The foam in the cuff must be flattened by withdrawing air before the tube is placed in the trachea. Once the tube is in place, the pilot tube is opened and the foam in the cuff returns to its original cylindrical shape and seals against the trachea at a low pressure of 20 mm Hg. A Fome cuff that is too small will not provide a seal, and one that is too large may seal with a pressure and one higher than 20 mm Hg.

(Q) Which of the following should be at the bedside of an intubated patient?

a. 25 mL syringe 428 B
b. pressure manometer 429 a
c. sterile endotracheal tube of the appropriate size 428 c

FRAME 226. LARYNGOSCOPES

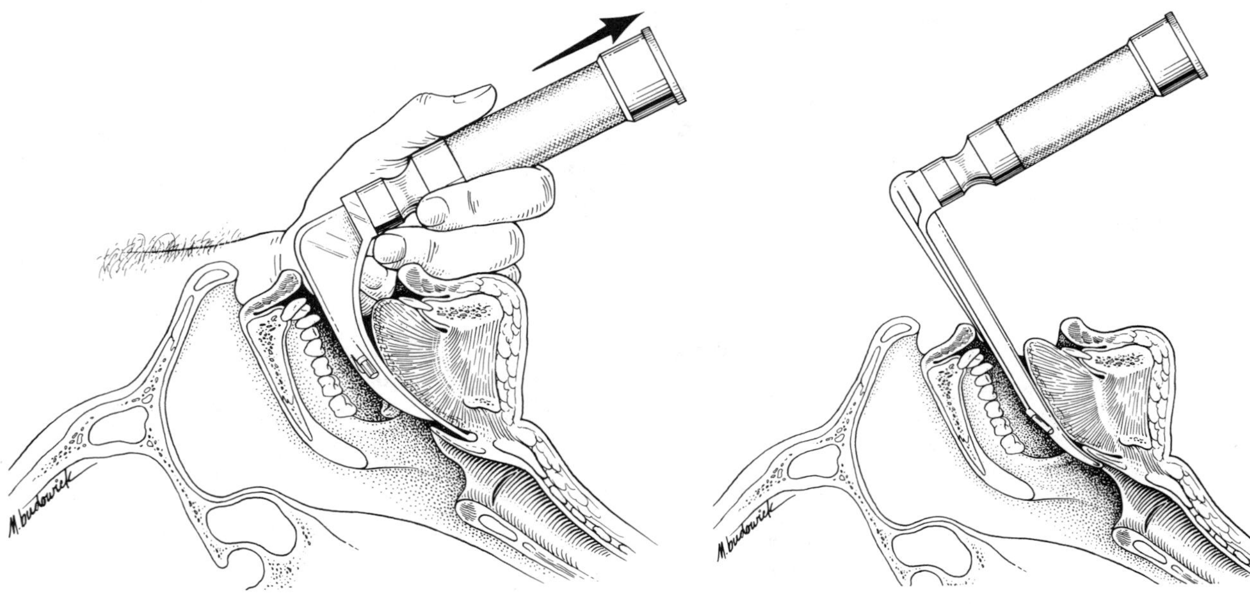

Figure 15–9 **Figure 15–10**

Figure 15–9 Direct laryngoscopy with curved (Macintosh) blade in vallecula. (Source: Finucane, BT and Santora, AH: Principles of Airway Management. FA Davis, Philadelphia, 1988. Used with permission.)

Figure 15–10 Direct laryngoscopy with straight (Miller) blade directly lifting epiglottis. (Source: Finucane, BT and Santora, AH: Principles of Airway Management. FA Davis, Philadelphia, 1988. Used with permission.)

One way to ensure that an endotracheal tube is placed in the trachea is to watch the tube pass through the vocal cords during intubation. The laryngoscope is a device used to assist intubation of the trachea by displacing soft tissue, providing a flange to help guide the tube, lifting the epiglottis directly (with a straight blade) or indirectly (with a curved blade), and illuminating the vocal cords. The handle of the laryngoscope blade has batteries that power a light at the end of the blade. A laryngoscope should always be checked to ensure that the batteries are fresh and that electrical contact between the handle and the blade is clean. Occasionally the bulb in the blade will burn out or vibrate loose and need to be replaced or tightened. The curved blade lifts the epiglottis when the tip of the blade is placed in the vallecula and the laryngoscope is pulled forward and upward using firm but steady pressure without rotating the wrist (Fig. 15–9). When a straight blade is used, the epiglottis is lifted directly (Fig. 15–10). A straight blade is preferred with small children and neonates because their larynx is located more superiorly and their epiglottis is more horizontal. The intubation tray should have various sizes of curved (Macintosh) and straight (Miller) blades, two handles, tongue depressor, oral and nasal airways, a variety of endotracheal tubes, needles and syringes, stylet (to mold the curve of the tube), tonsil sucker (Yankauer) and flexible suction catheter, Magill forceps (used for nasotracheal intubation), tape, local anesthetic solution or gel, and water-soluble gel.

(Q) Which of the following laryngoscope blades would be best for intubation of a 1-year-old child?

a. curved (Macintosh) size 3 428 D
b. straight (Miller) size 1 428 b
c. straight (Miller) size 3 429 C

FRAME 227. SUCTION CATHETERS

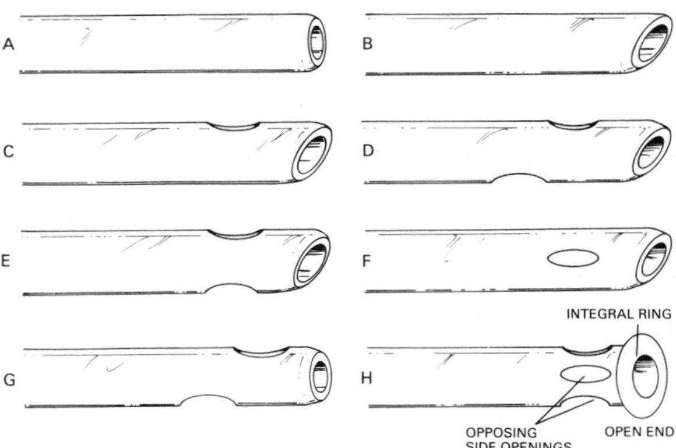

Figure 15–11 (*A*) open-end suction catheter with orifice perpendicular to long axis of catheter; (*B*) open-end suction catheter with angular cut; (*C*) Argyle whistle-tip catheter with angular end and single side opening; (*D*) Argyle whistle-tip catheter with angular end and two staggered side openings; (*E*) Travenol whistle-tip catheter with angular end and two side openings; (*F*) Portex whistle-tip suction catheter with angular end and single side opening; (*G*) Argyle DeLee tip catheter with open end perpendicular to long axis of catheter, with two staggered side openings; (*H*) Argyle Aero-Flo tip catheter with integral ring situated below four opposed eyes.

Several different types of suction catheters are available to meet specific clinical needs (Fig. 15–11). The most basic design has a single hole cut perpendicular to the length of the catheter. This type of catheter has the potential to grab onto the mucosal wall of the trachea, and the negative pressure being generated by the vacuum regulator will be exerted on that surface. Continuous negative pressure against the wall can damage the tracheal mucosa. Releasing the vacuum pressure by removing your thumb from the Y-connector each time the catheter is moved in the airway will reduce the damage done by this type of catheter to the airway mucosa. Catheters with a single hole cut at an angle increases the area that the negative pressure can be applied to and the precaution against continuous aspiration also applies to this design. Placing additional holes on the side of the suction catheter will minimize the damage done when the hole on the end of the catheter grabs onto the airway wall. The extra opening allows the negative pressure to be directed to the opening on the side when the hole on the end grabs the wall of the airway. The addition of two side-wall holes, either directly opposite (Travenol whistle-tip) or staggered (Argyle whistle-tip or DeLee tip), further reduces the damage when one of the three holes attaches to the airway wall. The Argyle Aero-Flo tip suction catheter has four side holes surrounding an integral ring that keeps the side holes from attaching to the airway wall and allows the secretions to move through any of the five openings.

(Q) Which of the following suction catheters presents the greatest risk of injuring the airway wall?

a. Argyle whistle-tip with two side holes — 429 D
b. Argyle DeLee tip — 428 a
c. Argyle Aero-Flo tip — 429 b

428A (from page 423, frame 223)
Wrong. A seizure pattern with sudden onset of unconsciousness and tonic contraction of muscles (including respiratory muscles) may cause the tongue to obstruct the airway. The nasal airway may allow the patient to breathe but will not prevent the tongue from being bitten. Return to page 423, frame 223, and select another answer.

428B (from page 425, frame 225)
Wrong. A syringe is needed to adjust the amount of air in the cuff of the endotracheal tube, but there is a more important piece of equipment to have at the bedside. Return to page 425, frame 225, and select another answer.

428C (from page 424, frame 224)
Wrong. Without the mask in place the air will leak out through the mouth and nose. Return to page 424, frame 224, and select another answer.

428D (from page 426, frame 226)
Wrong. A size 3 curved blade (Macintosh) is too long for use with a 1-year-old. A straight blade is preferred for intubation of infants because of the superior location of the larynx compared with that of older children and adults. Return to page 426, frame 226, and select another answer.

428a (from page 427, frame 227)
Wrong. The Argyle DeLee tip catheter has less surface area on the end cut, which makes it safer than the other two catheters. Return to page 427, frame 227, and select another answer.

428b (from page 426, frame 226)
Correct. The size 1 straight (Miller) blade would be best to intubate infants; the other blades are used with older children and adults. A straight blade is preferred for intubation of infants because of the superior location of the larynx compared with that of adults. Please continue on page 427, frame 227.

428c (from page 425, frame 225)
Correct. The endotracheal tube may need to be replaced because there is a large leak in the cuff, an obstruction in the tube, or a separation of the pilot tube from the cuff. A sterile endotracheal tube of the right size at the bedside will allow the tube to be replaced without delay and thereby minimize the risk of aspiration pneumonia or hypoventilation if the patient is being mechanically ventilated. Please continue on page 426, frame 226.

428d (from page 423, frame 223)
Correct. A seizure pattern with sudden onset of unconsciousness and tonic contraction of muscles (including respiratory muscles) may cause the tongue to obstruct the airway. The oral airway will allow the patient to breathe and may prevent the tongue from being bitten. Once the patient regains consciousness, the oral airway must be removed immediately so that gag and vomit reflexes are not triggered. Please continue on page 424, frame 224.

429A (from page 424, frame 224)
Correct. The trachea should be intubated with an endotracheal tube at the first opportunity because it is the emergency airway of choice and has fewer complications than an esophageal obturator airway. Please continue on page 425, frame 225.

429B (from page 423, frame 223)
Wrong. A seizure pattern with sudden onset of unconsciousness and tonic contraction of muscles (including respiratory muscles) may cause the tongue to obstruct the airway. The endotracheal tube may allow the patient to breathe but will not prevent the tongue from being bitten. The patient may bite down on the endotracheal tube and obstruct the airway. It is unlikely that an endotracheal tube can be placed before the tonic phase begins. Return to page 423, frame 223, and try again.

429C (from page 426, frame 226)
Wrong. A size 3 straight (Miller) blade is too long for use with a 1-year-old. Return to page 426, frame 226, and select another answer.

429D (from page 427, frame 227)
Correct. The Arygle whistle-tip is the most likely among the three suction catheters to cause trauma to the airway wall, since the angle cut on the end hole has a large surface area. The two side holes will help to minimize the chance of the catheter grabbing the airway wall and causing damage. Please continue on page 430, frame 228.

429a (from page 425, frame 225)
Wrong. Most respiratory care practitioners have their own pressure manometer for measuring cuff pressure. It usually is too expensive to have a pressure manometer at the bedside of all intubated patients. Return to page 425, frame 225, and select another answer.

429b (from page 427, frame 227)
Wrong. The Arygle Aero-Flo tip suction catheter is the least likely to cause trauma to the airway, since the integral ring keeps the four side holes from attaching to the mucosal wall. Return to page 427, frame 227, and select another answer.

429c (from page 424, frame 224)
Wrong. A nasogastric tube can be used to decompress the stomach before removing the esophageal obturator airway. However, there is a better way to protect airways from aspiration pneumonia. Return to page 424, frame 224, and select another answer.

FRAME 228. VACUUM REGULATORS

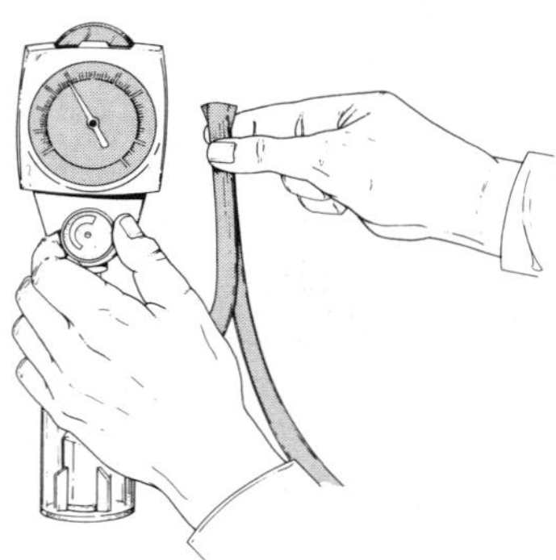

Figure 15–12

Some vacuum regulators have a selector knob for switching between three suctioning modes—suction off, regulated suction, and full suction. Full-line suction can provide flow as high as 110 L/min with the actual subatmospheric pressure and flow created in the suction catheter determined by internal diameter and length of the suction tube. If the flow is turbulent, the suction flow will be related to the square root of the pressure difference between the proximal and distal ends of the tube, and will be proportional when the flow is laminar. In the regulated suction mode subatmospheric pressure can be set between 0 and 200 mm Hg. Suction pressure is set with the outlet of the vacuum regulator occluded (Fig. 15–12). The safe vacuum level varies according to the size of the patient: neonatal, 60 to 80 mm Hg; pediatric, 80 to 100 mm Hg; and adults, 80 to 120 mm Hg.

Inability to suction secretions from the airway may be the result of one of the following: (1) kinked suction tubing, (2) disconnected suction tubing, (3) mucus plug in suction catheter, (4) the float of a full collection reservoir turning off the regulator, or (5) the catheter not coming in contact with secretions. In emergency situations such as vomiting when an esophageal obturator airway is removed, the suction catheter may become plugged. The appropriate action would be to clear the obstruction, use a tonsil sucker (Yankauer), or aspirate with the suction tubing. When suction stops because of thick secretions, tracheal instillation of normal saline may help thin the secretions so they will pass through the suction catheter. The volume instilled will vary with the size of the patient: neonatal, few drops to 0.33 mL; older children, 1 to 3 mL; and adults, 5 to 10 mL. The normal saline should be dispersed after injection into the tracheal tube by using a manual resuscitator to provide deep breathing. The resuscitator should deliver an inspired oxygen concentration of 1.00 except with neonates and infants younger than 6 months of age, who should receive an F_{IO_2} 0.10 higher than their regular oxygen therapy.

(Q) What is the appropriate amount of suction pressure to use when suctioning a 6-year-old child?

a. 60 to 80 mm Hg 436 A
b. 80 to 100 mm Hg 436 b
c. 80 to 120 mm Hg 437 C

FRAME 229. SPUTUM SPECIMEN COLLECTOR

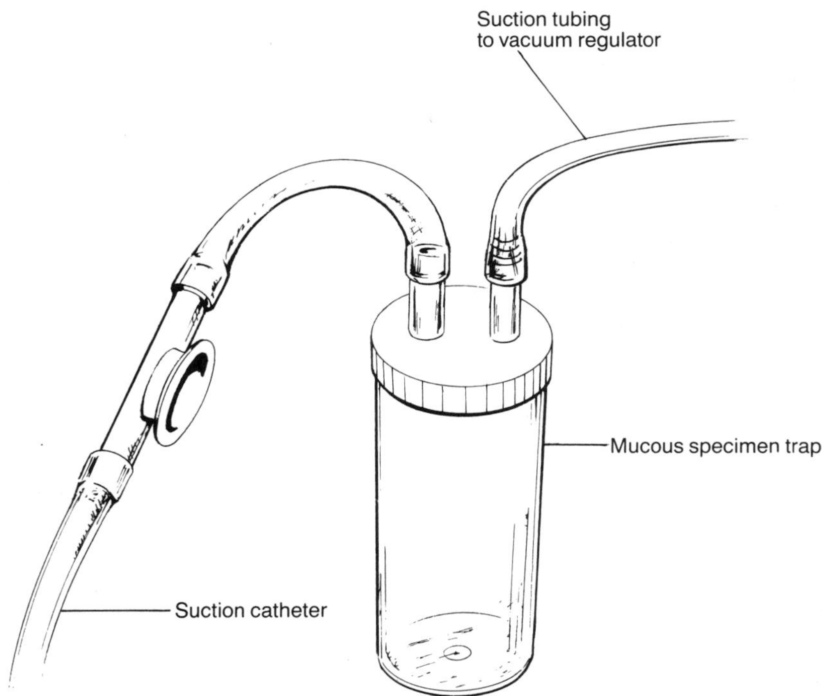

Figure 15–13 Mucus specimen trap.

Routine sputum cultures are frequently used to diagnose the etiology of a lower respiratory tract infection. The specimen cannot be collected from expectorated sputum because of the large number and variety of anaerobic flora in the normal mouth and oropharynx. A sterile sputum trap can be connected between the suction catheter and the suction tubing to collect a specimen from the trachea (Fig. 15–13). Great care must be taken to not contaminate the specimen as it is collected into the sterile sputum trap. Once the specimen is collected, the inlet and outlet of the trap are connected together with a small sterile piece of tubing to seal the container. Care must be taken not to aspirate into the sputum trap water or saline that is used to rinse the suction catheter. There is not a suitable transport medium for sputum and it must be brought in a dry, sterile container to the clinical laboratory immediately for bacterial and cytologic examination. Since the laboratory may have the capability to exam specimens during the day shift only, call the lab and check before obtaining the specimen; the sputum should not be collected during the evening or night shifts.

(Q) Which of the following steps should be taken when collecting a sputum specimen for bacterial and cytological examination from an intubated patient?

a. induce a cough with tracheal instillation of water 436 D
b. induce a cough with tracheal instillation of hypertonic saline 437 A
c. induce a cough by coaching and chest physiotherapy 437 b

FRAME 230. TRACHEOSTOMY TUBES AND BUTTONS

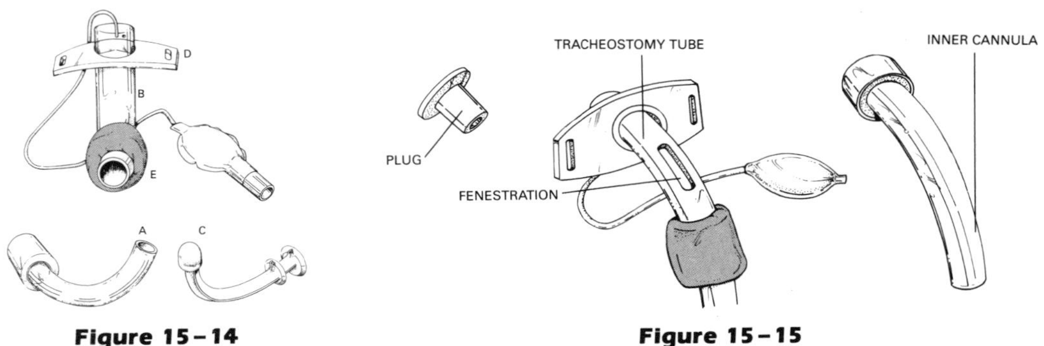

Figure 15–14

Figure 15–15

Figure 15–14 A standard tracheostomy tube showing (*A*) inner cannula, (*B*) outer cannula, (*C*) obturator, (*D*) flange, and (*E*) cuff.

Figure 15–15 Fenestrated tracheostomy tube with removable inner cannula and plug.

Tracheostomy tubes (Fig. 15–14) are used for long-term patients because they are easier to suction and stabilize, cause less resistance to airflow, easily attach to equipment, and allow the patient to eat. They reduce complications to the upper airway, glottis, and larynx. The inner cannula can be taken out and cleaned with a tracheostomy brush and hydrogen peroxide, and rinsed with sterile water. The obturator replaces the inner cannula of the tracheostomy tube when the tube is inserted into the stoma and immediately removed when the tube is in place. A spare tracheostomy tube of the same size should always be available at the bedside. Since the upper airways are bypassed, adequate humidification must be accomplished by continuous use of a nebulizer driven with air or oxygen. Although the cuff on a tracheostomy tube may not need to be inflated continuously, a high-volume low-pressure cuff should be used. The minimal leak technique should be used to inflate the cuff. Problems encountered immediately after a tracheotomy is done include (1) bleeding, (2) pneumothorax, (3) subcutaneous and mediastinal emphysema, and (4) air embolism. Late complications of tracheostomy tubes include (1) infection of the stoma, (2) airway obstruction from secretions or cuff overinflation, (3) hemorrhage, and (4) tracheoesophageal fistula.

Fenestrated tracheostomy tubes (Fig. 15–15) have an opening in the outer cannula that allows the patient to breathe through the upper airway when the tube is corked with the inner cannula removed and cuff deflated. The fenestrated tube can be useful for assessing the patient's ability to be extubated and to allow the patient to speak.

A *tracheal button* is used when there is some doubt about the patient's ability to permanently maintain a patent airway without a tracheostomy tube (Fig. 15–16). The tracheal button does not protrude into the trachea and the patient can breathe from the upper airway without increased resistance. The purpose of the button is to keep the stoma open for suctioning or emergency ventilation. The upper airway must be sealed if the stoma is used for emergency ventilation. The tracheal button allows the patient to talk, since air moves through the larynx.

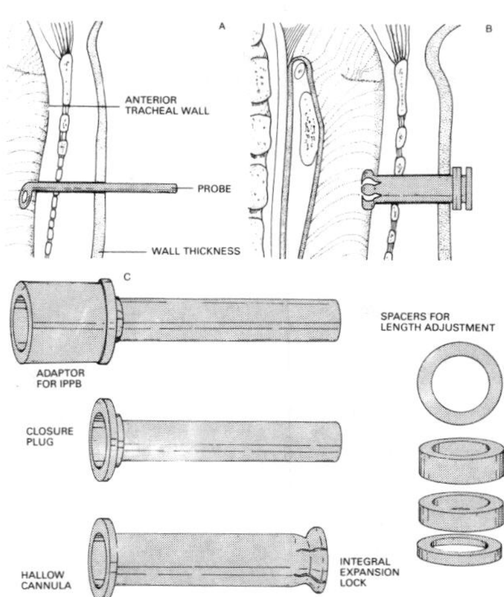

Figure 15–16 Tracheostomy button. (*A*) A probe is used to measure the length of button needed; (*B*) tracheostomy button in place; (*C*) parts of the tracheostomy button.

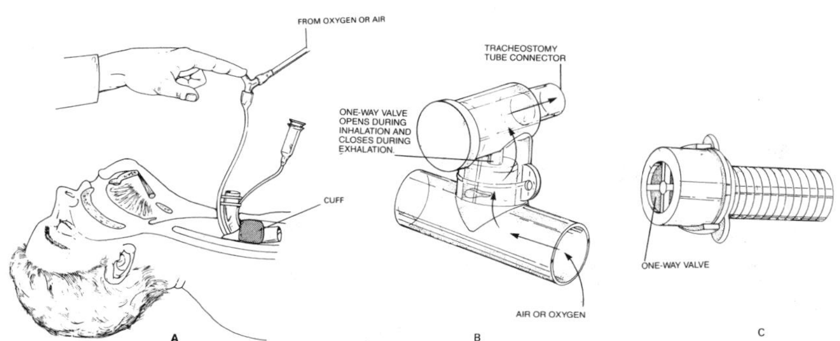

Figure 15–17 Various tubes to allow the patient to talk. (*A*) Pitt speaking tracheostomy tube; (*B*) Olympic Trach-Talk; (*C*) Kistner plastic tracheostomy tube.

The *Pitt speaking tube* (Fig. 15–17*A*) is designed with a small tube above the cuff that allows a low flow of oxygen or air to travel through the larynx when the patient wants to speak. The patient speaks by directing flow to his vocal cords by occluding a Y-connector. The lower airways remain protected from aspiration pneumonia by the inflated cuff, and speech becomes possible during mechanical ventilation or continuous positive-airway pressure (CPAP). The *Olympic Trach-Talk* (Fig. 15–17*B*) is a device that attaches to the outer cannula of a fenestrated tracheostomy tube (inner cannula is removed and cuff is deflated). The purpose of the Trach-Talk one-way valve is to allow the patient to breath in through the tracheostomy tube but not out; thus exhaled tidal volumes are forced through the upper airway. The flow to the upper airway helps the patient produce sufficient intrathoracic pressure to generate an effective cough. The *Kistner* tracheostomy tube (Fig. 15–17*C*) is another example of a one-way valve that directs exhaled tidal volumes through the upper airway. However, the Kistner tube replaces a tracheal button rather than attaching to the tracheostomy tube.

(Q) Which of the following tracheostomy tubes will facilitate the patient's ability to cough effectively without plugging the outer cannula?

a. Olympic Trach-Talk — 437 B
b. Pitt speaking tracheostomy tube — 436 a
c. Shiley fenestrated tracheostomy tube — 437 c

FRAME 231. INCENTIVE SPIROMETERS

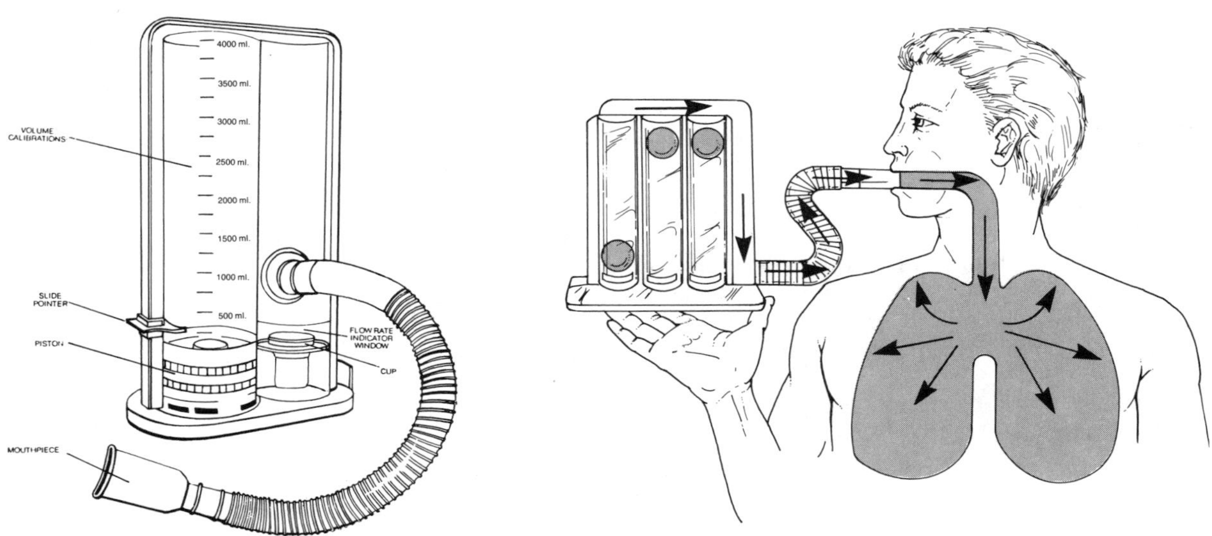

Figure 15–18 **Figure 15–19**

Figure 15–18 Voldyne volumetric deep-breathing exerciser.

Figure 15–19 Triflo II incentive breathing exerciser.

Incentive spirometers are used to encourage deep breathing and prevent atelectasis. Other devices that focus on inspiratory flow instead of tidal volume are also used to encourage sustained maximal inspirations. The purpose of having patients use these devices is to reinflate collapsed alveoli by increasing the transpulmonary pressure and functional residual capacity. The Voldyne volumetric deep-breathing exerciser is an example of an incentive spirometer that focuses on volume-oriented goals (Fig. 15–18). The procedure for its use includes the following steps: (1) exhale to the resting functional residual capacity (FRC) level, (2) create a tight seal around mouthpiece, (3) inspire slowly until the piston rises to the level of the slide pointer, and (4) remove mouthpiece from lips and exhale normally. The incentive spirometer should be used when awake with 10 deep breaths per hour as a minimum. Short rest periods should be taken between deep breaths so that hyperventilation does not occur.

The Triflo II incentive breathing exerciser is a device that can be used to encourage sustained maximal inspiration (Fig. 15–19). The number of balls that ascend will determine the magnitude of the inspiratory effort and the flow created. A flow of either 600 or 900 mL/sec (36 or 54 L/min) is recommended to enhance uniform distribution of the inspired gas. A flow of 1200 mL/sec (72 L/min) is considered too high for good distribution of inspired gas. The device is designed to indicate flow according to how many balls rise in the chambers, for example, 1 ball—600 mL/s, 2 balls—900 mL/s, and 3 balls—1200 mL/s. Regardless of the inspiratory flow generated the patient should be encouraged to suspend the balls at the top of the chambers for at least 3 seconds. The patient should be encouraged to keep the third ball at the bottom of the chamber; for example, all three balls should not rise to the top of chamber. Exhalation should be normal and the balls will fall to the bottom of the chamber as the mouthpiece is removed from the lips.

(Q) How is the incentive spirometry volume goal determined?

a. The patients ideal body weight is multiplied by 15 mL/kg. 436 d

b. The spontaneous tidal volume is multiplied by 3. 437 D

c. A maximal inspiratory capacity becomes the goal. 436 B

FRAME 232. CHEST PERCUSSORS

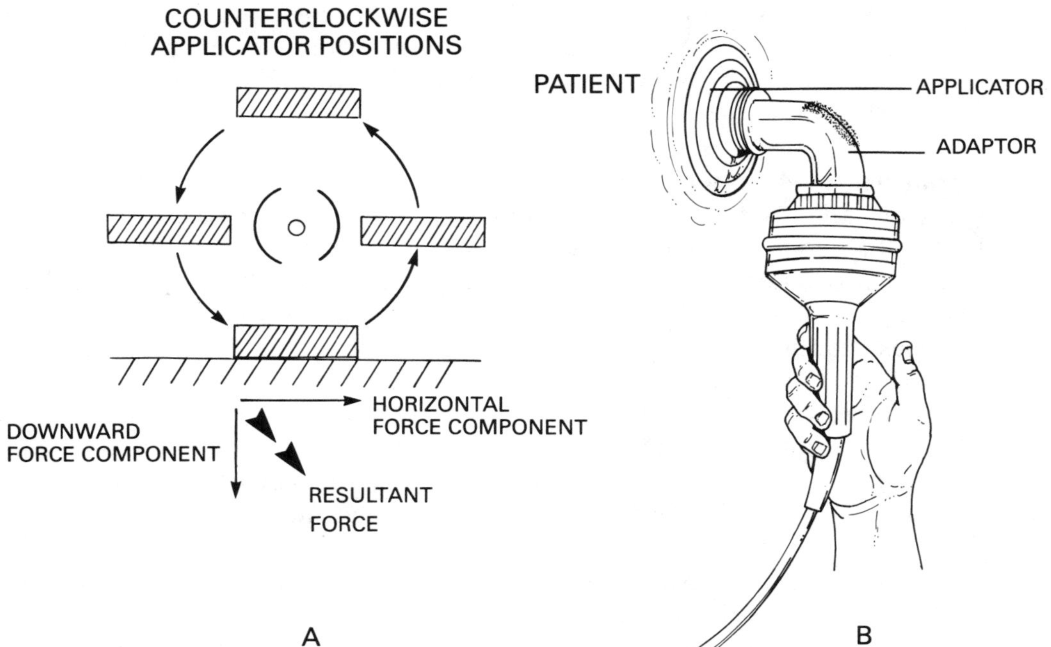

Figure 15–20 Vibramatic chest percussor: (*A*) horizontal and perpendicular force components of applicator; (*B*) technique for holding the handle of the percussor.

The illustrations (Fig. 15–20) above show an example of a chest percussor that can be used during bronchial hygiene therapy to help loosen and mobilize retained secretions. Care should be taken to apply the vibrator using the right technique and the following guidelines: (1) the adapters that connect the applicator to the directional stroking unit must be assembled correctly, (2) the applicator should be held on one location of the patient's chest for only 30 to 60 seconds, (3) the applicator should be held lightly with the fingers only so that no additional force is applied by the therapist's body weight, (4) the wrist and arm must be relaxed so that mechanical energy is not lost through the therapist's hand and arm, (5) low-frequency oscillations should be used on large patients and higher frequencies on smaller patients, and (6) the amount of percussive force should be assessed by placing a hand on the chest next to the applicator. Before the chest percussor is applied to the chest, the patient should be placed in the appropriate postural drainage position to facilitate removal of secretions. Adequate rest periods and time for coughing should be provided as the percussor is moved from one area of the chest to another.

(Q) Which of the following would be the best way to hold the applicator of a mechanical chest percussor?

a. hold loosely with the fingers of one hand — 436 C
b. hold tightly with both hands — 436 c
c. hold tightly with one hand — 437 a

436A (from page 430, frame 228)
Wrong. Suction pressure of 60 to 80 mm Hg is used for neonates. It is lower than that used with children because of the smaller lung volume of neonates and the greater risk of causing atelectasis and hypoxemia. Return to page 430, frame 228, and select another choice.

436B (from page 434, frame 231)
Correct. The patient's maximum achievable inspiratory capacity should be the initial goal. The goal may increase as atelectatic areas are inflated. It would be frustrating to the patient and result in noncompliance to set the goal higher than the patient can achieve. Using 15 mL/kg, a goal may fall below what the patient can do. Please continue on page 435, frame 232.

436C (from page 435, frame 232)
Correct. The applicator must be held loosely with the fingers of one hand so that the body weight of the therapist does not increase the force being delivered. If the applicator is held with two hands, a hand will not be available to assess the force being applied to the chest. Holding the applicator rigidly may diminish the force being delivered as energy is absorbed by the hand and arm. Please continue on page 438 and complete the chapter exercises.

436D (from page 431, frame 229)
Wrong. The water will dilute the sample and if suctioned into the trap may cause cells in the sample to burst due to differences in osmolality. This would damage the specimen for cytologic evaluation. Return to page 431, frame 229, and select another answer.

436a (from pages 432–433, frame 230)
Wrong. The Pitt speaking tube would have to be corked and the cuff deflated. Since the outer cannula is not fenestrated, exhalation would be against high resistance caused by the deflated cuff. Return to pages 432–433, frame 230, and select another answer.

436b (from page 430, frame 228)
Correct. The suction pressure used with small children is 80 to 100 mm Hg. A lower suction pressure of 60 to 80 mm Hg is used with neonates, and a higher pressure of 80 to 120 mm Hg for adults. Please continue on page 431, frame 229.

436c (from page 435, frame 232)
Wrong. If the applicator is held with two hands, a hand is not available to assess the force being applied to the chest. Return to page 435, frame 232, and select another answer.

436d (from page 434, frame 231)
Wrong. Using a goal of 15 mL/kg may fall below what the patient can do. Return to page 434, frame 231, and select another answer.

437A (from page 431, frame 229)
Wrong. The hypertonic saline, if suctioned into the trap, will dilute the sample and damage cells in the specimen. Return to page 431, frame 229, and select another answer.

437B (from pages 432–433, frame 230)
Correct. The Olympic Trach-Talk allows the patient to inhale from the tracheostomy tube but forces exhalation through the upper airways. A fenestrated tube with inner cannula removed and cuff deflated must be used with this one-way valve. Please continue on page 434, frame 231.

437C (from page 430, frame 228)
Wrong. This pressure would be too high for a 6-year-old. A suction pressure of 80 to 120 mm Hg is the range used for adults. Return to page 430, frame 228, and select another answer.

437D (from page 434, frame 231)
Wrong. It will be frustrating to the patient and result in noncompliance to set the goal higher than the patient can achieve. Return to page 434, frame 231, and select another answer.

437a (from page 435, frame 232)
Wrong. Holding the applicator rigidly may diminish the force being delivered as energy is absorbed by the hand and arm. Return to page 435, frame 232, and select another answer.

437b (from page 431, frame 229)
Correct. The sputum from the trachea should be aspirated into the trap without contaminating the specimen with water or hypertonic saline, which will damage cells. Please continue on pages 432–433, frame 230.

437c (from pages 432–433, frame 230)
Wrong. A fenestrated tube would have to be corked, the inner cannula removed, and the cuff deflated. Which tube allows inspiration to occur through the tracheostomy tube and forces exhaled tidal volumes through the upper airway? Return to pages 432–433, frame 230, and make another selection.

EXERCISES

1. Collect six different types of oropharyngeal and nasopharyngeal airways and compare and contrast the differences in design.
2. List the steps you would take prior to removing an esophageal obturator airway from a patient in the emergency room.
3. Intubate a mannequin with an endotracheal tube, inflating the cuff, and securing the tube in place with 1-in tape. Complete this exercise with a partner who is instructed to pull the tube from the trachea if it is left unattended prior to being taped in place.
4. Draw a picture of a laryngoscope with both straight and curved blades. Label the light source, electrical connection between handle and blade, guide flange, tip that lifts the epiglottis (straight blade), tip that is inserted in the vallecula (curved blade), and battery compartment.
5. Identify eight different designs for suction catheters and list the advantages and disadvantages of each one in terms of trauma to the airway.
6. Identify a situation that would justify increasing the suction vacuum above 120 mm Hg.
7. Describe the damage that would be done to a sputum specimen for bacterial and cytologic evaluation that has been mixed with water or hypertonic saline.
8. Identify the circumstances that would justify the use of the following types of tracheostomy tubes: standard design, fenestrated, tracheal button, Pitt speaking tube, Olympic Trach-Talk, and Kistner tube.
9. Collect three different types of disposable incentive spirometers and evaluate their design in terms of whether the focus is placed on volumetric goals or sustained maximal inspiratory flow.
10. Find a partner and practice applying chest percussion using a pneumatic or electrically driven percussor with special attention directed on evaluating the force being delivered by the applicator.

POSTTEST

This test is designed to evaluate what you have learned from completing Chapter 15. Check your answers on page 441 and review the topics where your answer is incorrect.

1. Which of the following would facilitate tracheal suctioning for a conscious patient *without* an endotracheal tube in place?
   A. Cath-Guide Guedel oral airway
   B. Berman oral airway
   C. nasopharyngeal airway
   D. Yankauer tonsil sucker
   E. Magill forceps
2. Long-term use of nasopharyngeal airways may cause which of the following?
   I. retention of secretions
   II. laryngospasm
   III. vomiting
   IV. nose bleeds
   V. tissue necrosis
   A. I and IV only
   B. II and III only
   C. I, II, and V only
   D. II, III, IV, and V only
   E. I, II, III, IV, and V
3. Which of the following is a clinical sign that an esophageal obturator airway is in the trachea?
   A. vomiting
   B. bleeding
   C. chest pain
   D. absence of breath sounds
   E. subcutaneous emphysema
4. Which of the following must be done to use a manual resuscitator with an esophageal obturator airway (EOA)?
   I. remove mask from manual resuscitator
   II. deflate cuff of EOA
   III. ensure a 15/22 mm connector is attached to outlet tube of EOA
   IV. ensure EOA mask makes a tight seal with face
   V. remove mask from EOA
   A. II and V only
   B. II and III only
   C. I, III, and IV only
   D. II, III, and V only
   E. I, II, III, and IV only
5. What size endotracheal tube is appropriate for an average adult male?
   A. 6.5 to 7.0
   B. 7.0 to 7.5
   C. 7.5 to 8.0
   D. 8.0 to 8.5
   E. 8.5 to 9.0
6. What is the average distance from the teeth to carina?
   A. 13 cm
   B. 17 cm
   C. 20 cm
   D. 27 cm
   E. 35 cm

7. Which of these facilitates endotracheal intubation by changing the curve of the tube?
   A. stylet
   B. Magill forceps
   C. use of a Miller blade
8. Which of these laryngoscope blades is best for intubating an average male?
   A. Macintosh 1
   B. Macintosh 3
   C. Miller 1
   D. Wis Hippie 1½
   E. Guedel 1
9. Which of the following suction catheters is *most* likely to apply the vacuum pressure to the airway wall?
   A. whistle-tip (one side hole)
   B. whistle-tip (two opposing side holes)
   C. straight-tip (without side holes)
   D. straight-tip (two opposing side holes)
   E. straight-tip (four opposing side holes)
10. How should vacuum pressure be applied to a suction catheter?
    I. constantly during passage into tracheal tube
    II. constantly during removal from tracheal tube
    III. intermittently during removal from tracheal tube
    IV. when the catheter is fully inserted into tracheal tube
    V. only when the catheter is inside tracheal tube
    A. I only
    B. I and II only
    C. I and III only
    D. I and V only
    E. III and IV only
11. What is the safe range of suction pressure to use with neonates?
    A. 60 to 80 mm Hg
    B. 80 to 100 mm Hg
    C. 80 to 120 mm Hg
    D. 100 to 140 mm Hg
    E. 140 to 180 mm Hg
12. How much normal saline should be instilled into the endotracheal tube of adults when secretions threaten to occlude the airway?
    A. ⅓ mL
    B. 1 to 3 mL
    C. 3 to 5 mL
    D. 5 to 10 mL
    E. 10 to 15 mL
13. A sputum specimen for bacterial and cytologic evaluation should be collected from the
    A. mouth.
    B. nasopharynx.
    C. oropharynx.
    D. laryngopharynx.
    E. trachea.
14. How should a sputum specimen be transported to the clinical lab?
    A. cooled in ice
    B. hydrated with normal saline
    C. hydrated with sterile water
    D. covered with hypertonic saline
    E. in a dry sterile container
15. Which of the following would be best to maintain the patency of a tracheal stoma and keep it open for suctioning or emergency ventilation?
    A. Pitt speaking tube
    B. tracheal button
    C. Olympic Trach-Talk
    D. fenestrated tracheostomy tube
    E. standard tracheostomy tube

16. Which of the following tracheostomy tubes uses low-flow oxygen or air to allow the patient to talk?
    A. Pitt speaking tube
    B. tracheal button
    C. Olympic Trach-Talk
    D. fenestrated tracheostomy tube
    E. standard tracheostomy tube
17. What is the maximum amount of inspiratory flow that a patient should generate with the Triflo II incentive breathing exerciser?
    A. 600 mL/s
    B. 900 mL/s
    C. 1200 mL/s
    D. 36 L/min
    E. 72 L/min
18. How should patients using incentive deep-breathing devices exhale?
    A. normally
    B. faster than normal
    C. slower than normal
    D. maximally done to residual volume
    E. faster than normal every other breath
19. A chest percussor when used with a 90-kg patient should have the percussion force increased by
    A. using a lower oscillation frequency.
    B. using a higher oscillation frequency.
    C. holding the applicator tightly with one hand instead of the fingers.
    D. holding the applicator with two hands instead of the fingers.
    E. by transferring therapist body weight to the applicator.
20. Which of the following is true regarding chest percussors?
    I. Higher oscillation frequencies are used with larger patients.
    II. The percussor applicator should be held firmly with one hand.
    III. The appropriate postural drainage position should be used.
    IV. The applicator should be held over one area for only 30 to 60 seconds.
    V. The percussor should be held loosely with two hands.
    A. I and III only
    B. II and IV only
    C. III and IV only
    D. II, IV, and V only
    E. I, III, IV, and V only

ANSWERS TO POSTTEST

1. C (F223)
2. D (F223)
3. D (F224)
4. C (F224)
5. D (F225)
6. D (F225)
7. A (F226)
8. B (F226)
9. C (F227)
10. E (F227)
11. A (F228)
12. D (F228)
13. E (F229)
14. E (F229)
15. B (F230)
16. A (F230)
17. B (F231)
18. A (F231)
19. A (F232)
20. C (F232)

BIBLIOGRAPHY

Barnes, TA: Respiratory Care Practice. Year Book Medical Publishers, Chicago, 1988.

Burton, GG and Hodgkin, JE: Respiratory Care: A Guide to Clinical Practice, ed 2. JB Lippincott, Philadelphia, 1984.

Eubanks, DH and Bone, RC: Comprehensive Respiratory Care, ed 2. CV Mosby, St. Louis, 1990.

Kacmarek, RM and Stoller, JK: Current Respiratory Care. BC Decker, Philadelphia, 1988.

McPherson, SP: Respiratory Home Care Equipment. Daedalus Enterprises, Dallas, 1988.

McPherson, SP: Respiratory Therapy Equipment, ed 4. CV Mosby, St. Louis, 1990.

Riggs, JH: Respiratory Facts. FA Davis, Philadelphia, 1989.

Surkin, HB and Parkman, AW: The Respiratory Care Workbook. FA Davis, Philadelphia, 1990.

16

Mechanical Ventilators

233. IPPB machines
234. Adjustment of IPPB machines
235. Troubleshooting IPPB machines
236. Volume-preset ventilators
237. Ventilator circuits
238. Control interaction
239. Troubleshooting ventilator malfunction
240. Ventilator alarm systems
241. Continuous-flow IMV systems
242. PEEP devices

PRETEST

This pretest is designed to measure what you already know about mechanical ventilators. Check your answer on page 445 and continue on page 446, frame 233.

1. What control affects the flow capability of the Bird Mark 7 ventilator?
   A. air mix
   B. sensitivity
   C. pressure
   D. expiratory time
   E. hand-timer rod

2. What is the maximum flow capability of the Bird Mark 7 ventilator?
   A. 40 L/min
   B. 55 L/min
   C. 65 L/min
   D. 80 L/min
   E. 95 L/min

3. Which of these controls on the Bird Mark 7 ventilator affect(s) inspiratory time?
   I. flow
   II. expiratory time
   III. pressure
   IV. sensitivity
   V. air mix
   A. I only
   B. I and III only
   C. III, IV, and V only
   D. I, III, IV, and V only
   E. I, II, III, IV, and V

4. Which of the following controls on the Bird Mark 7 ventilator affect(s) the cycle rate?
   I. flow
   II. expiratory time
   III. pressure
   IV. sensitivity
   V. air mix
   A. I only
   B. I and III only
   C. III, IV, and V only
   D. I, III, IV, and V only
   E. I, II, III, IV, and V

5. What is the most *common* cause of failure to cycle with IPPB machines?
   A. high cycling pressure
   B. low cycling pressure
   C. sensitivity
   D. leaks in the circuit
   E. inadequate inspiratory flow

6. Rapid cycling of an IPPB machine requires which control to be adjusted?
   A. pressure
   B. expiratory flow
   C. sensitivity
   D. air mix
   E. inspiratory flow

7. Which of the inspiratory flow patterns found on some volume-preset ventilators is closest to that seen with spontaneous breathing?
   A. sine
   B. square
   C. accelerating
   D. decelerating
   E. plateau

8. When secretions accumulate in the trachea of a patient, which parameter on a volume-preset ventilator will change?
   A. tidal volume
   B. peak inspiratory pressure
   C. plateau pressure
   D. positive end-expiratory pressure (PEEP)
   E. inspiratory time
9. What is the most *common* circuit-related problem with adult volume-preset ventilators?
   A. leaks
   B. condensate
   C. tubing compliance
   D. humidifier water levels
   E. infection
10. The average permanent ventilator circuit has a tubing compliance of
   A. 1 mL/cm H_2O.
   B. 3 mL/cm H_2O.
   C. 5 mL/cm H_2O.
   D. 7 mL/cm H_2O.
   E. 9 mL/cm H_2O.
11. Which of the following controls affect(s) the inspiratory-to-expiratory ratio (I:E ratio) on a volume-preset ventilator?
   I. flow
   II. F_{IO_2}
   III. tidal volume
   IV. cycle rate
   V. sensitivity
   A. I only
   B. III only
   C. I and IV only
   D. II, III, and V only
   E. I, III, and IV only
12. Which of the following may be affected if the pressure limit is reached on a volume-preset ventilator?
   I. flow
   II. tidal volume
   III. inspiratory time
   IV. I:E ratio
   V. cycle rate
   A. I only
   B. II only
   C. II, IV, and V only
   D. II, III, and IV only
   E. I, II, III, IV, and V
13. What pressure should be held in a ventilator circuit to check for leaks?
   A. 25 cm H_2O.
   B. 40 cm h_2O.
   C. 55 cm H_2O.
   D. 80 cm H_2O.
   E. 95 cm H_2O.
14. To check for an *internal* leak in a ventilator, system pressure should be measured with the circuit occluded
   A. after the exhalation valve.
   B. after the Y-connector.
   C. before the Y-connector.
   D. after the humidifier.
   E. before the humidifier.

15. What is the safest way to check an alarm system?
    A. Change alarm threshold and check response time.
    B. Simulate a threshold level and check response time.
    C. Visually verify threshold and delay controls.
    D. Time the deactivation period after pushing the delay button.
    E. Change the delay time until the alarm is triggered.
16. The low-pressure alarm threshold should be set
    A. 5 cm H_2O above PEEP.
    B. 10 cm H_2O above baseline.
    C. 10 to 20 cm H_2O above baseline.
    D. 2 to 3 cm H_2O below peak inspiratory pressure.
    E. 5 to 10 cm H_2O below peak inspiratory pressure.
17. A typical flow through a continuous-flow IMV system is
    A. 12 L/min.
    B. 18 L/min.
    C. 24 L/min.
    D. 40 L/min.
    E. 80 L/min.
18. The pressure release valve on a bag reservoir for an IMV system should be set
    A. 2 to 3 cm H_2O below peak inspiratory pressure.
    B. 5 to 10 cm H_2O below peak inspiratory pressure.
    C. 5 to 10 cm H_2O above baseline pressure.
    D. 5 to 10 cm H_2O above PEEP.
    E. 2 to 3 cm H_2O above PEEP.
19. Which of the following is an example of a flow-resistor PEEP device?
    A. spring-loaded valve
    B. calibrated weight valve
    C. magnetic valve
    D. adjustable clamp
    E. water column
20. Which of these factors determine whether a PEEP device is a threshold resistor?
    I. diameter of the outlet
    II. diameter of the inlet
    III. affect on mean airway pressure
    IV. need for continuous flow
    V. time it takes for peak inspiratory pressure to fall to PEEP level
    A. I and II only
    B. III and V only
    C. I, III, and IV only
    D. II, III, IV, and V only
    E. I, II, III, IV, and V

ANSWERS TO PRETEST

1. A (F233)
2. C (F233)
3. D (F234)
4. E (F234)
5. D (F235)
6. C (F235)
7. A (F236)
8. B (F240)
9. B (F237)
10. B (F237)
11. E (F238)
12. D (F238)
13. D (F239)
14. E (F239)
15. B (F240)
16. E (F240)
17. D (F241)
18. E (F241)
19. D (F242)
20. E (F242)

FRAME 233. IPPB MACHINES

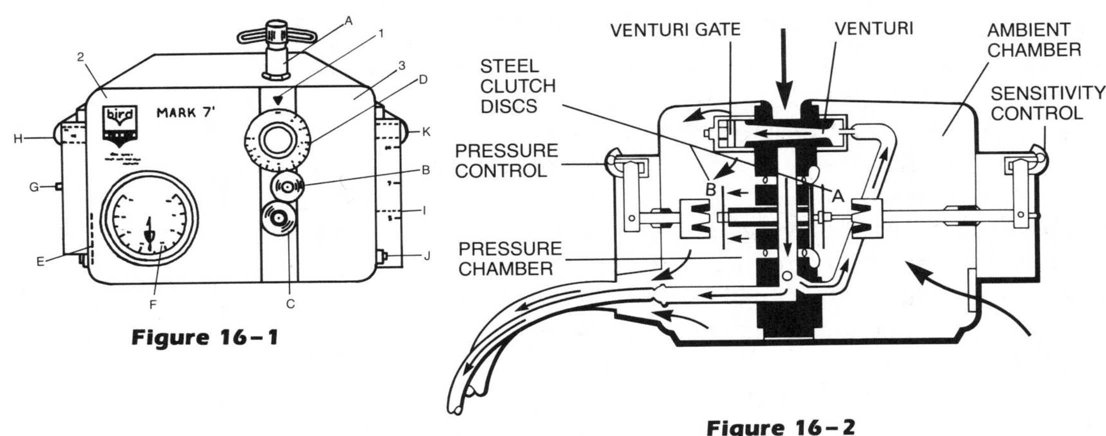

Figure 16–1

Figure 16–2

Figure 16–1 Bird Mark 7. (Source: Surkin, HB and Parkman, AW: The Respiratory Care Workbook. FA Davis, Philadelphia, 1990. Used with permission.)

Figure 16–2 Structure of Bird Mark 7.

The Bird Mark 7 (Fig. 16–1) is commonly used to deliver intermittent positive-pressure breathing (IPPB) and has three primary components: (1) the *center body* with (*A*) gas inlet, (*B*) air-mix control and Venturi, (*C*) expiratory timer, and (*D*) flow-rate control; (2) the *ambient compartment* with (*E*) metal filter for entrained air, (*F*) manometer, (*G*) hand-timer rod, and (*H*) sensitivity control; and (3) the *pressure compartment* with (*I*) connections for mainstream breathing circuit, (*J*) a single outlet to both nebulizer and exhalation valve, and (*K*) pressure control. The Mark 7 is pneumatically powered and controlled, pressure cycled, and small enough to be easily transported. The Mark 7 (Fig. 16–2) terminates inspiration when pressure on the master diaphragm overcomes the attractive force between the magnet and the metal clutch disc (*B*) in the pressure chamber.

The pressure-limit control is the major determinant of tidal volume, which will vary with the patient's pulmonary compliance and airway resistance. The inspiratory flow depends upon whether the air-mix control is set on 100% O_2 ("in" position) or the Venturi is operative ("out" position). The inspiratory flow control depends on the position of the air-mix control and ranges from 0 to 40 L/min on 100% O_2 and 0 to 65 L/min (against 15 cm H_2O) with the air mix Venturi active.

The sensitivity control moves the magnet away from the metal clutch disc (Fig. 16-2) in the ambient chamber. The metal clutch disc (*A*) is attached to the master diaphragm, which controls flow into the pressure chamber. The Bird Mark 7 will cycle rapidly on and off if the sensitivity control magnet is too far from the metal disc. The pressure manometer should be monitored to check the amount of inspiratory pressure required to trigger an assisted breath.

The Mark 7 can be used in the control mode of ventilation by turning on the expiratory timer, which automatically triggers a positive-pressure breath at a rate determined by the amount of time it takes for gas to bleed out of a cartridge that is pressurized during the inspiratory phase.

(Q) The Bird Mark 7 terminates inspiration when what happens?

a. Flow falls to a specified level. 452 A
b. Pressure overcomes the force of a magnet. 452 c
c. A preset-level tidal volume is delivered. 453 B

FRAME 234. ADJUSTMENT OF IPPB MACHINES

IPPB machines are pressure cycled and will *not* deliver a preset tidal volume. The pressure and flow controls are used to vary the size of the tidal volume delivered. If the inspiratory flow is too fast, more pressure will be used to move the gas through the airways and less driving pressure will be available to distend the lungs. Increasing the flow will shorten inspiratory time and may increase the respiratory rate when using control-mode ventilation (CMV). Decreasing the flow to a more appropriate level may increase the tidal volume delivered. If the flow is too low, the pressure manometer will rise very slowly and the inspiratory time will increase to an uncomfortable length. Increasing the pressure limit will increase the tidal volume and lengthen the inspiratory time unless the flow is increased concurrently.

The flow waveform and range will change dramatically when the Bird Mark 7 ventilator is switched from air mix to 100% O_2. The peak inspiratory flow achievable will drop by 38%, from 65 to 40 L/min, when the Venturi is turned off by pushing the air-mix control in. When the IPPB machine is set to deliver 100% source gas, it becomes a constant-flow generator because the flow control has a pressure of 50 pounds per square inch gauge (psig) on the inlet side. The air-mix Venturi and the pressure control will also affect the FIO_2 delivered, since pressure changes will affect the Venturi gate and alter the amount of air mixed with oxygen.

The sensitivity control may affect the peak inspiratory pressure generated by the Mark 7. The interaction of the magnets in the ambient and pressure compartments links both controls through the magnetic clutch system that cycles the ventilator. Increasing the sensitivity will raise the peak inspiratory pressure, and decreasing the sensitivity will drop the pressure limit.

(Q) Which controls on the Bird Mark 7 ventilator affect the tidal volume?

a. tidal volume, flow, and air mix 452 D

b. pressure, sensitivity, and expiratory timer 453 A

c. pressure, flow, and sensitivity 453 b

FRAME 235. TROUBLESHOOTING IPPB MACHINES

Common problems encountered when using IPPB machines include failure to pressure-cycle, inadequate inspiratory flow, highly variable F_{IO_2}, medication nebulizer failure, premature pressure cycling, rapid uncontrolled cycling, and control interaction. Failure to pressure-cycle usually is caused by a leak in the circuit from a defective exhalation valve or by gas escaping from a loose connection, such as a misthreaded medication nebulizer cup. Patients must be carefully instructed to make a tight seal with their lips around the mouthpiece of the breathing circuit and to breathe deeply so that gas does not leak from the mouth. A hand-held mask may be needed with certain geriatric patients who cannot maintain a seal around the mouthpiece. Some pressure-cycled IPPB machines have a supplemental flow device to compensate for the volume lost through small leaks so that pressure cycling occurs without delay.

Inadequate flow can be a problem when the air-mix control is set on 100% source gas, especially when the pressure control is set to a high level. It is rarely necessary to power IPPB machines with oxygen, and air can be substituted as a source gas. When powered with air, the Venturi can be activated, and the peak flow will be substantially increased. If the Bird Mark 7 is powered by oxygen, the F_{IO_2} will vary throughout the inspiration because the entrainment gate of the Venturi will be affected by back pressure. Powering an IPPB machine with air allows F_{IO_2} to be controlled by bleeding oxygen into a reservoir attached to the gas entrainment port.

Premature pressure cycling of IPPB machines occurs when the patient occludes the mouthpiece with the tongue or exhales before the pressure limit is reached. Patient instruction and coaching should resolve both of these problems. Rapid uncontrolled cycling will occur if the sensitivity control is adjusted so high that the gas flow through the circuit triggers the next breath before an inspiratory effort is made by the patient. Adjusting the sensitivity control using a rubber test lung will solve this problem.

When the medication nebulizer stops working, it is usually the result of a disconnected hose that powers the jet. Occasionally a problem with the nebulizer will be the result of the capillary down tube becoming disconnected. Finally control interaction (see frame 234) may result in a malfunction that can be corrected by readjusting the control that is adversely affected. Changing inspiratory flow will affect the inspiratory time and the tidal volume delivered. The pressure and sensitivity controls on the Bird Mark 7 interact because they are attached to magnets that attract a metal clutch plate that initiates and pressure-cycles the IPPB machine.

(Q) When the inspiratory time becomes too long after the pressure control on a Bird Mark 7 is increased, which control needs to be adjusted?

a. sensitivity — 452 a
b. expiratory timer — 453 c
c. inspiratory flow — 453 C

FRAME 236. VOLUME-PRESET VENTILATORS

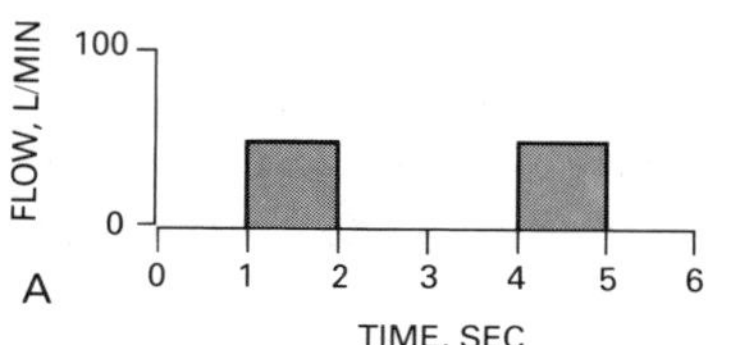

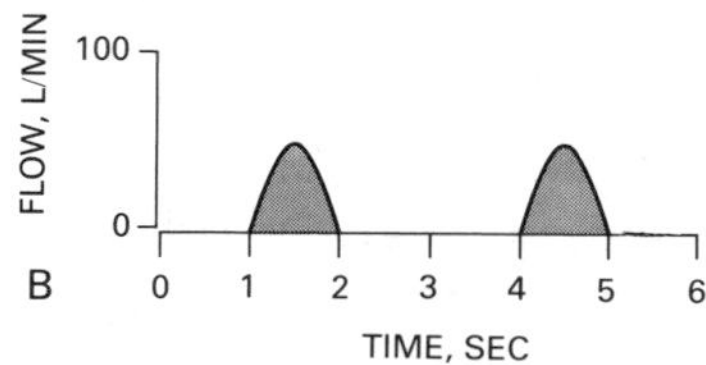

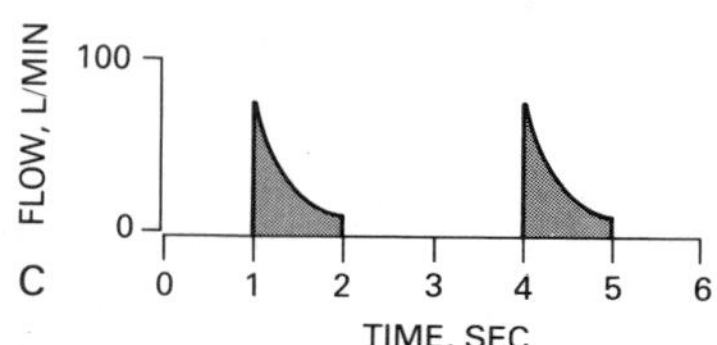

Figure 16–3 Common inspiratory waveforms.

A volume-cycled ventilator will terminate the inspiratory phase after delivering the preset tidal volume regardless of the peak airway pressure required. Since many ventilators have pressure- and time-limiting capabilities that terminate inspiration, most clinicians prefer to use the term *volume-preset* to describe volume-cycled ventilators. Volume-preset ventilators will guarantee delivery of the tidal volume within certain pressure and time limits. If the pressure limit is set 10 cm H_2O above the average peak inspiratory pressure, then small changes in airway resistance and pulmonary compliance will not affect delivery of the tidal volume.

Ventilators can be classified according to these functional characteristics: (1) mechanism for terminating inspiration (pressure-cycled, volume-cycled, flow-cycled, and time-cycled; (2) mechanism for initiating inspiration (controlled ventilation, assisted ventilation, assist-control, IMV, and SIMV; (3) single versus double circuit; (4) power source (pneumatic or electrical); (5) control source (electrical or fluidic); (6) inspiratory waveforms available (square, sine, accelerating, decelerating); (7) expiratory waveforms (retarding exhalation); and (8) ability to apply greater than ambient pressure to the airways during inspiratory and expiratory phases during all modes of ventilation (PEEP).

Some neonatal ventilators are time-cycled when a preset inspiratory time is reached. Tidal volume on such a ventilator will be determined by the pressure limit and the inspiratory time. The inspiratory pressure will rise to a preset level and remain constant until the ventilator is time-cycled into the expiratory phase.

Some ventilators are time-cycled into the expiratory phase when the inspiratory flow drops to a certain level during pressure-support ventilation (pressure is held constant and flow decreases throughout the inspiratory phase). The shape of the inspiratory waveform is an important functional characteristic of volume-preset ventilators (Fig. 16–3). The sine wave flow is the closest to that seen with normal spontaneous breathing. Constant-flow generators can generate a square wave and develop a high driving pressure (100 to 4000 cm H_2O) across a high internal resistance. Since the change in pressure needed to move the tidal volume into the lungs is usually less than 50 cm H_2O, the high internal pressure on the distal side of the (ventilator) side of the orifice ensures a constant flow and delivery of a preset tidal volume. Inspiratory time will be determined by the flow rate and the size of the tidal volume.

(Q) The best way to increase the tidal volume on a neonatal ventilator is to

a. increase the inspiratory time. 452 B

b. decrease the inspiratory time. 452 d

c. decrease the pressure limit. 453 a

FRAME 237. VENTILATOR CIRCUITS

A ventilator breathing circuit serves as a conduit for gas flow between the ventilator and lungs. It must be flexible so that tension is not placed on the tracheal tube, yet strong enough not to tear, develop leaks, or kink. The circuit must have ports for monitoring several important parameters such as (1) proximal airway pressure, (2) proximal gas temperature, and (3) inspired oxygen concentration. Several critical components direct gas flow, control the humidity and temperature of the inspired gas, and establish a baseline of pressure (PEEP or continuous positive-airway pressure [CPAP]) during both inspiratory and expiratory phases.

Some of the preset tidal volume delivered by a ventilator never reaches the lungs because it is used to fill the extra volume created in the ventilator circuit as it distends during the inspiratory phase. In addition to the circuit stretching, high pressure during inspiration will cause gas molecules to move closer together and more gas will be required to fill the circuit. This is especially a problem when mainstream humidifiers with large reservoirs are allowed to operate with the water level close to the fill line. The amount of tidal volume lost in the circuit during inspiration is calculated using the tubing compliance factor. This factor is determined for each circuit and reported in milliliters of volume lost per centimeter H_2O of pressure. The average permanent (nondisposable) circuit has a compliance factor of approximately 3 mL/cm H_2O, which means a change in the circuit pressure of 40 cm H_2O (peak airway pressure—PEEP or baseline pressure) would result in 120 mL of tidal volume being lost in the circuit. The volume lost in the circuit becomes a critical factor in the ventilation of neonates and small children.

Ventilators such as the Bennett 7200a automatically compensate for the volume lost in the circuit and actually deliver all of the preset tidal volume to the lungs. If a ventilator that *does not compensate* for volume lost in the circuit is replaced with one that *does compensate,* the preset tidal volume must be decreased accordingly. Switching to a ventilator that compensates for volume lost in the circuit without reducing preset tidal volume is especially a problem with adult respiratory disease syndrome, in which peak inspiratory pressure may be above 60 cm H_2O.

If the heated humidifier is working properly, the gas in the inspiratory circuit will cool on the way to the patient and water will collect in the tubing. Accumulation of water in the circuit can affect peak airway pressure and delivered tidal volume. Circuits should include water traps or be drained frequently. The water should always be drained away from the humidifier to prevent pathogens from contaminating the reservoir.

(Q) If the tubing compliance factor is 4 mL/cm H_2O, peak inspiratory pressure is 50 cm H_2O, PEEP is 10 cm H_2O, and preset tidal volume is 1000 mL; what is the tidal volume delivered to the lungs by a volume-preset ventilator?

a. 800 mL 452 C
b. 840 mL 452 b
c. 960 mL 453 D

ANSWERS TO FRAMES

452A (from page 447, frame 233)
Wrong. The Bird Mark 7 is not flow-cycled. Return to page 447, frame 233, and review Figure 16-2; then select another answer.

452B (from page 450, frame 236)
Correct. A time-cycled and pressure-limited ventilator is commonly used with neonates. Increasing the inspiratory time will allow a larger tidal volume to be delivered while a sustained preset inspiratory pressure is held constant. Please continue on page 451, frame 237.

452C (from page 451, frame 237)
Wrong. You neglected to subtract the baseline PEEP from the peak inspiratory pressure. PEEP keeps the circuit stretched throughout the entire respiratory cycle and must be considered when the change in pressure during inspiration is calculated. Return to page 451, frame 237, and select another answer.

452D (from page 448, frame 234)
Wrong. IPPB machines are pressure-cycled and do not have a tidal volume control. The tidal volume delivered will depend on the patient's pulmonary compliance and airway resistance. The flow control may affect the tidal volume delivered. The air-mix control will change the range of flow that can be achieved. Return to page 448, frame 234, and try again.

452a (from page 449, frame 235)
Wrong. The sensitivity control may need to be readjusted, since the pressure-limit magnet is closer to the metal clutch plate. However, this would cause the inspiratory time to become too long. Return to page 449, frame 235, and select another answer.

452b (from page 451, frame 237)
Correct. The volume lost to the circuit is determined by calculating the change in pressure during inspiration (peak inspiratory pressure — PEEP) and multiplying by the circuit compliance factor. Delivered tidal volume is determined by subtracting volume lost in the circuit from the preset tidal volume ($1000 - 160 = 840$ mL). Please continue on page 454, frame 238.

452c (from page 447, frame 233)
Correct. The Bird Mark 7 is pressure-cycled from inspiration to expiration. The flow when delivering 100% O_2 will be constant (square waveform) and flow will not drop substantially throughout inspiration. When the Venturi is active, the flow will decrease throughout inspiration but the machine will still be pressure-cycled into expiration. Please continue on page 448, frame 234.

452d (from page 450, frame 236)
Wrong. A time-cycled and pressure-limited ventilator is commonly used with neonates. Decreasing the inspiratory time while a sustained preset inspiratory pressure is held constant will result in a smaller tidal volume being delivered. Return to page 450, frame 236, and select another answer.

453A (from page 448, frame 234)
Wrong. The expiratory timer will have no effect on tidal volume. Return to page 448, frame 234, and select another answer.

453B (from page 447, frame 233)
Wrong. IPPB machines like the Bird Mark 7 are not volume-cycled ventilators. The tidal volume they deliver will depend on the patient's pulmonary compliance and airway resistance and on pressure, flow, and sensitivity controls. Return to page 447, frame 233, and select another answer.

453C (from page 449, frame 235)
Correct. Increasing the cycling pressure without raising the inspiratory flow rate will lengthen the inspiratory time. Adjustment of the inspiratory flow control should solve this problem. Please continue on page 450, frame 236.

453D (from page 451, frame 237)
Wrong. You calculated the pressure change in the circuit correctly but forgot to multiply by the compliance factor to determine the volume lost in the circuit. Return to page 451, frame 237, and select another answer.

453a (from page 450, frame 236)
Wrong. A time-cycled and pressure-limited ventilator is commonly used with neonates. Decreasing the sustained preset inspiratory pressure will result in a smaller tidal volume being delivered. Return to page 450, frame 236, and select another answer.

453b (from page 448, frame 234)
Correct. Pressure, flow, and sensitivity controls all affect the tidal volume delivered by a Bird Mark 7 IPPB machine. High flow may decrease tidal volume. The peak inspiratory pressure and sensitivity controls interact with each other to affect the tidal volume. Please continue on page 449, frame 235.

453c (from page 449, frame 235)
Wrong. Adjusting the expiratory timer will not solve this problem and this control is usually not used for IPPB treatments. Return to page 449, frame 235, and select another answer.

FRAME 238. CONTROL INTERACTION

Respiratory care practitioners need to understand the functional characteristics of volume-preset ventilators well enough to be able to predict which controls will interact with each other. Increasing the inspiratory flow on a constant-flow generator will decrease the inspiratory time and decrease the inspiratory-to-expiratory (I:E) ratio (the I:E ratio decreases when the fraction gets smaller, e.g., 1:3, 1:4, 1:5). Conversely, decreasing the inspiratory flow will lengthen the inspiratory time and increase the I:E ratio. If the inspiratory flow is held constant and the tidal volume is increased, the inspiratory time will increase.

The delivery of tidal volume by a volume-preset ventilator is guaranteed only if the pressure limit is not exceeded. Reaching the pressure limit on a volume-preset ventilator commonly cycles the ventilator into the expiration in order to protect the lungs from high pressure. The pressure limit should be set 10 cm H_2O higher than the average peak inspiratory pressure (PIP) so that the pressure limit does not interfere with delivery of the preset tidal volume when small changes in PIP occur. The pressure limit should be set close to the peak inspiratory pressure so that increases in airway resistance or decreases in pulmonary compliance will trigger a high-pressure alarm. The sounding of a high-pressure alarm may alert practitioners to unnoticed changes in pulmonary dynamics.

Changing the mandatory cycling rate on a volume-preset ventilator will affect the expiratory time and the I:E ratio. Increasing the rate will decrease the total cycle time (sum of inspiratory and expiratory phases), shorten the expiratory phase, and increase the I:E ratio. Only the expiratory phase changes when the total cycle time is decreased, because the inspiratory time on a volume-preset ventilator will be preset or determined by the inspiratory flow. To maintain an appropriate I:E ratio when the mandatory rate is increased, the inspiratory flow may need to be increased because the preset tidal volume will usually fall within a narrow range of 10 to 15 mL/kg.

The appropriate way to calculate the I:E ratio is to determine the total cycle time by dividing 60 seconds by the ventilator cycling rate. The inspiratory time is calculated from preset tidal volume and preset inspiratory flow settings, or taken directly from time-cycled ventilators. The expiratory time is determined by subtracting the inspiratory time from the total cycle time.

The control interaction on a neonatal pressure-limited time-cycled ventilator is different from that of an adult volume-preset ventilator. The neonatal time-cycled ventilator has a continuous flow that travels through the patient circuit during inspiration and expiration. During inspiration the exhalation valve closes and gas is directed into the lungs as pressure in the circuit rises to a preset pressure limit, at which time gas begins to flow from a pressure popoff valve. Inspiratory time is preset and controls the opening of the exhalation valve. The tidal volume delivered is determined by the inspiratory time, the gas flow, and the pressure limit.

(Q) Which of the following controls on a volume-preset ventilator may affect the inspiratory time?

a. flow, tidal volume, and pressure limit 460 A
b. mandatory rate, sensitivity, and expiratory retard 461 D
c. flow, tidal volume, and sensitivity 461 c

FRAME 239. TROUBLESHOOTING VENTILATOR MALFUNCTION

A knowledge of the functional characteristics of volume-preset ventilators will help the practitioner deal with the problems encountered during mechanical ventilation. A manual resuscitator with an oxygen reservoir attached and PEEP capability should be at the bedside whenever a mechanical ventilator is in use. A leak in the ventilator circuit should be suspected when there is a sudden drop in peak inspiratory pressure and a decrease in exhaled tidal volume. The source of the leak should be found while the patient is ventilated with a manual resuscitator. Leaks occur at the following locations: (1) where the circuit attaches to the humidifier and other points of connection, (2) at the exhalation valve when the diaphragm tears or develops a pinhole, or (3) where small holes have developed in the large-bore tubing of the circuit. A test for leaks involves setting the high-pressure alarm at maximum, setting the tidal volume at 1000 mL, and occluding the patient connection and the exhalation valve. The ventilator and patient circuit is tight if 80 cm H_2O can be held for 2 to 4 seconds. If the peak pressure rapidly falls from its maximum when the system is occluded, a leak exists. If an internal leak is suspected, the machine outlet (before the humidifier) should be occluded with a manometer in line to check if a peak pressure of 80 cm H_2O can be held for 2 to 4 seconds.

Providing adequate humidity during mechanical ventilation requires that gas be delivered at 80% to 100% relative humidity at 32° to 37°C (90° to 99°F). The temperature must be monitored closely and enough heat must be provided to the water in the humidifier to saturate the gas passing through with water vapor. The gas must be heated to a higher temperature before leaving the humidifier to compensate for the cooling that occurs during transit along the length of the circuit (4 to 6 ft). The output temperature of a cascade humidifier may be 50°C and contain 84 mg/L water vapor (twice the absolute humidity required). If the room air temperature is 22°C, the warmed gas will cool as it moves through the tubing to the patient connection. The temperature at the Y-connector is usually maintained between 32° and 37°C. The temperature drop along the circuit will cause condensation of water vapor, and the absolute humidity drops from 84 to 44 mg/L. One half of the original vapor produced will collect in the inspiratory side of the circuit (40 mg/L). Adequate humidification is provided to the airway, since 100% relative humidity at 37°C requires only 44 mg/L of absolute humidity. However, a patient with a minute volume of 10 L will have 24 mL/h collect in the circuit (10 L/min × 40 mg/L × 60 min/h = 24,000 mg/h = 24 mL/h). Accordingly, troubleshooting an increase in peak inspiratory pressure should start with ensuring that condensed water has been emptied from the breathing circuit. Very large and sudden increases in peak inspiratory pressure usually result from an airway obstruction, the tracheal tube slipping into the right main-stem bronchus, or a tension pneumothorax.

(Q) If the spirometer on a Bennett MA-1 ventilator rises during inspiration, which of the following is the problem?

a. internal leak before the humidifier 460 B
b. leak located where water reservoir attaches to the humidifier 460 c
c. leak at the exhalation valve 461 C

FRAME 240. VENTILATOR ALARM SYSTEMS

The function of a ventilator alarm system is to alert the practitioner to a change in ventilation parameters. The most important principle to remember is that *inoperative or improperly adjusted alarms are dangerous.* Alarm systems should monitor the following critical ventilation parameters: (1) peak inspiratory pressure, (2) exhaled tidal volume, (3) inspired oxygen concentration, (4) PEEP level, and (5) I:E ratio.

The alarm may sound as the result of a change in the patient's condition, such as high system pressure caused by secretions in the airways. Alarms will also indicate a mechanical or electrical failure. Alarms on ventilators should be tested prior to patient use, every time a ventilator is checked, and after administering respiratory care. The best way to confirm the proper function of an alarm system is to simulate changes in ventilation parameters while the ventilator is connected to a test lung. If a PEEP alarm is supposed to sound within 10 seconds when the end-expiratory level drops by more than 3 cm H_2O, the PEEP level should be dropped by 4 cm H_2O to check the alarm's sensitivity and the response time. Whenever alarm thresholds are changed, the alarm sensitivity and response time should be checked.

Monitoring of PIP involves two alarm thresholds—high pressure and low pressure—which should be set 10 cm H_2O above and 5 to 10 cm H_2O below average PIP, respectively. The high-pressure alarm may have to be set higher than 10 above PIP when the patient is agitated and peak inspiratory pressure fluctuates widely. Some ventilators have independent controls for the high-pressure alarm and pressure release, and the alarm threshold should be set 2 to 3 cm H_2O below the pressure at which gas is vented from the circuit. Setting the alarm threshold higher than the pressure at which gas is vented from the circuit may result in a substantial decrease in ventilation if a majority of the tidal volume is vented. This may result in the patient being hypoventilated and exposed to high airway pressure without the alarm being triggered. The low-pressure alarm is designed to detect leaks and to sound a warning if the patient becomes disconnected from the ventilator circuit. The alarm threshold should be set 5 to 10 cm H_2O below the average peak inspiratory pressure so that flow through a disconnected circuit or large leak will not create enough pressure to recycle the alarm.

Tidal and minute volume alarms should have their thresholds set to detect a 10% to 20% decrease in exhaled volume. The F_{IO_2} should be monitored continuously and the alarm thresholds should be set at ± 0.05 of the desired inspired oxygen concentration. Oxygen monitors should have their alarm functions checked by exposing the sensor probe to increased and decreased concentrations of oxygen.

A safe alarm system is one that has its thresholds set properly so that it does not provide a series of false alarms. Alarms must not be easily turned off, but a 1- or 2-minute delay function needs to be provided to deactivate the alarm when the patient is disconnected from the ventilator for short periods, such as during suctioning.

(Q) On a ventilator that has independent controls for the high-pressure alarm and pressure release, the high-pressure alarm threshold should be

a. 2 to 3 cm H_2O below the pressure-release threshold. 460 a
b. 2 to 3 cm H_2O above the pressure-release threshold. 461 B
c. equal to the pressure-release threshold. 461 a

FRAME 241. CONTINUOUS-FLOW IMV CIRCUITS

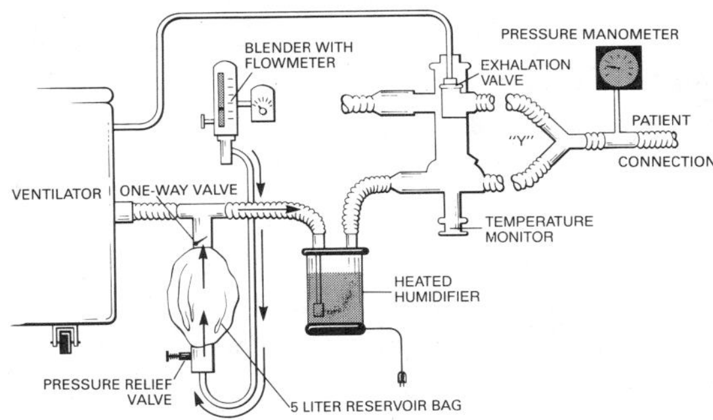

Figure 16–4 Continuous-flow-through reservoir bag IMV system.

When it is necessary to modify a ventilator circuit to provide IMV, the following should be provided: (1) a source of humidified gas for spontaneous breathing that has the same fractional oxygen concentration as that provided by mandatory breaths from the ventilator, (2) gas for spontaneous breathing that is delivered at a flow rate that exceeds the patient's peak inspiratory flow (gas for spontaneous breathing should be available without requiring a large inspiratory effort and the response time should be short), (3) a low-resistance one-way valve should be used between the spontaneous gas source (reservoir bag), (4) a device for lowering the ventilator rate to 2 per minute. The continuous-flow system with a 5-L reservoir bag (Fig. 16–4) is connected to the inspiratory side of the ventilator circuit at the inlet to the heated humidifier. Gas from an air-oxygen blender enters and distends the bag, then flows through a one-way valve into the cascade humidifier, continues through the circuit past the patient connection, and exits through the exhalation valve.

If the flow through the circuit does not match the patient's peak inspiratory flow, gas can be taken from the bag. When mandatory IMV breaths are delivered, the one-way valve between the bag and the ventilator circuit prevents continuous flow from entering the circuit and prevents the mandatory tidal volume from entering the bag. If a small stiff bag is used and the inspiratory flow delivered by the ventilator is less than the continuous flow, the one-way valve may open during the delivery of mandatory breaths and increase the size of the tidal volume.

The continuous flow through the circuit should exceed the patient's peak inspiratory flow in order to reduce the work required to breathe spontaneously. Typically the flow through the circuit may be 40 to 60 L/min or higher and may raise the baseline pressure in the circuit by 2 to 5 cm H_2O. The high flow through the circuit may cause resistance to exhalation as gas rushes out of the distended 5-L bag following the delivery of a mandatory tidal volume from the ventilator. The expiratory resistance is caused as the exhaled tidal volume, gas from the bag, and continuous high flow try to pass through the exhalation valve at one time. The use of an adjustable pressure-relief valve set to a pressure slightly higher than PEEP (2 to 3 cm H_2O above) but less than peak inspiratory pressure will limit the gas that collects in the bag when mandatory breaths are delivered by the ventilator. The use of a large, easily distensible, 5-L anesthesia bag will further reduce the pressure that builds during IMV breaths.

(Q) During continuous-flow IMV, the Bennett MA-1 ventilator should be set to deliver a flow that

a. is less than the continuous flow. 460 C
b. is equal to four times the minute volume. 460 b
c. equals or exceeds the continuous flow. 461 b

FRAME 242. PEEP DEVICES

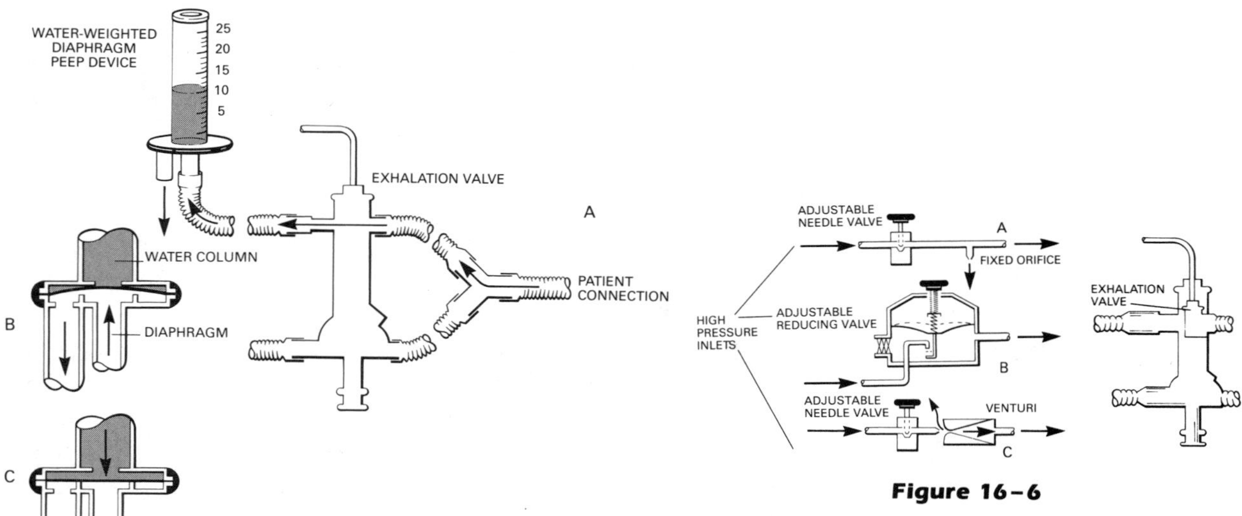

Figure 16–6

Figure 16–5

Figure 16–5 Water-weighted diaphragm PEEP device: (*A*) typical ventilator circuit; (*B*) diaphragm moves up when airway pressure is higher than that generated by the water column and exhaled gas passes out of the circuit; (*C*) when pressures equalize, the diaphragm seats and expiratory flow ceases.

Figure 16–6 Added pressure in exhalation valve balloon can be used to generate PEEP in the patient circuit. *A*, *B*, and *C*, illustrate three ways gas pressure within the balloon is controlled.

The use of a water-weighted diaphragm (Fig. 16–5) to create positive end-expiratory pressure is an example of a *threshold*-resistor PEEP device that is relatively free of back pressure at moderate flow-rate conditions. The airway pressure needed to lift the diaphragm off the exhalation port must be greater than the force created by the column of water that sits on top of the diaphragm. The height of the water column determines the level of PEEP created. This type of device can be applied distal to the exhalation valve of most volume-preset ventilators to control PEEP. If positive pressure is applied to the top of the water column during inspiration, the device can be used as an exhalation valve. This device is used as an exhalation valve and to regulate PEEP on the Emerson 3-MV ventilator.

The use of a pressurized exhalation valve balloon (Fig. 16-6) to create positive end-expiratory pressure is an example of a PEEP device that may be flow dependent. The pressure in the balloon will be lower than the pressure in the circuit because of the differences in the surface area between the balloon and the smaller area of the exhalation valve outlet. PEEP devices are best described according to the degree that they are flow dependent. If the entry and exit channels are small in diameter, high resistance will cause back pressure, and peak inspiratory pressure may take longer to return to the baseline (PEEP level). Ventilators that have threshold PEEP devices will have a lower mean-system pressure because the valve creates less resistance to exhalation than a flow resistor.

(Q) A threshold resistor creates PEEP by

a. restricting flow with a clamp. 460 D

b. using a water column, spring tension, or calibrated weight. 461 A

c. varying the size of an exhalation valve orifice. 460 d

EXERCISES

1. Identify on a Bird Mark 7 ventilator the following primary components: (1) *center body* with gas inlet, air-mix control, Venturi, expiratory timer, and flow control; (2) *ambient compartment* with metal filter for entrainment air, manometer, hand-timer rod, sensitivity control; and (3) *pressure compartment* with connections for mainstream breathing circuit and a single outlet to both nebulizer and exhalation valve, and the pressure control.
2. Connect a Bird Mark 7 ventilator to a test lung and adjust it to deliver a tidal volume of 700 mL at a rate of 10/min. Increase the settings, one at a time, on the following controls: pressure, flow, sensitivity, expiratory time, and observe the effect on tidal volume, inspiratory time, peak inspiratory pressure, respiratory rate, inspiratory flow, and I:E ratio. Repeat the exercise, decreasing each control setting one at a time, and observe what happens to the ventilation parameters.
3. Connect a Bird Mark 7 ventilator to a test lung with an oxygen analyzer probe in the inspiratory line. Monitor the FIO_2 at different cycling pressures with the Mark 7 set to entrain air. Switch from air mix to 100% oxygen and observe the change in inspiratory time and flow.
4. Classify the Bird Mark 7 and the Bennett MA-1 ventilators, identifying the following functional characteristics: mechanisms for terminating and initiating inspiration, power source, control source, inspiratory waveforms, expiratory waveforms, PEEP capability, and single or double circuit.
5. List five locations on a ventilator circuit that are likely to be the source of a leak.
6. Identify the controls on a volume-preset ventilator that will affect the I:E ratio.
7. Describe how to check a volume-preset ventilator and its circuit for leaks. Explain how to locate the source of the leak.
8. Attach a volume-preset ventilator to a test lung. Adjust all the alarm systems and check for threshold sensitivity and response time by simulating the condition that will trigger each alarm.
9. Adapt a Bennett MA-1 ventilator for IMV by attaching a continuous-flow system using a reservoir bag, one-way valve, blender, and pressure-release valve. Adjust the continuous flow through the circuit so that PEEP is not lost during spontaneous breathing. Ensure that the one-way valve stays closed during delivery of mandatory breaths by adjusting the ventilator flow to match or exceed the continuous flow through the circuit and by adjusting the pressure-release valve to slightly higher than the PEEP level.
10. Locate several flow-resistor and threshold-resistor PEEP devices and place them one at a time in a continuous-flow IMV system. Adjust the PEEP to 10 cm H_2O with a flow of 40 L/min through the circuit; then increase the flow to 60 L/min and check the PEEP created by each type of device.

460A (from page 454, frame 238)
Correct. Inspiratory flow, tidal volume, and pressure limit may all affect the inspiratory time. Most volume-preset ventilators will terminate the inspiratory phase when the pressure limit is reached. Please continue on page 455, frame 239.

460B (from page 455, frame 239)
Wrong. An internal leak would not cause the spirometer on the Bennett MA-1 to rise during inspiration. Return to page 455, frame 239, and select another answer.

460C (from page 457, frame 241)
Wrong. If the flow from the ventilator is less than the continuous flow, the one-way valve from the bag will open when a mandatory breath is delivered. The tidal volume delivered by the ventilator will be increased with gas from the bag. Return to page 457, frame 241, and try again.

460D (from page 458, frame 242)
Wrong. A threshold resistor does not require a continuous flow through the circuit to create PEEP. Return to page 458, frame 242, and select another answer.

460a (from page 456, frame 240)
Correct. The high-pressure alarm should be set to sound before part of the tidal volume is lost from the circuit; otherwise the practitioner may not be aware of the decrease in ventilation and increase in airway pressure. This is especially critical with right main-stem bronchial intubation and tension pneumothorax. Please continue on page 457, frame 241.

460b (from page 457, frame 241)
Wrong. Flow from the ventilator that is four times the minute volume may be less than the continuous flow. In that case the tidal volume delivered by the ventilator will be increased with gas from the bag. Return to page 457, frame 241, and try again.

460c (from page 455, frame 239)
Wrong. A leak at the humidifier would not cause the spirometer on the Bennett MA-1 to rise during inspiration. Return to page 455, frame 239, and select another answer.

460d (from page 458, frame 242)
Wrong. A device that varies back pressure by varying the orifice of an exhalation valve requires a continuous flow through the circuit to create PEEP. A threshold resistor is not flow dependent. Return to page 458, frame 242, and select another answer.

461A (from page 458, frame 242)
Correct. A threshold resistor does not require a continuous flow to create PEEP. A water column, calibrated weight, a spring-loaded valve, and a magnetic valve are all examples of threshold-resistor PEEP devices. Please continue on page 459 and complete the chapter exercises.

461B (from page 456, frame 240)
Wrong. The high-pressure alarm should be set to sound before part of the tidal volume is lost from the circuit. Return to page 456, frame 240, and select another answer.

461C (from page 455, frame 239)
Correct. The Bennett spirometer rises during inspiration because there is gas leaking though the exhalation valve. A small tear or pinhole in the diaphragm of the exhalation valve will prevent an adequate seal and gas will leak into the spirometer during inspiration. Please continue on page 456, frame 240.

461D (from page 454, frame 238)
Wrong. Changing the mandatory rate will alter the length of the respiratory cycle but will not change the inspiratory time. An expiratory retard will increase the time it takes for exhalation but will have no effect on inspiratory time. The sensitivity control on a volume-preset ventilator will have no effect on inspiratory time. On some ventilators a high-trigger sensitivity setting may cause the unit to cycle on and off without delivering the preset tidal volume. Return to page 454, frame 238, and select another answer.

461a (from page 456, frame 240)
Wrong. The high-pressure alarm should be set to sound before part of the tidal volume is lost from the circuit. Return to page 456, frame 240, and select another answer.

461b (from page 457, frame 241)
Correct. If the flow from the ventilator is less than the continuous flow, the one-way valve from the bag will open when a mandatory breath is delivered. Setting the flow on the ventilator higher than continuous flow will ensure that the one-way valve closes so that the tidal volume delivered by the ventilator will not be increased with gas from the bag. Please continue on page 458, frame 242.

461c (from page 454, frame 238)
Wrong. Changes in flow and tidal volume will change the inspiratory time. However, the sensitivity control on a volume-preset ventilator will have no effect on inspiratory time. On some ventilators a high-trigger sensitivity setting may cause the unit to cycle on and off without delivering the preset tidal volume. Return to page 454, frame 238, and select another answer.

POSTTEST

This test is designed to evaluate what you have learned from completing Chapter 16. Check your answers on page 464 and review the topics where your answer is incorrect.

1. The Bird Mark 7 ventilator when set to deliver 100% oxygen, has a maximum flow of
   A. 40 L/min.
   B. 55 L/min.
   C. 65 L/min.
   D. 80 L/min.
   E. 95 L/min.
2. The tidal volume on an IPPB machine is increased by adjusting which control?
   A. inspiratory time
   B. inspiratory flow
   C. peak inspiratory pressure
   D. sensitivity
   E. expiratory time
3. If the inspiratory flow on an IPPB machine set is too high, which ventilation parameter will be adversely affected?
   A. tidal volume
   B. peak inspiratory pressure
   C. mean airway pressure
   D. trigger sensitivity
   E. FIO_2 will be decreased
4. Which action will increase peak inspiratory pressure on the Bird Mark 7 ventilator?
   A. increasing flow
   B. increasing sensitivity
   C. decreasing expiratory time
   D. setting air mix on 100% O_2
   E. decreasing inspiratory time
5. If the pressure manometer on a Bird Mark 7 ventilator drops below zero during the first part of inspiration, and rises very slowly to the peak inspiratory pressure, which of the following controls needs to be adjusted?
   A. pressure
   B. sensitivity
   C. flow
   D. expiratory time
   E. cycle rate
6. To control the FIO_2 on IPPB machines, which of the following should be done?
   I. Power the machine with air.
   II. Add a gas-entrainment reservoir.
   III. Power the machine with a blender.
   IV. Turn off Venturi
   V. Titrate O_2 into gas-entrainment reservoir.
   A. I only
   B. V only
   C. III and IV only
   D. I, II, and V only
   E. I, IV, and V only
7. A ventilator that is a constant-flow generator has an inspiratory flow waveform best described as
   A. sine.
   B. square.
   C. accelerating.
   D. decelerating.
   E. sigmoidal.

8. A ventilator that has a sine wave inspiratory flow pattern has
   A. high flow at the beginning of inspiration.
   B. high flow at the end of inspiration.
   C. high flow in the middle of inspiration.
   D. high flow throughout inspiration.
   E. low flow throughout inspiration.

9. If water collects in the inspiratory limb of a circuit of a volume-preset pressure-limited ventilator, which of the following may decrease?
   A. mandatory cycle rate
   B. tidal volume
   C. peak inspiratory pressure
   D. inspiratory flow
   E. FIO_2

10. A leak in the circuit of a volume-preset ventilator is suspected when which of the following occur(s)?
    I. Exhaled tidal volume increases.
    II. Peak inspiratory pressure decreases.
    III. Inspiratory time increases.
    IV. Low-pressure alarm is triggered.
    V. PEEP alarm is triggered.
    A. I only
    B. II only
    C. II and III only
    D. I, II, and IV only
    E. II and IV only

11. If a volume-preset ventilator does not have a inspiratory flow control, which of the following actions will increase flow?
    A. decrease tidal volume
    B. increase I:E ratio
    C. decrease inspiratory time
    D. increase IMV rate
    E. decrease expiratory time

12. To correct an I:E ratio alarm (I:E > 1:1), which of the following actions might be taken on a volume-preset ventilator?
    I. decrease inspiratory time
    II. increase inspiratory flow
    III. increase the CMV rate
    IV. decrease the inspiratory pause
    V. decrease the high-pressure limit
    A. I only
    B. II only
    C. III and IV only
    D. I, II, and IV only
    E. I, II, III, IV, and V

13. If PEEP decreases by 5 cm H_2O with each spontaneous breath during continuous-flow IMV, which of the following actions will maintain the PEEP level?
    A. increase PEEP by 5 cm H_2O
    B. increase flow through the circuit
    C. decrease the size of IMV reservoir bag
    D. increase IMV rate
    E. replace exhalation valve

14. If water in the inspiratory limb of a ventilator obstructs inspiratory flow, which of the following actions should be taken?
    A. Turn heated humidifier to a lower setting.
    B. Drain the circuit at frequent intervals.
    C. Increase the pressure-release limit and alarm threshold.
    D. Increase the inspiratory flow rate.
    E. Decrease the tidal volume.

15. Provided a ventilator patient is not agitated, the PEEP alarm threshold should be set
   A. 1 cm H_2O below PEEP level.
   B. 3 cm H_2O below PEEP level.
   C. 5 cm H_2O below PEEP level.
   D. 1 cm H_2O above PEEP level.
   E. 3 cm H_2O above PEEP level.

16. Oxygen monitor-alarm functions should be checked by
   A. exposing the sensor probe to increased and decreased F_{IO_2}.
   B. decreasing the high F_{IO_2} threshold to less than 5% variance.
   C. decreasing the low F_{IO_2} threshold to less than 5% variance.
   D. exposing the probe to 100% oxygen.
   E. ensuring that the probe is tightly inserted in the circuit.

17. The inspiratory flow during mandatory breaths with a continuous-flow IMV system should be set to
   A. 20 L/min.
   B. 25 L/min.
   C. 30 L/min.
   D. 35 L/min.
   E. equal to continuous flow through the circuit.

18. Where should a low-resistance one-way valve used with continuous-flow IMV be placed?
   A. between the Y-connector and the inspiratory limb
   B. after the exhalation valve
   C. between the reservoir bag and the inspiratory limb
   D. between the ventilator outlet and the humidifier
   E. immediately after the humidifier

19. Which of the following is characteristic of flow-resistor PEEP devices?
   A. They are flow dependent.
   B. They regulate PEEP by height of a water column.
   C. They have low-resistance inlet and outlet valves.
   D. They create PEEP with a spring-loaded valve.
   E. They are used with demand-valve IMV systems.

20. A balloon-type exhalation valve can be characterized as a flow-resistor or threshold-type PEEP device according to its effect on
   A. mean airway pressure.
   B. inspiratory time.
   C. tidal volume.
   D. inspiratory flow.
   E. I:E ratio.

ANSWERS TO POSTTEST

1. A (F233)
2. C (F233)
3. A (F234)
4. B (F234)
5. C (F235)
6. D (F235)
7. B (F236)
8. C (F236)
9. B (F237)
10. E (F237)
11. C (F238)
12. D (F238)
13. B (F239)
14. B (F239)
15. B (F240)
16. A (F240
17. E (F241)
18. C (F241)
19. A (F242)
20. A (F242)

BIBLIOGRAPHY

Barnes, TA: Respiratory Care Practice. Year Book Medical Publishers, Chicago, 1988.

Burton, GG and Hodgkin, JE: Respiratory Care: A Guide to Clinical Practice, ed 2. JB Lippincott, Philadelphia, 1984.

Eubanks, DH and Bone, RC: Comprehensive Respiratory Care, ed 2. CV Mosby, St. Louis, 1990.

Kacmarek, RM and Stoller, JK: Current Respiratory Care. BC Decker, Philadelphia, 1988.

Kirby, RR, Smith, RA, and Desautels, DA: Mechanical Ventilation. Churchill Livingstone, New York, 1985.

Koff, PB, Eitzman, DV, and Neu, J: Neonatal and Pediatric Respiratory Care. CV Mosby, St. Louis, 1988.

McPherson, SP: Respiratory Therapy Equipment, ed 4. CV Mosby, St. Louis, 1990.

McPherson, SP: Respiratory Home Care Equipment. Daedalus Enterprises, Dallas, 1988.

Pilbeam, SP and Youtsey, JW: Mechanical Ventilation-Physiological and Clinical Applications. Multi-Media Publishing, St. Louis, 1986.

Riggs, JH: Respiratory Facts. FA Davis, Philadelphia, 1989.

Surkin, HB and Parkman, AW: The Respiratory Care Workbook. FA Davis, Philadelphia, 1990.

17

Summative Exam

This exam is designed to measure what you have learned from Chapters 1 through 16. Check your answers on pages 501–502 and review the topics where your answer is incorrect.

1. The structure that covers the opening to the larynx is called the
   A. cricoid cartilage.
   B. epiglottis.
   C. cricothyroid cartilage.
   D. vallecula.
   E. uvula.
2. The functional units of the lungs are called
   A. main-stem bronchi.
   B. lobar bronchi.
   C. segmental bronchi.
   D. respiratory bronchioles.
   E. alveoli.
3. The average length of an adult trachea is
   A. 2.5 to 5.0 cm.
   B. 5.0 to 7.5 cm.
   C. 7.5 to 10.0 cm.
   D. 10.0 to 12.5 cm.
   E. 12.5 to 15.0 cm.
4. Which of the following airways has alveoli on the walls?
   A. lobar bronchi
   B. segmental bronchi
   C. segmental bronchioles
   D. terminal bronchioles
   E. respiratory bronchioles
5. Which of the following structures are located in the mediastinum?
   I. trachea
   II. esophagus
   III. heart
   IV. inferior and superior venae cava
   V. lymph nodes
   A. I and III only
   B. IV and V only
   C. III, IV, and V only
   D. II, III, IV, and V only
   E. I, II, III, IV, and V

6. The central part of the diaphragm is made of a membrane called the
   A. xiphoid process.
   B. crura bundle.
   C. central tendon.
   D. lumbar tendon.
   E. crus tendon.

7. All of the following will increase respiratory rate *except*
   A. emotional excitement.
   B. hypothermia.
   C. increased metabolic rate.
   D. exercise.
   E. hyperthyroidism.

8. The right ventricle pumps blood into the
   A. pulmonary artery.
   B. pulmonary vein.
   C. superior vena cava.
   D. left atrium.
   E. pulmonary capillaries.

9. Anatomical dead-space ventilation in a 150-lb adult at rest is
   A. 1.2 L/min.
   B. 1.8 L/min.
   C. 2.4 L/min.
   D. 4.2 L/min.
   E. 5.4 L/min.

10. A normal inspiratory capacity for a young healthy male is
    A. 1200 mL.
    B. 2400 mL.
    C. 2900 mL.
    D. 3600 mL.
    E. 4800 mL.

11. The functional residual capacity is comprised of which of the following?
    I. residual volume
    II. inspiratory reserve volume
    III. expiratory reserve volume
    IV. tidal volume
    A. I and II only
    B. II and IV only
    C. II and III only
    D. I and III only
    E. II, III, and IV only

12. An abnormally fast breathing rate is called
    A. hyperventilation.
    B. hypoventilation.
    C. hypopnea.
    D. tachypnea.
    E. bradypnea.

13. What is a normal mixed-venous carbon dioxide tension?
    A. 6 mm Hg
    B. 40 mm Hg
    C. 46 mm Hg
    D. 50 mm Hg
    E. 60 mm Hg

14. A normal mixed-venous oxygen saturation is
   A. 40%.
   B. 60%.
   C. 75%.
   D. 97%.
   E. 100%.

15. Hypoxemia resulting from inhalation of carbon monoxide results from
   A. reduced alveolar oxygen tension.
   B. reduced arterial venous-oxygen tension.
   C. impaired alveolar capillary diffusion.
   D. hemoglobin deficiency.
   E. histotoxic problems.

16. How much oxygen will dissolve in 100 mL of blood if the Po_2 is 100 mm Hg?
   A. 0.003 mL
   B. 0.030 mL
   C. 0.30 mL
   D. 1.34 mL
   E. 4.50 mL

17. A patient with severe hypoxemia may have all of the following clinical signs *except*
   A. unconsciousness.
   B. restlessness.
   C. apnea.
   D. asystole.
   E. bradycardia.

18. Localized hypoxemia is associated with
   A. rotating tourniquets.
   B. congestive heart failure.
   C. fever.
   D. tissue trauma.
   E. shock.

19. Which of the following are *true* about the oxyhemoglobin dissociation curve?
   I. It shifts right with fever.
   II. It shifts right with hypothermia.
   III. It shifts right with a pH of 7.50.
   IV. It shifts left with a $Paco_2$ of 30 mm Hg.
   V. It shifts right in venous blood.
   A. I, IV, and V only
   B. II, III, and V only
   C. I, II, and III only
   D. II, III, IV, and V only
   E. I, II, III, IV, and V

20. The steeper portion of the oxyhemoglobin dissociation curve has a $Pa{O_2}$ range of
   A. 10 to 40 torr.
   B. 40 to 70 torr.
   C. 70 to 100 torr.
   D. 100 to 130 torr.
   E. 130 to 160 torr.

21. To maintain acid-base balance in body fluids the ratio of bicarbonate to dissolved CO_2 is
   A. 1:1.
   B. 20:1.
   C. 100:1.
   D. 800:1.
   E. 1000:1.

22. The hydrogen ion is a single proton in the nucleus of a hydrogen atom that has lost
   A. a cation.
   B. a single electron.
   C. CO_2.
   D. O_2.
   E. a buffer.

23. Which of the following pH ranges is considered acidemia?
   A. 7.30 to 7.35
   B. 7.35 to 7.40
   C. 7.40 to 7.45
   D. 7.45 to 7.50
   E. 7.50 to 7.55

24. All of the following substances prevent marked alterations in pH when a strong acid or alkali is introduced or removed from body fluids *except*
   A. hemoglobin-oxyhemoglobin.
   B. bicarbonate-carbonic acid.
   C. normal saline.
   D. protein.
   E. phosphate.

25. For every molecule of CO_2 excreted by the lungs, a hydrogen is converted to
   A. HCO_3^-.
   B. H_2O.
   C. CO_2.
   D. HC1.
   E. H_2SO_4.

26. The increased depth and rate of breathing observed during exercise is caused by
   A. increased body temperature.
   B. decreased Pa_{O_2}.
   C. decreased Pa_{CO_2}.
   D. increased Pa_{CO_2}.
   E. decreased $P\bar{v}_{CO_2}$.

27. Which of the following regulate acid-base balance?
   I. kidneys
   II. lungs
   III. buffers
   IV. heart
   V. lymph system
   A. I and III only
   B. II and IV only
   C. III and V only
   D. I, II, and III only
   E. I, II, III, and V only

28. Carbon dioxide is carried from the tissues to the lungs in all of the following forms *except*
   A. bicarbonate.
   B. carbamino.
   C. carbonic anhydrase.
   D. carbonic acid.
   E. when dissolved in blood.

29. Which of the following is the most common protein form that combines with NH_2 to carry CO_2 from the tissues to the lungs?
   A. oxyhemoglobin
   B. reduced hemoglobin
   C. HCO_3^-
   D. H_2CO_3
   E. albumin

30. Respiratory compensation of metabolic alkalosis occurs over
   A. a few minutes.
   B. a few hours.
   C. 6 to 12 hours.
   D. 24 hours.
   E. several days.

31. The proportion of nitrogen in the atmosphere is
   A. 0.03%.
   B. 0.93%.
   C. 20.95%.
   D. 78.08%.
   E. 85.30%.

32. The molecular activity of oxygen in a cylinder can be described as
A. static activity.
B. potential energy.
C. kinetic energy.
D. energy in motion.
E. entropy in motion.

33. When a piston compresses gas in a cylinder all of the following are true *except*
A. heat is produced.
B. pressure increases.
C. potential energy decreases.
D. temperature is increased.
E. molecular collisions increase.

34. The amount of pressure exerted by a gas in a mixture is determined by which of the following?
I. atmospheric pressure
II. humidity
III. temperature
IV. molecular weight
V. fractional concentration
A. I and III only
B. II and IV only
C. I, II, and IV only
D. I, II, III, and V only
E. I, II, III, IV, and V

35. If temperature and mass are held, what will the final volume be given the following data? $P_1 = 500$ mm Hg, $P_2 = 1000$ mm Hg, $V_1 = 2000$ mL.
A. 500 mL
B. 1000 mL
C. 1500 mL
D. 2000 mL
E. 2500 mL

36. If volume and mass are held constant, what will the final temperature be given the following data? $P_1 = 760$ torr, $P_2 = 380$ torr, $T_1 = 100°C$
A. 50°C
B. 100°C
C. 187°K
D. 373°K
E. 746°K

37. If mass remains constant, what will the final pressure be given the following data? $T_1 = 100°C$, $T_2 = 224°C$, $V_1 = 2$ L, $V_2 = 1.5$ L, $P_1 = 760$ torr.
A. 452 torr
B. 1350 torr
C. 1464 torr
D. 2270 torr
E. 2722 torr

38. Gas volumes recorded in a spirometer must be corrected to
   A. ATPS.
   B. STPD.
   C. BTPS.
   D. ATPD.
   E. BTPD.

39. The comparison of absolute humidity to the amount of water that is held in saturated gas at body temperature is called
   A. relative humidity.
   B. body humidity.
   C. vaporization index.
   D. water-vapor tension.
   E. temperature deficit.

40. Given the following data, what will airway resistance be? Flow 30 L/min, peak airway pressure 40 cm H_2O, plateau pressure 30 cm H_2O.
   A. 5 cm H_2O/L/s
   B. 10 cm H_2O/L/s
   C. 15 cm H_2O/L/s
   D. 20 cm H_2O/L/s
   E. 25 cm H_2O/L/s

41. Which of the following humidifiers and nebulizers is most likely to be contaminated with pathogens?
   A. bubble humidifiers
   B. cascade humidifiers
   C. air-entrainment nebulizers
   D. medication nebulizers
   E. jet humidifier

42. Which of the following environmental factors enhance or inhibit the growth of microorganisms?
   I. temperature
   II. moisture
   III. osmotic pressure
   IV. pH
   V. barometric pressure
   A. I and IV only
   B. II and III only
   C. I, II, and V only
   D. I, II, IV, and V only
   E. I, II, III, IV, and V

43. The best way to determine what pathogens may be contaminating respiratory care equipment is to culture the devices
   A. before use.
   B. before being removed from the patient.
   C. after being removed from the patient.
   D. immediately before being cleaned.
   E. after being cleaned.

44. The most common cause of nosocomial infections is
   A. respiratory care nebulizers.
   B. random handwashing.
   C. improper handwashing.
   D. close proximity of hospital beds.
   E. inadequate number of precaution rooms.

45. Which of the following sterilizing techniques is affected by high altitude?
   A. gas sterilization
   B. steam autoclaving
   C. boiling
   D. liquid disinfectants
   E. iodophor solutions

46. The final step in disinfecting contaminated respiratory care equipment with ethylene oxide is to
   A. place in drier.
   B. soak in a detergent.
   C. reassemble.
   D. seal in a plastic bag.
   E. place in aerator.

47. The temperature maintained during ethylene oxide sterilization is
   A. 30° to 40°F.
   B. 40° to 50°F.
   C. 50° to 60°F.
   D. 100° to 140°F.
   E. 190° to 212°F.

48. Which of the following is true regarding an incomplete disinfectant?
   A. It inhibits only bacterial growth.
   B. It destroys only vegetative forms of microorganisms.
   C. It destroys only the spore form of microorganisms.
   D. Given enough time, it will sterilize equipment.
   E. It inactivates spores.

49. To determine if pathogens are located in the reservoir of a nebulizer, a culture specimen should be taken from
   A. water in the reservoir.
   B. condensate from the inspiratory limb of the breathing circuit.
   C. condensate from the expiratory limb of the breathing circuit.
   D. the nebulizer inlet.
   E. the nebulizer outlet.

50. Equipment coming from a contagious precautions room should be
   A. cleaned in the room.
   B. stored in the hallway next to the room.
   C. returned to the department in a double bag.
   D. boiled for 30 minutes before reuse.
   E. steam autoclaved.

51. Which of the following patient information is necessary when determining if an order for a change in tidal volume delivered by a ventilator is appropriate?
   I. gender
   II. age
   III. height
   IV. weight
   V. $Paco_2$
   A. I and III only
   B. II and IV only
   C. IV and V only
   D. III, IV, and V only
   E. I, II, III, IV, and V

52. Which of the following indicates a need to integrate two or more forms of bronchial hygiene therapy?
   A. strong cough
   B. dried retained secretions
   C. thin, watery sputum
   D. chronic cough
   E. blood-tinged sputum

53. The volume of air that can be exhaled after a maximal inspiration is called the
   A. tidal volume.
   B. inspiratory reserve volume.
   C. residual volume.
   D. vital capacity.
   E. functional capacity.

54. The normal $FEV_1/FVC\%$ is
   A. 50%.
   B. 65%.
   C. 83%.
   D. 97%.
   E. 100%.

55. The maximal volume that a patient can breathe per minute is normally measured over what period of time?
   A. 5 to 12 seconds
   B. 12 to 30 seconds
   C. 30 to 60 seconds
   D. 1 to 2 minutes
   E. 2 to 5 minutes

56. Patients with emphysema commonly have a $FEV_1/FEV\%$ of
   A. < 25%.
   B. < 50%.
   C. < 70%.
   D. < 83%.
   E. < 97%.

57. Which of the following is typically lower than predicted with the restrictive pattern of pulmonary disease?
   A. FVC
   B. MVV
   C. $FEV_1/FVC\%$
   D. $FEV_3/FVC\%$
   E. RV

58. All of the following may decrease with the restrictive pattern of pulmonary disease *except*
   A. VC.
   B. IC.
   C. TLC.
   D. MVV.
   E. FRC.

59. All of the following are factors that affect a patient's ability to breathe at sustained high velocity *except*
   A. muscular force available.
   B. height of the patient.
   C. compliance of the lungs.
   D. airway resistance.
   E. patient cooperation.

60. A meaningful improvement in FEV_1 resulting from the administration of a bronchodilator requires a *minimum* increase of
   A. 10%.
   B. 15%.
   C. 20%.
   D. 25%.
   E. 50%.

61. Ordering a "stat" x-ray will provide information leading to all of the following interventions *except*
   A. repositioning a chest suction catheter.
   B. decreasing FIO_2.
   C. continuing IPPB treatments.
   D. pulling back an endotracheal tube.
   E. inserting a chest tube.

62. Irregular tidal volumes that may be slow and deep or rapid and shallow, and are often accompanied by periods of apnea, are called
    A. ataxic.
    B. Biot's.
    C. Cheyne-Stokes.
    D. apneustic.
    E. eupnea.

63. If a victim of an upper airway obstruction collapses to the floor, which of the following actions should be taken?
    A. Lift victim off floor and apply Heimlich maneuver.
    B. Turn victim onto his stomach and apply thrust between scapula.
    C. Turn victim onto his back and apply thrust well below the xiphoid process.
    D. Locate a Magill forcep.
    E. Begin an emergency tracheotomy.

64. Which of the clinical entities are associated with sputum that is purulent, fetid, and bloody?
    A. bronchial asthma
    B. pulmonary edema
    C. bronchiectasis
    D. cystic fibrosis
    E. bronchitis

65. Which of the following can be used to ensure that the trachea is midline?
    I. chest x-ray
    II. arterial blood-gas study
    III. palpation
    IV. percussion
    V. auscultation
    A. I and III only
    B. II and IV only
    C. II and V only
    D. I, III, IV, and V only
    E. I, II, III, IV, and V

66. Low-pitched continuous breath sounds associated with rapid airflow through an obstructed airway caused by excess sputum and bronchospasm are called
    A. wheezes.
    B. rhonchi.
    C. crackles.
    D. sibilant rales.
    E. crepitations.

67. A patient who can walk a mile at his own pace without dyspnea but cannot keep pace on a level with a normal person has a dyspnea class of
    A. I.
    B. II.
    C. III.
    D. IV.
    E. V.

68. Maximum inspiratory pressure should be measured with the airway occluded for
A. 10 seconds.
B. 15 seconds.
C. 20 seconds.
D. 25 seconds.
E. 30 seconds.

69. A patient on the CMV mode of ventilation at a rate of 10/min and a minute volume of 7.5 L will have tidal volume of
A. 500 mL.
B. 600 mL.
C. 750 mL.
D. 900 mL.
E. 1000 mL.

70. What is the acid-base status of a patient with the following blood-gas data? pH 7.32, $Paco_2$ 30 torr, HCO_3^- 17 mEq/L
A. uncompensated respiratory acidosis
B. compensated metabolic alkalosis
C. partially compensated metabolic acidosis
D. compensated respiratory acidosis
E. compensated respiratory alkalosis

71. Which of the following is an example of a low-flow variable-performance oxygen therapy device?
A. Venturi mask
B. mechanical ventilator
C. non-rebreathing mask
D. air-entrainment nebulizer
E. oxyhood

72. Which of the following are advantages of high-flow oxygen therapy devices?
I. ability to match the patient's peak inspiratory flow
II. increased aerosol density when compared with low-flow devices
III. the best device to administer low-density Helox mixtures
IV. the best device to deliver oxygen to COPD patients at home
V. accurate control of FIO_2
A. I and IV only
B. II and III only
C. IV and V only
D. I and V only
E. I, III, and V only

73. Which of the following is an indication that *optimal* PEEP may have been exceeded?
A. Pao_2 continues to rise.
B. Intrapulmonary shunting decreases.
C. Urine output drops to 10 mL/h.
D. Static compliance increases.
E. Airway resistance increases.

74. Which of the following ventilator changes should be made for a 50-kg ventilator patient, given the following data? F_{IO_2} 0.50, PEEP 10 cm H_2O, V_T 750 mL, SIMV 8/min, Pa_{O_2} 55 torr, Pa_{CO_2} 38 torr, pH 7.36.
A. Increase F_{IO_2} to 1.00.
B. Increase F_{IO_2} to 0.60.
C. Increase V_T to 1000 mL.
D. Increase PEEP to 15 cm H_2O.
E. Increase SIMV rate to 10/min.

75. Which of the following is a clinical sign that a patient has become hypoxemic during tracheal suctioning?
A. coughing episode
B. premature ventricular contractions
C. hyperpnea
D. restlessness
E. tachypnea

76. To deliver a total flow of 15 L/min of a 70%/30% helium-oxygen mixture, an oxygen flowmeter would be set at
A. 6 L/min.
B. 8 L/min.
C. 10 L/min.
D. 12 L/min.
E. 15 L/min.

77. A patient in congestive heart failure will be most comfortable in which of the following positions?
A. supine
B. prone
C. Fowler's
D. semi-Fowler's
E. Trendelenburg's

78. Which of the following would benefit from long-term oxygen therapy?
I. cor pulmonale
II. polycythemia
III. pulmonary hypertension
IV. chronic congestive heart failure
V. cardiac arrhythmias with chronic hypoxemia
A. I and IV only
B. II and V only
C. II and III only
D. I, III, IV, and V only
E. I, II, III, IV, and V

79. All of the following may improve when a COPD patient is given low-flow oxygen therapy *except*
   A. a decrease in hematocrit.
   B. Pao_2 increased to 80 torr.
   C. a lower pulmonary vascular resistance.
   D. improved right heart function.
   E. improved appetite.

80. All of the following are hazards of the use of high oxygen concentrations *except*
   A. increase in alveolar type I cells.
   B. hemorrhage.
   C. inactivation of surfactant.
   D. atelectasis.
   E. oxygen-induced hypoventilation with COPD patients.

81. Which of the following are true regarding humidity therapy?
   I. A humidifier must heat gas to 37°C.
   II. Cold aerosols decrease airway resistance.
   III. A heated humidifier is needed for intubated patients.
   IV. Only cool gas mixtures should be delivered to infants.
   V. A nasal cannula is humidified when O_2 flow exceeds 4 L/min.
   A. I and III only.
   B. III and V only.
   C. II and IV only.
   D. I, III, IV, and V only.
   E. I, II, III, IV, and V.

82. Which of the following humidifiers would have a beneficial effect on post-extubation edema?
   A. unheated mainstream nebulizer
   B. heated cascade humidifier
   C. heated air-entrainment nebulizer
   D. heated pass-over humidifier
   E. ultrasonic nebulizer

83. What size aerosol droplet will be most effective in delivering a mucolytic to the main-stem bronchi?
   A. 0.1 to 1 μm
   B. 1 to 5 μm
   C. 5 to 10 μm
   D. 10 to 15 μm
   E. 15 to 20 μm

84. To increase aerosol deposition in the peripheral airways, inspiratory flow should be
   A. 25 L/min.
   B. 30 L/min.
   C. 35 L/min.
   D. 40 L/min.
   E. 50 L/min.

85. To compensate for loss of humidity in the inspiratory tubing, the absolute humidity of gas leaving the outlet of a heated humidifier should be
   A. 22 mg/L.
   B. 30 mg/L.
   C. 44 mg/L.
   D. 66 mg/L.
   E. 84 mg/L.

86. Heat-moisture exchangers provide absolute humidity that does not *exceed*
   A. 20 mg/L.
   B. 25 mg/L.
   C. 30 mg/L.
   D. 35 mg/L.
   E. 40 mg/L.

87. To produce a strong cough the tidal volume should be at least
   A. 7 mL/kg.
   B. 10 mL/kg.
   C. 13 mL/kg.
   D. 15 mL/kg.
   E. 20 mL/kg.

88. Which of the following are true regarding the use of water and weak electrolyte solutions to reduce the viscosity of sputum?
   I. Mucus gel layer is relatively impenetrable to water.
   II. Bland aerosols may trigger reflex mucus production.
   III. Bland aerosols may trigger a cough.
   IV. Bland aerosols may decrease airway resistance.
   V. Results seen are similar to those observed with sputum induction.
   A. I and III only.
   B. II and IV only.
   C. III, IV, and V only.
   D. I, II, III, and V only.
   E. I, II, III, IV, and V.

89. Which of the following bronchoactive MDI aerosol medications is *not* appropriate to treat acute bronchospasm?
   A. cromolyn sodium
   B. metaproterenol
   C. terbutaline
   D. isoetharine
   E. albuterol

90. Which of the following are physiologic effects of adrenergic bronchodilators stimulating *beta-1* receptors?
   I. tachycardia
   II. flushing of skin
   III. palpitation
   IV. tremor
   V. decrease in airway resistance
   A. I only
   B. I and II only
   C. I and III only
   D. I, II, III, and IV only
   E. I, II, III, IV, and V

91. Which of the following is the *prophylactic* treatment of choice to prevent atelectasis from developing?
   A. IPPB
   B. aerosol therapy
   C. incentive spirometry
   D. chest physiotherapy
   E. bronchial hygiene therapy

92. The proper length of a nasopharyngeal airway may be estimated by
   A. measuring from the tip of nose to tragus of ear plus 1 in.
   B. measuring from the tip of nose to tragus of ear plus 2 in.
   C. measuring from the tip of nose to posterior angle of the chin.
   D. one half the length of the appropriate size endotracheal tube.
   E. doubling the age in centimeters.

93. The appropriate size endotracheal tube for use with an adult female is
   A. 6.0 mm.
   B. 6.5 mm.
   C. 7.0 mm.
   D. 8.0 mm.
   E. 9.0 mm.

94. If an end-tidal CO_2 monitor reads 3 mm Hg immediately after intubation, the tube is located in the
   A. trachea.
   B. left main-stem bronchus.
   C. right main-stem bronchus.
   D. larynx.
   E. esophagus.

95. The intracuff pressure for a tracheal tube should not exceed
   A. 15 mm Hg.
   B. 18 mm Hg.
   C. 25 mm Hg.
   D. 30 mm Hg.
   E. 35 mm Hg.

96. What is the appropriate suction catheter to use with a size 6 endotracheal tube?
   A. 10 Fr
   B. 12 Fr
   C. 14 Fr
   D. 16 Fr
   E. 18 Fr

97. When administrating bronchial hygiene therapy, which of the following should be done first?
   A. IPPB
   B. aerosol therapy
   C. incentive spirometry
   D. cough instruction and evaluation
   E. posutral drainage

98. *Prophylactic* chest physiotherapy is usually reserved for all of the following patients *except*
   A. high-risk abdominal surgery.
   B. high-risk thoracic surgery.
   C. ventilator patients.
   D. high pack-per-year smoking history.
   E. abnormal pulmonary function values postoperatively.

99. Which of the following are true regarding chest percussion and vibration?
   I. During percussion the clavicles should be avoided.
   II. During vibration the spine should be avoided.
   III. Percussion is done throughout inspiration and expiration.
   IV. Vibration is done throughout inspiration and expiration.
   V. During percussion wrists should be held stiff.
   A. I and II only
   B. III and IV only
   C. I, II, and III only
   D. I, III, IV, and V only
   E. I, II, III, IV, and V

100. Which postural drainage position would be best to drain the anterior basal segments of both lower lobes?
   A. prone Trendelenburg's
   B. supine Trendelenburg's
   C. modified sideways with left-side down
   D. semi-Fowler's
   E. Fowler's

101. Which of the following would be best to mobilize retained secretions for a patient with recent rib fractures?

I. chest percussion
II. chest vibration
III. aerosol therapy
IV. IPPB
V. postural drainage

A. I and II only
B. II and IV only
C. II, III, and V only
D. I, II, III, and IV only
E. I, II, III, IV, and V

102. The use of large tidal volumes, inspiratory pause, and adequate exhalation will limit IPPB rate to

A. 4 to 6/min.
B. 6 to 8/min.
C. 8 to 10/min.
D. 12 to 14/min.
E. 14 to 16/min.

103. The incidence of pneumothorax during IPPB is increased when which of the following happens?

A. cycling pressure over 30 cm H_2O
B. high inspiratory flow
C. coughing
D. high cycling rate
E. slow inspiratory flow

104. How should the size of the tidal volume be determined for IPPB therapy?

A. 100% of spontaneous tidal volume
B. 100% of limited vital capacity
C. 200% of predicted tidal volume
D. 7 mL/kg
E. 10 mL/kg

105. During IPPB, if the patient complains of dizziness, headache, and a tingling sensation in the fingers, what action should be taken?

A. Increase cycling pressure.
B. Increase the breaths per minute.
C. Increase the frequency of rest periods.
D. Decrease the inspiratory flow.
E. Increase the F_{IO_2}.

106. Which of the following would cause an IPPB machine to terminate inspiration prematurely?
   A. the patient exhaling prematurely
   B. failure of the patient to make a tight seal around the mouthpiece
   C. inspiratory flow set too high
   D. air-mix Venturi not operating
   E. expiratory time too short

107. Decreasing transpulmonary pressure leads to
   I. alveolar inflation and expansion.
   II. lung and alveolar collapse.
   III. decreased expiratory reserve.
   A. I only
   B. II only
   C. III only
   D. I and II only
   E. II and III only

108. Which of the following is the *best* indication for incentive spirometry?
   A. retained secretions
   B. FVC that is 50% of predicted
   C. FVC of 12 mL/kg
   D. infection
   E. substantial alveolar collapse

109. The *minimum* length of sustained inspiratory flow during incentive spirometry should be
   A. 1 to 2 seconds.
   B. 2 to 3 seconds.
   C. 3 to 4 seconds.
   D. 4 to 5 seconds.
   E. 5 to 6 seconds.

110. The breathing exercise that directs increased ventilation to a specific area of the chest identified by pressure of the therapist's hand is called
   A. pursed-lip breathing.
   B. diaphragmatic breathing.
   C. relaxation exercises.
   D. lateral costal breathing.
   E. segmental breathing.

111. All of the following indicate that mechanical ventilation may be needed *except*
   A. a/A ratio < 0.45.
   B. $P(A\text{-}a)O_2$ on 100% $O_2 > 250$ mm Hg.
   C. $V_D/V_T > 0.60$.
   D. maximal inspiratory pressure < 20 cm H_2O.
   E. respiratory rate > 30/min.

112. All of the following are typical findings of adult respiratory distress syndrome *except*
A. acute hypoxemia.
B. increased lung water.
C. increased FRC.
D. acute hypercapnia.
E. increased pulmonary capillary permeability.

113. The mode of ventilation that holds pressure constant at a preset level throughout inspiration and controls the rate of mandatory ventilator delivered breaths is called
A. controlled mandatory ventilation.
B. assisted mandatory ventilation.
C. synchronized intermittent mandatory ventilation.
D. pressure-support ventilation.
E. pressure-control ventilation.

114. All of the following ventilator modes are subject to variation in minute volume as a result of the patient's spontaneous rate *except*
A. assisted mandatory ventilation.
B. assisted-controlled mandatory ventilation.
C. intermittent mandatory ventilation.
D. pressure-support ventilation.
E. pressure-control ventilation.

115. The lowest mean intrathoracic pressure will occur with which of the following ventilation parameters?
A. SIMV 12/min, PEEP 15 cm H_2O
B. CMV 10/min, PEEP 10 cm H_2O
C. AMV 12/min, PEEP 10 cm H_2O
D. IMV 12/min, PEEP 10 cm H_2O
E. AMV-CMV 10/min, PEEP 15 cm H_2O

116. What type of ventilator would be best to ventilate an ARDS patient?
A. constant-flow generator, pressure-cycled
B. constant-pressure generator, time-cycled
C. nonconstant-flow generator, pressure-cycled
D. nonconstant-flow, pressure-preset, flow-cycled
E. constant-flow generator, pressure-limited, volume-cycled

117. What inspiratory flow is needed with the following ventilation parameters? CMV 15/min, V_T 0.750 L, I:E 1:3.
A. 25 L/min
B. 30 L/min
C. 35 L/min
D. 40 L/min
E. 45 L/min

118. In adults, increases in the PEEP level should be made in increments of
   A. 1 to 2 cm H_2O.
   B. 2 to 3 cm H_2O.
   C. 3 to 5 cm H_2O.
   D. 5 to 7 cm H_2O.
   E. 7 to 10 cm H_2O.

119. In order to achieve inspiratory flow of 45 L/min with a Siemens 900C ventilator set to deliver a V_T of 750 mL, SIMV 12/min will require a inspiratory time setting of
   A. 20%.
   B. 25%.
   C. 33%.
   D. 50%.
   E. 67%.

120. Which of the following ventilation parameters should be changed for a 60-kg patient given the following data? SIMV 10/min, V_T 900 mL, PEEP 15 cm H_2O, PaO_2 65 torr, $PaCO_2$ 32 torr, pH 7.50, HCO_3^- 24 mEq/L.
   A. Add 5 cm H_2O of PEEP.
   B. Increase FIO_2 to 1.0.
   C. Decrease the tidal volume.
   D. Decrease rate to 8/min.
   E. Increase the inspiratory flow.

121. A ventilator patient on the SIMV mode with continuous flow has wide swings of the PEEP level. Which of the following actions should be taken?
   A. Increase the inspiratory flow of mandatory tidal volumes.
   B. Increase continuous flow through the circuit.
   C. Decrease PEEP by 5 cm H_2O.
   D. Increase the tidal volume.
   E. Adjust the sensitivity.

122. An indication that a patient is ready to be weaned from mechanical ventilation is maximum inspiratory pressure within 20 seconds of
   A. $>$ 20 cm H_2O.
   B. $>$ 25 cm H_2O.
   C. $>$ 30 cm H_2O.
   D. $>$ 35 cm H_2O.
   E. $>$ 40 cm H_2O.

123. In adults, which of the following actions is best to confirm a cardiac arrest?
   A. Palpate radial artery.
   B. Palpate brachial artery.
   C. Palpate carotid artery.
   D. Check pupil size.
   E. Auscultate for apical pulse.

124. Thrusts to the abdomen when using the Heimlich maneuver to clear an upper airway obstruction should be applied
    A. inward and upward.
    B. inward and downward.
    C. slowly only twice.
    D. directly over xiphoid process.
    E. above the xiphoid process.

125. Which of the maneuvers should be used to open the airway when a cervical spine injury is suspected?
    A. modified jaw thrust
    B. triple airway
    C. head tilt/chin lift
    D. chin lift
    E. head tilt

126. Mouth-to-mask rescue breathing for an adult, with one rescuer, should be done at a rate of
    A. 8/min.
    B. 10/min.
    C. 12/min.
    D. 15/min.
    E. 20/min.

127. Chest compressions during CPR for an infant should be delivered at a rate of
    A. 70/min.
    B. 80/min.
    C. 90/min.
    D. 100/min.
    E. 110/min.

128. Which of the following are true regarding the protocol for single-rescuer CPR for an adult victim?
    I. The ratio of chest compressions to ventilation is 15:1.
    II. The first step is to establish unresponsiveness.
    III. When starting rescue breathing give five large breaths.
    IV. If a pulse is absent, begin chest compressions at 80 to 100/min.
    V. Assess patient for pulse and breathing after 10 cycles.
    A. I and III only
    B. II and IV only
    C. I, III, and IV only
    D. II, IV, and V only
    E. I, II, III, IV, and V

129. Which of the following is (are) true regarding the protocol for two-rescuer CPR for an adult victim?
   I. The compression-to-ventilation ratio is 5:2.
   II. The second person to arrive begins chest compressions at once.
   III. A switch in responsibilities calls for a 5:1 compression-to-ventilation ratio.
   IV. The rescuer moving to the head begins ventilation at once.
   A. I only
   B. II only
   C. III only
   D. III and IV only
   E. I, III, and IV only

130. What size tidal volume will a practitioner with an average-size hand deliver with a manual resuscitator if only one hand is used?
   A. 500 mL
   B. 600 mL
   C. 700 mL
   D. 800 mL
   E. 900 mL

131. The oxygen flow to a manual resuscitator used for rescue breathing during CPR should be set at
   A. 5 L/min.
   B. 10 L/min.
   C. 15 L/min.
   D. 20 L/min.
   E. flush (maximum flow).

132. How long should chest compressions be interrupted to check for a carotid pulse?
   A. 5 seconds
   B. 10 seconds
   C. 15 seconds
   D. 20 seconds
   E. 30 seconds

133. When collecting an arterial blood sample from the radial artery, the first action after withdrawing the needle is
   A. pulling back on the plunger.
   B. rolling the syringe between the hands.
   C. sealing the syringe.
   D. compressing the puncture site.
   E. expelling air bubbles.

134. During acute respiratory acidosis the expected metabolic compensation for a Pa_{CO_2} of 70 mm Hg will be
   A. an increase of 2 mEq/L of HCO_3^-.
   B. an increase of 4 mEq/L of HCO_3^-.
   C. an increase of 12 mEq/L of HCO_3^-.
   D. a decrease of 2 mEq/L of HCO_3^-.
   E. a decrease of 12 mEq/L of HCO_3^-.

135. A neonate should have oxygenation supported to produce a pulse-oximeter reading of
   A. 60%.
   B. 70%.
   C. 80%.
   D. 90%.
   E. 100%.

136. The presence of wrinkles in the cuff of a tracheal tube means that
   A. the tube is too small.
   B. the tube is too large.
   C. intracuff pressure is < 25 mm Hg.
   D. no more volume can be added.
   E. the trachea is distended.

137. What is the resistance of a patient-ventilator system for a constant-flow generator given the following data? Inspiratory flow 60 L/min, peak inspiratory pressure 40 cm H_2O, plateau pressure 30 cm H_2O, PEEP 10 cm H_2O, V_T 1.0 L.
   A. 5 cm H_2O/L/s
   B. 10 cm H_2O/L/s
   C. 15 cm H_2O/L/s
   D. 20 cm H_2O/L/s
   E. 25 cm H_2O/L/s

138. Goals for IPPB include all of the following *except*
   A. decreasing intracranial pressure.
   B. increasing vital capacity above 15 mL/kg.
   C. improving cough.
   D. mobilizing secretion.
   E. treating pulmonary edema.

139. Beta-1 and beta-2 side effects of adrenergic bronchodilators include all of the following *except*
   A. tremors.
   B. tachycardia.
   C. somnolence.
   D. flushing of the skin.
   E. palpitation.

140. What is the color of sputum that may result as a response to an allergic or infectious process?
A. white
B. yellow
C. bright red
D. pink
E. brown

141. Static compliance correlates closely with lung disorders that produce changes in which of the following?
A. timed vital capacity
B. functional residual capacity
C. airway resistance
D. residual volume
E. minute volume

142. The reduction of urine output that may be seen with mechanical ventilation may be the result of
A. increased right ventricular preload.
B. decreased intra-alveolar pressure.
C. increased intrathoracic pressure.
D. decreased functional residual capacity.
E. increased FIO_2.

143. Which of the following are important when evaluating the home of a respiratory home care patient?
I. the number of floors
II. the number of electrical outlets
III. the air conditioning and heating systems
IV. the ease with which daily living activities can be accomplished
V. delivery access for oxygen cylinders or liquid O_2 reservoirs
A. I and III only
B. II and IV only
C. I, III, and V only
D. I, II, IV, and V only
E. I, II, III, IV, and V

144. A respiratory home care patient and his or her family need instruction on all of the following *except*
A. the anatomy and pathophysiology of the patient's disease.
B. how to use a disposable manual resuscitator.
C. benefits and dangers of oxygen therapy.
D. transfilling portable liquid oxygen systems.
E. transfilling portable oxygen tanks.

145. Which of the following actions should be taken if a respiratory home care patient becomes less active due to dyspnea?
A. Teach the patient how to complete daily activities by noon.
B. Encourage the patient not to dress in the morning.
C. Review the principles of work simplification.
D. Suggest that the bed be moved into the family room.
E. Suggest a quick shower rather than use of a bathtub.

146. All of the following are likely to encourage the nutritional status of a respiratory home care patient *except*
A. fluid intake of 3 to 4 L/day.
B. exercise program with oxygen if necessary.
C. limiting meals to two per day.
D. pharmacologic control of pain.
E. use of oxygen during meals.

147. How long will a 14-lb portable liquid oxygen system last at 2 L/min?
A. 2 hours
B. 4 hours
C. 8 hours
D. 12 hours
E. 24 hours

148. With evidence of damage to other organs from hypoxemia the *alternate* Medicare criteria for low-flow continuous long-term oxygen therapy are an Sao_2 of
A. 70 to 74%.
B. 75 to 79%.
C. 80 to 84%.
D. 85 to 89%.
E. 90 to 94%.

149. Oxygen may be used during rehabilitation programs for respiratory home care patients if their Sao_2 during exercise drops below
A. 75%.
B. 80%.
C. 85%.
D. 90%.
E. 97%.

150. Which of the following are true regarding maintenance of oxygen concentrators?
   I. Oxygen flow should be checked at regular intervals.
   II. Air intake filters should be cleaned weekly.
   III. Backup oxygen cylinders must be checked at regular intervals.
   IV. An alternating noise every 30 seconds means service is needed.
   V. Internal malfunctions can greatly reduce oxygen concentration.
   A. I and II only
   B. III and V only
   C. I, II, and IV only
   D. I, II, III, and V only
   E. I, II, III, IV, and V

151. Which of the following adrenergic bronchodilators has the shortest duration?
   A. albuterol or salbutamol (Proventil, Ventolin)
   B. isoproterenol (Isuprel)
   C. terbutaline (Brethine, Bricanyl)
   D. metaproterenol (Alupent, Metaprel)
   E. isoetharine (Bronkosol, Dilabron)

152. All of the following are clinical signs of a pulmonary infection *except*
   A. fever.
   B. hyperresonance to percussion.
   C. change in color of sputum.
   D. change in viscosity of sputum.
   E. increasing dyspnea.

153. What is the cylinder duration of an E-cylinder with 1000 psig at a flow of 10 L/min?
   A. 16 minutes
   B. 28 minutes
   C. 2 hours, 40 minutes
   D. 4 hours, 40 minutes
   E. 5 hours

154. What is the best method for determining if an oxygen regulator is leaking?
   A. Listen for a hissing noise.
   B. Spray regulator release valves with a petroleum lubricant.
   C. Spray regulator release valves with soapy water.
   D. Increase pressure into regulator valve inlet to 3000 psig.
   E. Connect regulator to a Helox mixture.

155. A Thorpe tube flowmeter can be checked to see if it compensates for back pressure by
   A. pressurizing Thorpe tube with outlet valve open to flush.
   B. pressurizing Thorpe tube with outlet valve closed.
   C. pressurizing Thorpe tube and turning it to a horizontal position.
   D. checking to see if the needle valve comes before the Thorpe tube.
   E. checking the accuracy with a Helox mixture.

156. Which of the following may happen if a check valve on the oxygen inlet of a blender fails?
   A. The pressure on the oxygen inlet will drop.
   B. The pressure on the air inlet will drop.
   C. The F_{IO_2} delivered by the blender may increase.
   D. The F_{IO_2} delivered by the blender may decrease.
   E. Water will condense in the oxygen inlet.

157. Which of the following oxygen therapy devices is best for short periods such as emergency medical transport of a trauma victim?
   A. nasal cannula
   B. simple mask
   C. partial rebreathing mask
   D. non-rebreathing mask
   E. face tents

158. The oxygen flow to a nasal cannula for a COPD patient usually should not exceed
   A. 1 L/min.
   B. 2 L/min.
   C. 3 L/min.
   D. 4 L/min.
   E. 6 L/min.

159. Which of the following are disadvantages of a partial rebreathing mask?
   I. They are relatively uncomfortable.
   II. Air dilution is likely to occur.
   III. F_{IO_2} will vary with ventilation pattern and is hard to predict.
   IV. There is a potential for aspiration.
   V. The maximum F_{IO_2} that can be achieved is 0.40.
   A. I and III only
   B. I and IV only
   C. II and V only
   D. I, II, III, and IV only
   E. I, II, III, IV, and V

160. The oxygen flow necessary to achieve an F_{IO_2} of 0.55 to 0.70 with a disposable non-rebreathing mask during quiet breathing is
   A. 2 to 4 L/min.
   B. 4 to 6 L/min.
   C. 6 to 8 L/min.
   D. 8 to 10 L/min.
   E. enough flow to keep the reservoir bag full during inspiration.

161. The total flow from an air-entrainment nebulizer set to deliver an FIO_2 of 0.40 with an oxygen flow of 10 L/min is
A. 20 L/min.
B. 30 L/min.
C. 40 L/min.
D. 50 L/min.
E. 60 L/min.

162. Which of the following will occur when a 50% air-entrainment mask with oxygen flow of 12 L/min is used with a patient who has a peak inspiratory flow of 45 L/min?
A. Total flow of 48 L/min will deliver an FIO_2 of 50%.
B. Total flow of 33 L/min will deliver an FIO_2 of less than 50%.
C. Total flow of 24 L/min will deliver an FIO_2 of greater than 50%.
D. The O_2 flow must be limited to $\leq$ 10 L/min with this mask.
E. Humidifier will limit the FIO_2 that can be delivered.

163. When an oxyhood is used inside an isolette that has an ambient temperature of 37°C, the gas to the oxyhood should have an inlet temperature of
A. 22°C.
B. 30°C.
C. 32°C.
D. 37°C.
E. 40°C.

164. An oxyhood is used inside an isolette when the FIO_2 needed exceeds
A. 0.30.
B. 0.40.
C. 0.50.
D. 0.60.
E. 0.70.

165. The Air-Shields Croupette model D for infants with an oxygen flow of 8 to 10 L/min produces an FIO_2 with a range of
A. 0.30 to 0.35.
B. 0.35 to 0.40.
C. 0.40 to 0.45.
D. 0.45 to 0.55.
E. 0.50 to 0.60.

166. The minimum flow necessary for a low-resistance CPAP system usually exceeds
A. 20 L/min.
B. 30 L/min.
C. 40 L/min.
D. 60 L/min.
E. 80 L/min.

167. The bag of a self-inflating manual resuscitator used to ventilate infants using a mask should have a minimum volume of
A. 50 mL.
B. 100 mL.
C. 200 mL.
D. 300 mL.
E. 600 mL.

168. When a Bird Mark 7 ventilator is switched from air mix to 100% source gas, which of the following controls must be increased?
A. flow
B. pressure
C. expiratory time
D. sensitivity
E. inspiratory time

169. Which of the following are advantages of using pulse-oximeters?
I. real-time data
II. no calibration necessary
III. ease of application
IV. accurate when dysfunctional hemoglobin is present
V. not affected by bilirubin concentrations < 20 mg/L
A. I and III only
B. II and IV only
C. I, II, and III only
D. I, II, III, and V only
E. I, II, III, IV, and V

170. All of the following are common reasons why polarographic oxygen analyzers fail to calibrate *except*
A. low battery charge.
B. light bulb needs replacement.
C. low amount of electrolyte.
D. torn membrane.
E. probe placed in a wet part of ventilator circuit.

171. All of the following will affect the absolute humidity delivered by pass-over humidifiers *except*
A. inspiratory time.
B. high gas flow.
C. ambient temperature.
D. water-reservoir dead space.
E. water-reservoir temperature.

172. Which of the following may cause a jet humidifier to whistle or click?
I. excessive oxygen flow
II. air entrainment
III. kinked delivery tubing
IV. obstruction in delivery tubing
V. empty water reservoir
A. I and II only
B. III and V only
C. I, III, and IV only
D. II, IV, and V only
E. I, II, III, IV, and V

173. What is the purpose of the tower in a cascade humidifier?
    A. to monitor water temperature
    B. to hold the heating element rods
    C. to filter bacteria from the mainstream gas
    D. to increase the surface area between gas and water
    E. to increase the laminar flow of gases

174. What temperature at the proximal probe will turn a Bird wick humidifier off?
    A. 32° to 34°C
    B. 34° to 36°C
    C. 36° to 38°C
    D. 38° to 40°C
    E. 40° to 42°C

175. How long does it take to nebulize 3 to 5 mL of solution in a small-volume disposable sidestream nebulizer if the source gas flow is 5 to 10 L/min?
    A. 3 to 5 minutes
    B. 5 to 10 minutes
    C. 10 to 15 minutes
    D. 15 to 20 minutes
    E. 20 to 25 minutes

176. To deliver medication from a metered-dose inhaler to the periphery of the lung, the inspiratory flow should be
    A. 25 L/min.
    B. 30 L/min.
    C. 35 L/min.
    D. 40 L/min.
    E. 60 L/min.

177. All of the following are signs that water has accumulated in the delivery tubing of an air-entrainment nebulizer *except*
    A. aerosol exiting from tubing in small puffs.
    B. decrease in total flow from the tubing.
    C. decrease in F_{IO_2} of gas exiting from tubing.
    D. a gurgling sound from the tubing.
    E. decrease in noise from air-entrainment port.

178. All of the following will lower the aerosol density delivered by an ultrasonic nebulizer *except*
    A. baffling and condensation in the tubing.
    B. temperature of liquid in the solution cup.
    C. residue from soaps or plastics in the solution cup.
    D. decreased fluid in the couplant chamber.
    E. decrease in flow of carrier gas.

179. The Solo-Sphere nebulizer utilizes which of the following principles?
    A. Babington
    B. piezo-electric
    C. dew point
    D. convection
    E. kinetic activity

180. Which of the following would be the best to provide humidification to an intubated patient during transport to another local hospital?
    A. cascade humidifier
    B. heat-moisture exchanger
    C. pass-over humidifier
    D. ultrasonic nebulizer
    E. hydronamic nebulizer

181. Which of the following airways helps to guide the suction catheter to the trachea of a conscious patient who is too weak to raise retained secretions but is expected to recover within 24 hours?
    A. oropharyngeal airway
    B. nasopharyngeal airway
    C. oral endotracheal tube
    D. nasal endotracheal tube
    E. esophageal obturator airway

182. Which of the following are true about the esophageal obturator airway?
    I. A skilled practitioner is needed to place the EOA.
    II. Subcutaneous emphysema is a sign of esophageal rupture.
    III. The cuff of the EOA holds about 30 mL of air.
    IV. The EOA is advanced until the 27-cm mark is seen.
    V. The EOA should be suctioned after the tube is placed.
    A. I and II only.
    B. II and IV only.
    C. III and V only.
    D. II and III only.
    E. I, II, III, IV, and V.

183. What is the appropriate size endotracheal tube for an average male?
    A. 6.5 to 7.0
    B. 7.0 to 7.5
    C. 7.5 to 8.0
    D. 8.0 to 8.5
    E. 8.5 to 9.0

184. Which of the following devices may be used during a nasotracheal intubation but usually is not needed with orotracheal tubes?
    A. Yankauer tonsil sucker
    B. Magill forceps
    C. Wis-Hippie laryngoscope blade
    D. Miller laryngoscope (straight blade)
    E. Macintosh laryngoscope (curved blade)

185. Which of the following will reduce the trauma caused by a suction catheter?
   I. applying suction pressure to catheter for only 20 seconds at one time
   II. releasing suction pressure when moving catheter in the airway
   III. applying and releasing pressure when catheter is not moving
   IV. oxygenating the patient before and after suctioning the trachea
   V. using an Arygle Aero-Flo suction catheter
   A. I and III only
   B. II and IV only
   C. I, II, and III only
   D. II, III, IV, and V only
   E. I, II, III, IV, and V

186. What is the maximum suction pressure that can be generated in the regulated mode of most suction regulators?
   A. 100 mm Hg
   B. 120 mm Hg
   C. 140 mm Hg
   D. 160 mm Hg
   E. 200 mm Hg

187. Sputum expelled from the throat or lungs cannot be used for bacteriologic examination because
   A. the volume collected may be too small.
   B. of the large variety of flora in the mouth and oropharynx.
   C. exposure to 21% oxygen will kill anaerobic bacteria.
   D. saliva pH is too acidic.
   E. saliva will dilute the concentration of pathogens in the sample.

188. Which of the following are true regarding tracheostomy tubes?
   I. Tracheostomy tubes will allow the patient to eat.
   II. The cuff on the tube should stay inflated continuously.
   III. Tracheostomy tubes reduce complications to the larynx.
   IV. The cuff on the tube should have a low volume.
   V. Humidification is not needed if the cuff is deflated.
   A. I and III only
   B. II and IV only
   C. III and V only
   D. I, II, IV, and V only
   E. I, II, III, IV, and V

189. How often should an incentive breathing device be used after upper abdominal surgery?
   A. every hour while patient is awake
   B. every 2 hours
   C. every 4 hours
   D. TID
   E. BID

190. Which of the following is *not* true regarding chest percussors?
   A. Hold the applicator loosely with the fingers of one hand.
   B. The appropriate postural drainage position should be used.
   C. Percussor should be held over one area for 2 to 5 minutes.
   D. Lower oscillation frequencies are used with larger patients.
   E. The therapist should never apply body weight to the applicator.

191. The expiratory time on a Bird Mark 7 ventilator is controlled by
   A. magnets.
   B. Venturi.
   C. pressurized cartridge.
   D. master diaphragm.
   E. metal clutch disc.

192. Which of the following controls on a Bird Mark 7 affect(s) the F_{IO_2}?
   I. flow
   II. pressure
   III. air mix
   IV. expiratory timer
   A. I only
   B. II only
   C. III only
   D. I and IV only
   E. I, II, and III only

193. All of the following are likely to cause a prolonged inspiration when a Bird Mark 7 ventilator is used for an IPPB treatment *except*
   A. leaks around the mouthpiece.
   B. a decrease in sensitivity.
   C. an air mix set on 100% source gas.
   D. a loose connection in the inspiratory line.
   E. an inspiratory flow that is too low.

194. Most neonatal ventilators are cycled from inspiration to expiration when which of the following occurs?
   A. A pressure limit is reached.
   B. A preset tidal volume is delivered.
   C. A minimum flow is reached.
   D. A preset inspiratory time elapses.
   E. A piston travels a preset distance.

195. Which of the following determines whether peak inspiratory pressure or plateau pressure is used to calculate the volume lost in the circuit of a volume-preset ventilator?
   A. inspiratory pause time
   B. magnitude of the peak inspiratory pressure
   C. PEEP level
   D. tubing compliance factor
   E. I:E ratio

196. All of the following may trigger the pressure limit alarm on a volume-preset ventilator *except*
   A. right main-stem intubation.
   B. increase in compliance.
   C. acute bronchospasm.
   D. water in the inspiratory line.
   E. increase in airway secretions.

197. Which of the following may decrease the tidal volume delivered by a volume-preset ventilator that has water in the inspiratory limb?
   A. inspiratory flow set too high
   B. pressure limit set higher than the pressure-release valve
   C. sensitivity set too low
   D. low-pressure alarm set too low
   E. leaking exhalation valve

198. The threshold on an I:E ratio alarm on a volume-preset ventilator is usually set at
   A. 1:1.
   B. 1:2.
   C. 1:3.
   D. 2:1.
   E. 3:1.

199. Continuous flow through an IMV circuit should be set according to
   A. inspiratory time of IMV breaths.
   B. inspiratory time of spontaneous tidal volumes.
   C. peak inspiratory flow of spontaneous tidal volumes.
   D. minute volume.
   E. IMV rate.

200. Which of the following characteristics of an exhalation valve used to create PEEP determine whether it is a threshold or flow resistor?
   A. pressure applied to valve diaphragm
   B. response time of balloon deflation
   C. diameter of inlet and outlet ports
   D. vertical or horizontal position
   E. temperature of exhaled gas

ANSWERS TO SUMMATIVE EXAM

1. B (F3)
2. E (F4)
3. D (F5)
4. E (F6)
5. E (F9)
6. C (F13)
7. B (F15)
8. A (F19)
9. B (F22)
10. D (F26)
11. D (F28)
12. D (F34)
13. C (F36)
14. C (F38)
15. D (F39)
16. C (F40)
17. B (F40)
18. A (F41)
19. A (F43)
20. B (F43)
21. B (F44)
22. B (F45)
23. A (F46)
24. C (F47)
25. B (F48)
26. D (F49)
27. D (F50)
28. C (F53)
29. B (F54)
30. A (F58)
31. D (F60)
32. B (F62)
33. C (F63)
34. D (F67)
35. B (F69)
36. C (F70)
37. B (F71)
38. C (F72)
39. B (F73)
40. D (F74)
41. C (F80)
42. E (F82)
43. B (F85)
44. B (F87)
45. C (F88)
46. E (F89)
47. C (F89)
48. B (F90)
49. A (F91)
50. C (F92)
51. D (F93)
52. B (F94)
53. D (F95)
54. C (F96)
55. B (F97)
56. B (F98)
57. A (F99)
58. D (F100)
59. B (F101)
60. B (F102)
61. B (F103)
62. B (F104)
63. C (F105)
64. C (F106)
65. A (F107)
66. B (F108)
67. C (F109)
68. C (F110)
69. C (F111)
70. C (F112)
71. C (F113)
72. D (F114)
73. C (F115)
74. D (F116)
75. B (F117)
76. C (F118)
77. C (F119)
78. E (F120)
79. B (F121)
80. A (F122)
81. B (F123)
82. A (F124)
83. C (F125)
84. A (F126)
85. E (F127)
86. C (F128)
87. D (F129)
88. D (F130)
89. A (F131)
90. C (F132)
91. C (F133)
92. A (F134)
93. D (F135)
94. E (F136)
95. B (F137)
96. A (F138)
97. D (F139)
98. E (F140)
99. C (F141)
100. B (F142)

101. C (F143)
102. B (F144)
103. C (F145)
104. B (F146)
105. C (F147)
106. A (F148)
107. E (F149)
108. B (F150)
109. B (F151)
110. E (F152)
111. B (F153)
112. C (F154)
113. E (F155)
114. E (F156)
115. B (F157)
116. E (F158)
117. E (F159)
118. C (F160)
119. A (F161)
120. D (F162)
121. B (F163)
122. A (F164)
123. C (F165)
124. A (F166)
125. A (F167)
126. C (F168)
127. D (F169)
128. B (F170)
129. C (F171)
130. B (F172)
131. C (F173)
132. A (F174)
133. D (F175)
134. A (F176)
135. D (F177)
136. C (F178)
137. B (F179)
138. A (F180)
139. C (F181)
140. B (F182)
141. B (F183)
142. C (F184)
143. E (F185)
144. E (F186)
145. C (F187)
146. C (F188)
147. D (F189)
148. D (F190)
149. C (F191)
150. D (F192)
151. B (F193)
152. B (F194)
153. B (F195)
154. C (F196)
155. B (F197)
156. C (F198)
157. B (F199)
158. B (F200)
159. D (F201)
160. E (F202)
161. C (F203)
162. B (F204)
163. D (F205)
164. A (F206)
165. D (F207)
166. D (F208)
167. D (F209)
168. A (F210)
169. C (F211)
170. B (F212)
171. A (F213)
172. C (F214)
173. D (F215)
174. D (F216)
175. B (F217)
176. A (F218)
177. C (F219)
178. E (F220)
179. A (F221)
180. B (F222)
181. B (F223)
182. D (F224)
183. D (F225)
184. B (F226)
185. D (F227)
186. E (F228)
187. B (F229)
188. A (F230)
189. A (F231)
190. C (F232)
191. C (F233)
192. E (F234)
193. B (F235)
194. D (F236)
195. A (F237)
196. B (F238)
197. B (F239)
198. A (F240)
199. C (F241)
200. C (F242)

Index

A page number followed by a "t" indicates a table; a page number in italic indicates a figure.